1987 Nursing Events

APRIL

1-5
National Student Nurses Association Annual Congress. Hyatt Regency Hotel, Chicago. Contact: NSNA (212) 581-2211.

5-10
Annual AORN Congress. Atlanta. Contact: AORN, (303) 755-6300.

6-9
Cardiac Critical Care Nursing Symposium. Stouffer Inn on the Square, Cleveland. Contact: Center for CME, the Cleveland Clinic Educational Foundation, (800) 762-8172 or 8173.

9-10
Annual Psychiatric Nursing Conference. Quality Inn, Towson, Md. Contact: School of Nursing Continuing Education Program, University of Maryland, (301) 528-3767.

"Neonatal Nursing: The Infant, the Family, and the Caregiver." Hyatt Regency Hotel, Nashville, Tenn. Contact: Nursing Continuing Education, Vanderbilt University Hospital, (615) 322-2081.

11-26
Australia–New Zealand '87 Nursing Study Tour. Contact: Professional Nursing Seminars, (800) 237-3762.

27-29
Nursing Management Congress and Exposition. New York City. Contact: Nursing Management Seminars, (312) 341-1014.

27-5/1 and 5/4-8
"Diabetes Education Update." Hilton Inn East, Wichita, Kan. Contact: Center for Continuing Health Education, Wichita State University, (316) 689-3628.

28
"Improving the Work Climate Through Small Group Interaction." Nashville, Tenn. Contact: Nursing Continuing Education, Vanderbilt University Hospital, (615) 322-2081.

MAY

1-2
"Computers in the OR: Advanced." San Francisco. Contact: AORN, (303) 755-6300.

2
"Trauma Victims: A Perioperative Challenge." Detroit. Contact: AORN, (303) 755-6300.

3-7
American Association of Neuroscience Nurses' Annual Meeting. Registry Hotel, Dallas. Contact: AANN, (312) 823-9850.

4-5
"Enterostomal Therapy." Cleveland. Contact: Center for CME, the Cleveland Clinic Educational Foundation, (800) 762-8172 or 8173.

4-7
AACN Annual National Teaching Institute. New Orleans. Contact: AACN (714) 644-9310, ext. 320.

6-9
Oncology Nursing Society's Annual Congress. Denver. Contact: ONS, (412) 344-3899.

14-17
American Geriatrics Society and American Federation for Aging Research Joint Annual Meeting. Hyatt Regency Hotel, New Orleans. Contact: AGS, (212) 308-1414.

16-18
American Nephrology Nurses' Association National Symposium. Marriott Marquis Hotel, New York City. Contact: ANNA, (609) 589-2187.

20-22
Nurse Theorist Conference. Pittsburgh. Contact: Discovery International, (412) 391-8471.

31-6/4
National Orthopedic Nurses Association Annual Congress. Baltimore Convention Center. Contact: NAON (609) 582-1011.

JUNE

8-12
"Effective Staff Development." Denver. Contact: AORN, (303) 755-6300.

8-26
"Physical Assessment for RNs." Cincinnati. Contact: Continuing Education, College of Nursing and Health, University of Cincinnati, (513) 872-5554.

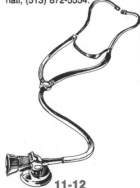

11-12
National Nursing Symposium on Home Health Care. Ann Arbor, Mich. Contact: School of Nursing, University of Michigan, (313) 763-3210.

14-18
"Nursing's Vital Links in the New Environment." Washington, D.C. Contact: National League for Nursing, (212) 582-1022.

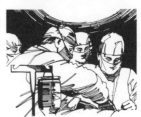

15-19
"OR Management: Building an Effective Team." Denver. Contact: AORN, (303) 755-6300.

27-7/1
National Association of School Nurses Annual Conference. Chicago. Contact: NASN, (207) 883-2117.

NURSE'S REFERENCE LIBRARY®

Nursing
Yearbook87

NURSING87 BOOKS™
SPRINGHOUSE CORPORATION
Springhouse, Pennsylvania

NURSING87 BOOKS™

SPRINGHOUSE CORPORATION BOOK DIVISION

Chairman
Eugene W. Jackson

Vice-Chairman
Daniel L. Cheney

President
Warren R. Erhardt

Vice-President and Director
Timothy B. King

Vice-President, Book Operations
Thomas A. Temple

Vice-President, Production and Purchasing
Bacil Guiley

Program Director, Reference Books
Stanley E. Loeb

NURSING YEARBOOK87

Editorial Director
Helen Klusek Hamilton

Clinical Director
Barbara McVan, RN

Art Director
Sonja E. Douglas

Staff for this volume

Editors: June Gomez, Kevin J. Law, June Norris

Clinical Editor: Sandra Ludwig Nettina, RN, MSN

Contributing Clinical Editors: Diane Cochet, RN, BSN, Joanne Patzek DaCunha, RN, BS, Julie Tackenberg, RN, MA

Acquisitions: Margaret L. Belcher, RN, BSN

Drug Information Manager: Larry Neil Gever, RPh, PharmD

Editorial Services Manager: David R. Moreau

Copy Editors: Diane M. Labus, Doris Weinstock, Debra Young

Production Coordinator: Sally Johnson

Designers: Carol Cameron-Sears, Thomas R. Chinnici, Ann M. Croft

Illustrators: Michael Adams, Dimitrios Bastas, Neesa Becker, Denise Brunkus, John Cymerman, Design Management, Marie Garafano, Jean Garner, John Gist, Tom Herbert, Jesse Hulse, Robert Jackson, Mark Mancini, Taylor Oughton, Pat Perlebery, Robert Phillips, George Retseck, Eileen Rudnick, Doug Smock, Bea Weidner

Art Production Manager: Robert Perry III

Art Assistants: Donald Knauss, Mark Marcin, Robert Wieder

Typography Manager: David C. Kosten

Typographers: Elizabeth A. DiCicco, Diane Paluba, Nancy Wirs

Senior Production Manager: Deborah C. Meiris

Assistant Production Managers: Pat Dorshaw, Tim A. Landis

Indexer: Barbara Hodgson

Researcher: Nancy Lange

Editorial Assistants: Maree E. DeRosa, Marlene C. Rosensweig

Special thanks to Carlos Lummus, who assisted in preparation of this volume.

© 1987 by Springhouse Corporation, 1111 Bethlehem Pike, Springhouse, Pa. 19477

Printed in the United States of America.

NRLYB-020187
ISBN 0-87434-085-3

Nursing Yearbook87

This volume is the second of an annual series conceived by the publishers of *Nursing87®* magazine. Gathered with the aid of a panel of experts from every area of nursing and medical practice, information in each volume will provide an annual update of the most significant developments in health care. Covering all areas of nursing practice, from clinical information to career and professional considerations, this new series brings today's nurse the timely information she needs to practice nursing with skill and confidence.

Other publications:

NURSE'S REFERENCE LIBRARY®
Diseases
Diagnostics
Drugs
Assessment
Procedures
Definitions
Practices
Emergencies
Signs & Symptoms

NEW NURSING SKILLBOOK™ SERIES
Giving Emergency Care Competently
Monitoring Fluid and Electrolytes Precisely
Assessing Vital Functions Accurately
Coping with Neurologic Problems Proficiently
Reading EKGs Correctly
Combatting Cardiovascular Diseases Skillfully
Nursing Critically Ill Patients Confidently
Dealing with Death and Dying
Managing Diabetes Properly
Giving Cardiovascular Drugs Safely

NURSING PHOTOBOOK™ SERIES
Providing Respiratory Care
Managing I.V. Therapy
Dealing with Emergencies
Giving Medications
Assessing Your Patients
Using Monitors
Providing Early Mobility
Giving Cardiac Care
Performing GI Procedures
Implementing Urologic Procedures
Controlling Infection
Ensuring Intensive Care
Coping with Neurologic Disorders
Caring for Surgical Patients
Working with Orthopedic Patients
Nursing Pediatric Patients
Helping Geriatric Patients
Attending Ob/Gyn Patients
Aiding Ambulatory Patients
Carrying Out Special Procedures

NURSING NOW™ SERIES
Shock
Hypertension
Drug Interactions
Cardiac Crises
Respiratory Emergencies
Pain

NURSE'S CLINICAL LIBRARY®
Cardiovascular Disorders
Respiratory Disorders
Endocrine Disorders
Neurologic Disorders
Renal and Urologic Disorders
Gastrointestinal Disorders
Neoplastic Disorders
Immune Disorders

***Nursing87* DRUG HANDBOOK™**

MediQuik Cards™

CLINICAL POCKET MANUAL™ SERIES
Diagnostic Tests
Emergency Care
Fluids and Electrolytes
Signs and Symptoms
Cardiovascular Care
Respiratory Care
Critical Care
Neurologic Care
Surgical Care

NURSE REVIEW™ SERIES
Cardiac Problems
Respiratory Problems
Gastrointestinal Problems
Neurologic Problems
Vascular Problems
Genitourinary Problems
Endocrine Problems

Contents

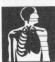

Advisory board, clinical consultants, and contributors

At the time of publication, the advisors, clinical consultants, and contributors held the following positions:

Advisory board

Debra C. Broadwell, RN, ET, PhD, Associate Professor, Emory University School of Nursing, Atlanta

Karin M. Byrne, RN, MS, JD, Associate, Morrison, Mahoney & Miller, Boston

A. Bruce Campbell, MD, PhD, Attending Physician (Hematology/Oncology), Scripps Memorial Hospital, La Jolla, Calif.

Brian B. Doyle, MD, Clinical Professor of Psychiatry and of Family and Community Medicine, Georgetown University School of Medicine, Washington, D.C.

Stephen C. Duck, MD, Director, Endocrinology and Metabolism, Milwaukee Children's Hospital; Associate Professor of Pediatrics, Medical College of Wisconsin, Milwaukee

John J. Fenton, PhD, DABCC, Professor of Clinical Chemistry, West Chester (Pa.) University; Director of Chemistry, Crozer-Chester Medical Center, Chester, Pa.

Mary Lillian "Lillee" Gelinas, RNC, MSN, (former) Director of Nursing, Memorial Hospital of Burlington County, Mount Holly, N.J.

A. Hadi Hakki, MD, FRCS, Assistant Professor of Surgery, Hahnemann University Hospital, Philadelphia; Associate Attending Surgeon, Bryn Mawr (Pa.) Hospital

Nancy M. Holloway, RN, MSN, CCRN, CEN, Consultant, Critical Care and Emergency Nursing, Nancy Holloway & Associates, Oakland, Calif.

Ruth S. Kitson, RN, BAAN, MBA, Director of Nursing—Critical Care Services, Toronto Western Hospital

Brenda Marion Nevidjon, RN, BSN, MSN, Providence CancerCare Manager/Clinical Nurse Specialist, Providence Medical Center, Seattle

John J. O'Shea, MD, Senior Staff Fellow, Cell Biology and Metabolism Branch, National Institute of Child Health and Human Development, National Institutes of Health, Bethesda, Md.

Susan Jane Rumsey, BSN, MPH, Perinatal Outreach Education Coordinator, Wake Area Health Education Center, Raleigh, N.C.

Barbara L. Solomon, RN, DNSc, Research Associate, Walter Reed Army Medical Center, Washington, D.C.

June L. Stark, RN, BSN, CCRN, Critical Care Instructor/Renal Nurse Consultant, New England Medical Center Hospitals, Boston

John Kimmel Wiley, MD, FACS, Neurosurgeon, Miami Valley Neurosurgery, Inc., Dayton, Ohio

Clinical consultants

Barbara Gross Braverman, RN, MSN, CS, Instructor of Psychiatry, Medical College of Pennsylvania, Philadelphia

June M. Buckle, RN, MSN, Assistant Director for Clinical Practice, The Johns Hopkins Hospital Department of Medicine, Baltimore

Karen E. Burgess, RN, MSN, Neurologic/Orthopedic/Rehabilitation Clinical Nurse Specialist, Huntington Memorial Hospital, Pasadena, Calif.

Mimi Callanan, RN, MSN, Epilepsy Clinical Specialist, Mid-Atlantic Regional Epilepsy Center, Philadelphia

A. Bruce Campbell, DO, PhD, Attending Physician (Hematology/Oncology), Scripps Memorial Hospital, La Jolla, Calif.

Karen Gruber D'Andrea, RNC, MS, Nurse Practitioner in Gynecology, Endocrinology, and Infertility, Brookline, Mass.

Brian B. Doyle, MD, Clinical Professor of Psychiatry and of Family and Community Medicine, Georgetown University School of Medicine, Washington, D.C.

Thaddeus P. Dryja, MD, Assistant Professor of Ophthalmology, Harvard Medical School/Massachusetts Eye and Ear Infirmary, Boston

Stephen C. Duck, MD, Director, Endocrinology and Metabolism, Milwaukee Children's Hospital; Associate Professor of Pediatrics, Medical College of Wisconsin, Milwaukee

Paul A. Epstein, MD, Diplomate, American Board of Internal Medicine; Fellow in Endocrinology and Diabetes, Hospital of the University of Pennsylvania, Philadelphia

June M. Fry, MD, PhD, Associate Professor of Neurology; Director, Sleep Disorders Center; and Chief, Division of Somnology, Medical College of Pennsylvania, Philadelphia

Mary Ann Gardiner, RN, BSN, Nurse Clinician, Travacare–Travenol Laboratories, Deerfield, Ill.

Barbara S. Henzel, RN, BSN, GIA, Clinical Nurse Supervisor, GI Endoscopy Suite, Hospital of the University of Pennsylvania, Philadelphia

Nancy M. Holloway, RN, MSN, CCRN, CEN, Critical Care and Emergency Nursing Consultant, Nancy Holloway & Associates, Oakland, Calif.

Mark P. Jacobson, DO, Assistant Professor of Pediatrics, University of Medicine and Dentistry of New Jersey, School of Osteopathic Medicine, Stratford, N.J.

Cynthia Ann LaSala, RN, BSN, Clinical Nurse, Emergency Department, University Hospital, Boston

Peter G. Lavine, MD, Director, Coronary Care Unit, Crozer-Chester Medical Center, Chester, Pa.

Patricia W. McAlary, RN, MS, Clinical Assistant to Director, Boston Pain Center–Spaulding Rehabilitation Hospital, Boston

Chris Platt Moldovanyi, RN, MSN, Director of Nursing Education—Operating Room/Endocrinology Clinical Nurse Specialist, Cleveland Clinic Foundation

John J. O'Shea, Jr., MD, Senior Staff Fellow, Cell Biology and Metabolism Branch, National Institute of Child Health and Human Development, National Institutes of Health, Bethesda, Md.

Yechiam Ostchega, RN, MSN, Clinical Nurse Specialist—Research, Medicine Branch/Cancer Nursing, National Cancer Institute, National Institutes of Health, Bethesda, Md.

Patricia A. Payne, BSN, MPH, CNM, Program Nurse Specialist, Low Birthweight Prevention Program, Department of OB/GYN, Medical University of South Carolina, Charleston

Mary Faut Rodts, RN, MS, Clinical Specialist in Orthopaedics, Rush–Presbyterian–St. Luke's Medical Center, Chicago

Gizell Maria Rossetti, MD, Staff Neurologist, Nicolet Clinic, Neenah, Wis.

Eric Silfen, MD, Director, Emergency Medical Services, Reston (Va.) Hospital Center

June L. Stark, RN, BSN, CCRN, Critical Care Instructor/Renal Nurse Consultant, New England Medical Center, Boston

Richard W. Tureck, MD, Assistant Professor of OB-GYN, University of Pennsylvania School of Medicine, Philadelphia; Director, In Vitro Fertilization and Embryo Transfer Program, Hospital of the University of Pennsylvania, Philadelphia

Contributors

Kathleen Gainor Andreoli, DSN, FAAN, Vice-President for Educational Services, Interprofessional Education, and International Programs, and Professor of Nursing, The University of Texas Health Science Center at Houston

Catherine Bast, RN, MSN, Assistant Professor of Medical-Surgical Nursing, Amarillo (Tex.) College

Joan M. Baumann, RN, BSN, Staff Nurse, Emergency Department, Holy Cross Hospital of Silver Spring (Md.)

John M. Bertoni, MD, PhD, Associate Professor of Neurology, Thomas Jefferson University, Philadelphia

Barbara Gross Braverman, RN, MSN, CS, Instructor of Psychiatry, Medical College of Pennsylvania, Philadelphia

Debra C. Broadwell, RN, ET, PhD, Associate Professor, Emory University School of Nursing, Atlanta

Laurie Shepherd Brown, RN, MSN, Nurse Practitioner–Health Services, Middlebury College, Vermont

June M. Buckle, RN, MSN, Assistant Director for Clinical Practice, Department of Medicine, The Johns Hopkins Hospital, Baltimore

Karen E. Burgess, RN, MSN, Neurologic/Orthopedic/Rehabilitation Clinical Nurse Specialist, Huntington Memorial Hospital, Pasadena, Calif.

Jennifer Burks, RN, MSN, Nurse Consultant, Germantown, Md.

Raynell J. Clark, MT, BA, Research Technician, Clinical Immunology Research and Development, Mayo Clinic, Rochester, Minn.

Diane Cochet, RN, BSN, Clinical Research Associate, Centocor, Malvern, Pa.

Roberta M. Conti, RN, MS, FAAN, CNAA, Nurse Consultant, Fairfax, Va.

F. Susan Cowchock, MD, Associate Professor of Medicine, Obstetrics, and Gynecology/Director of NTD Laboratory and Pregnancy Loss Center, Thomas Jefferson University, Philadelphia

Joanne Patzek DaCunha, RN, BS, Clinical Editor, Springhouse Corporation, Springhouse, Pa.

Carol Solomon Dalglish, RN, MSN, Clinical Specialist, Center for Fertility and Reproductive Research, Vanderbilt University Medical Center, Nashville, Tenn.

Patricia M. Dedrick, RN, MS, NP, Cardiovascular Nurse Practitioner, Kaiser Permanente Medical Center, San Diego

Jacqueline Dienemann, RN, PhD, Assistant Professor of Nursing, George Mason University, Fairfax, Va.

Gloria Ferraro Donnelly, RN, PhD, FAAN, Chairman, Department of Nursing, La Salle University, Philadelphia

Brian B. Doyle, MD, Clinical Professor of Psychiatry and of Family and Community Medicine, Georgetown University School of Medicine, Washington, D.C.

Mahmoud A. ElSohly, PhD, Research Professor, Research Institute of Pharmaceutical Sciences, University of Mississippi, University

Judith Ricciardi Errickson, RN, MS, Assistant Professor, College of Nursing, Villanova (Pa.) University

Madeline E. Fassler, RN, BSN, CEN, President, Creative Education Resources, Inc., San Leandro, Calif.

Deborah C. Foisie, RN, BS, Oncology Research Nurse/Data Manager, University of Washington Hospital, Seattle

Larry Neil Gever, RPh, PharmD, Drug Information Manager, Springhouse Corporation, Springhouse, Pa.

Lauren A. Giannakopoulos, RN, Staff Nurse, Burn/Plastic Unit, Strong Memorial Hospital, University of Rochester (N.Y.)

Christine Grady, RN, MSN, CS, Clinical Nurse Specialist, National Institutes of Health, Bethesda, Md.

Debra Haire-Joshu, RN, MSEd, MSN, Research Instructor in Medicine/Coordinator for Professional Education, Diabetes Research and Training Center, Washington University School of Medicine, St. Louis

Pat Hayes, RN, BS, Head Nurse, High Plains Baptist Hospital, Amarillo, Tex.

Barbara S. Henzel, RN, BSN, GIA, Clinical Nurse Supervisor, GI Endoscopy Suite, Hospital of the University of Pennsylvania, Philadelphia

Henry A. Homburger, MD, Codirector, Clinical Immunology, Mayo Clinic, Rochester, Minn.

Carol A. Huneke, RN, ET, Enterostomal Therapy Nurse, Veterans Administration Medical Center, Albany, N.Y.

Terry E. Jaros, RNC, BSN, Staff Nurse, Veterans Administration Medical Center, Albany, N.Y.

Jerry A. Katzmann, PhD, Laboratory Director, Clinical Immunology Laboratory, Mayo Clinic, Rochester, Minn.

Sherry L. Keramidas, PhD, Associate Medical Director, Cystic Fibrosis Foundation, Rockville, Md.

Jeananne Krejci, RN, BA, Cardiology Nurse Clinician, Hennepin County Medical Center, Minneapolis

Joyce A. Kunkel, RN, MS, CNRN, Clinical Nurse Specialist, Neurosurgery, Miami Valley Neurosurgery, Inc., Dayton, Ohio

Cynthia Ann LaSala, RN, BSN, Clinical Nurse, Emergency Department, University Hospital, Boston

Dennis E. Leavelle, MD, Consulting Pathologist/Assistant Professor, Mayo Medical Laboratories, Mayo Clinic, Rochester, Minn.

Carol Lorenzo, RN, Supervisor, GI Procedure Lab, Buffalo (N.Y.) General Hospital

Brenda L. Lyon, RN, DNS, Associate Professor and Chairperson, Graduate Department of Nursing of Adults with Biodissonance; Director and Private Practitioner, School of Nursing Office for Nursing Practice; and Adjunct Clinical Associate Professor, Indiana University Hospitals, Indiana University School of Nursing, Indianapolis

Ann Marriner, RN, PhD, Professor, Indiana University School of Nursing, Indianapolis

Margaret Fisk Mastal, RN, MSN, CNAA, Administrative Director, Professional Development and Research, Washington (D.C.) Hospital Center

Edwina A. McConnell, RN, MS, Independent Nurse Consultant, Madison, Wis.

Harry G. McCoy, PharmD, Clinical Director, MEDTOX Laboratories, Inc., St. Paul

Patricia A. McLaughlin, RN, BSN, Research Coordinator, Radiation Therapy, Albert Einstein Medical Center, Northern Division, Philadelphia

Chris Platt Moldovanyi, RN, MSN, Director of Nursing Education—Operating Room/Endocrinology Clinical Nurse Specialist, Cleveland Clinic Foundation

Scarlott K. Mueller, RN, BSN, MPH, Head Nurse/Clinical Associate, Duke University Medical Center, Durham, N.C.

Terri C. Murrell, RN, MSN, Cardiovascular Clinical Nurse Specialist, Scripps Clinic, La Jolla, Calif.

Marianne Nettina, RN, BS, (former) Staff Nurse, Operating Room, Mercy Hospital, Portland, Me.

Brenda Marion Nevidjon, RN, BSN, MSN, Providence CancerCare Manager/Clinical Nurse Specialist, Providence Medical Center, Seattle

Sharon C. Nilsen, RN, BSN, Assistant Director for Institutional Resources/Systems Nurse, University Hospital—Stony Brook (N.Y.)

Patricia Nornhold, RN, MSN, Clinical Director, *Nursing87* and *NursingLife,* Springhouse Corporation, Springhouse, Pa.

Whyte G. Owen, PhD, Consultant, Mayo Clinic/Foundation, Rochester, Minn.

Elise Robinson Pizzi, RN, MSN, Assistant Professor, College of Nursing, Villanova (Pa.) University

Jean Rabinow, BA, JD, Partner, McMillan & Rabinow, Trumbull, Conn.

Terri Rosenberg, RN, BSN, Staff Nurse, Hospital of the University of Pennsylvania, Philadelphia

Susan Rumsey, BSN, MPH, Perinatal Outreach Coordinator, Wake Area Health Education Center, Raleigh, N.C.

Susan E. Shapiro, RN, MS, CEN, Manager, Emergency Services, Marin General Hospital, Greenbrae, Calif.

William Simonson, PharmD, Associate Professor of Pharmacy, Oregon State University, Corvallis

Barbara L. Solomon, RN, DNSc, CCNS, Research Associate, Walter Reed Army Medical Center, Department of Endocrinology, Washington, D.C.

Alan Sturm, RN, GNC, Gerontologic Nurse Clinician/Consultant, Cofounder and Codirector, CARE-ED, The Genesee Hospital, Rochester, N.Y.

Julie N. Tackenberg, RN, MA, CNRN, Clinical Consultant, Springhouse Corporation, Springhouse, Pa.

Kathie Thompson, RN, BBA, Head Nurse, Cancer Control Agency of British Columbia, Vancouver

Beverly Vincent, RN, MSN, Oncology Clinical Nurse Specialist, University Hospital, University of Washington, Seattle

Robert Wharton, MD, Instructor, Pediatrics, Harvard Medical School, Cambridge, Mass.; Director, Weight Control Program, Children's Hospital, Boston; Associate Physician, Joslin Diabetes Center, Boston

Alice A. Whittaker, RN, MS, CCRN, Director, Nursing Planning, University Medical Center, Tucson, Ariz.

John K. Wiley, MD, FACS, Neurosurgeon, Miami Valley Neurosurgery, Inc., Dayton, Ohio

Lana M. Wilhelm, BSN, CNSN, Nutritional Support Nurse, University Hospital, St. Louis

Monica M. Ziegler, RN, Staffing Coordinator, University Hospital, The Milton S. Hershey Medical Center, Pennsylvania State University, Hershey, Pa.

Foreword

All things change, as we well know. But few things have changed as rapidly and with such pervasive and far-reaching effects as the current health care environment. Every day brings new demands on you to absorb new medical information and to adapt your nursing practice to new ideas and new responsibilities. For example, if you're not yet using computers at work, you surely will be before long. You can expect to share responsibility for your nursing unit's costs and budgets, as well as your hospital's efforts to attract patients and to develop and market new and profitable services. As a professional, you're expected to keep up with and adapt to all of these new developments—of course, while continuing to provide high-quality patient care.

But patient care isn't getting any easier—and not just because of exploding technology. The demographic shift to an older population means growing numbers of elderly patients will need special care. And, although fewer patients are being hospitalized, those who are tend to be acutely ill, needing ever more complex care. Care of ambulatory patients is being displaced from hospitals to specialized treatment centers. At the same time, growing numbers of knowledgeable consumers require health care providers to satisfy higher expectations of effective care.

How can nurses adapt to such rapid, all-encompassing change? Information is the key. Knowledge facilitates adaptation to change; rapid change requires easy access to reliably updated information. *Nursing Yearbook87* provides such access. This volume, second in an annual series, is designed to provide a yearly update of the most significant developments in health care.

Each volume in this series is divided into six sections representing major areas of special interest to nurses: Emergency Care; Diagnostic Tests; Diseases; Drugs; Law, Ethics, and Professional Practice; and Nursing Procedures. In this year's volume the section on Emergency Care updates the information about cardiopulmonary resuscitation, emergency triage, and two complex techniques—SvO_2 monitoring and ultrafiltration. The section on Diagnostic Tests includes several test panels that explain how antibodies and autoantibodies are used to detect or monitor disease. The next section, Diseases, updates the treatment of diabetes, AIDS, and cancer. For example, several entries offer information on treating cancer with monoclonal antibodies, radiation, lasers, and biologic response modifiers. And the Drugs section updates the use of recombinant DNA technology and provides recommendations for safer use of drugs in elderly patients.

Next, in the section on Law, Ethics, and Professional Practice, discussion of management and career issues offers practical and timely advice for dealing with the nonclinical aspects of nursing that are so important today for professional advancement. The final section, Nursing Procedures, offers guidelines for dealing with several new and complex aspects of patient care.

Nursing Yearbook87 offers nurses a convenient way to keep up with significant changes in health care. With this information, they can more easily maintain the high level of practice the nursing profession requires today.

KATHLEEN GAINOR ANDREOLI,
DSN, FAAN
Vice-President for Educational Services,
Interprofessional Education, and International Programs; Professor of Nursing,
The University of Texas
Health Science Center at Houston

ADVANCES AND ADJUSTMENTS
THE YEAR IN REVIEW

"Health care professionals may have witnessed more advances and made more adjustments than in any other year in recent history."

BY GLORIA FERRARO DONNELLY, RN, PHD, FAAN

Throughout the health care system survived another year of wrenching change. In fact, health care professionals may have witnessed and sustained more change and made more adjustments to it than in any other year in recent history. We're now living with the difficult realities of fiscal conservatism, an aging society, and exploding technology. The resulting constraints have challenged every sector of health care and are changing the way we practice nursing. Let's take a closer look at these major changes and professional adjustments as they relate to economic factors, shifting demographics, advancing technology, and new entrepreneurial ventures.

1

Economic adjustments

As health care institutions continued to absorb the financial constraints resulting from prospective reimbursement based on Diagnosis-Related Groups (DRGs), serious problems surfaced. Reports that seriously ill patients had been discharged prematurely—simply dumped "quicker and sicker"—prompted dramatic coverage by the media. A resulting U.S. Senate investigation led to the drafting of legislation calling for special monitoring to detect and prevent cost-related abuse of patients' rights and welfare. Such efforts to guarantee health care consumers their rights are certain to intensify

in the future and may eventually ease some of the fiscal pressure on those who provide health care for the acutely ill.

In the meantime, nurses continue their struggle to function as patient advocates, fiscal pressures notwithstanding. In acute care settings, this struggle places ever greater demands on nurses. First of all, it demands a high level of clinical expertise—sharply honed skills of assessment and intervention that cope efficiently with clinical complexity, and a continuously expanding knowledge base to underpin nursing judgments and actions on behalf of patients and their families. Such advocacy requires the confidence and the savvy to function effectively in situations that have enormous potential for conflict. It also requires a certain kind of self-advocacy. Consider, for example, working in the intensive care unit in a hospital where budget cuts have reduced the nursing staff and the funds for inservice training. The nurse who finds herself in this situation, overworked and undertrained in the use of new equipment, must protect herself and her patients by insisting on adequate staffing and adequate training. In other words, before she can be an effective advocate for the patient, today's nurse must have a solid grasp of her own personal and professional rights and an appropriate assertiveness for claiming them.

The prospective payment system has also had dramatic impact on hospitals. It has caused dramatic declines in inpatient occupancy rates, a reduction in the number of hospital beds, and numerous hospital closings. At the same time, the growing demand for post-acute, chronic care has multiplied the number of home health care agencies and hospice nursing services. This shift to chronic care settings will continue to grow in response to the graying of American society. *(continued)*

2

Adjustments to changing demographics

Current statistics project that by the year 2000, approximately 40% of the United States population will be over age 50, and of these, more than 12% will be over age 65. With an aging population, chronic illness will become the nation's dominant health care problem. Consequently, health care delivery will continue its shift from hospitals to extended care facilities and the patient's home. Nurses long accustomed to working in acute care settings have begun adjusting to this shift; many nurses displaced from hospital practice have moved to chronic care institutions and home care.

Home care, which is no longer just a matter of providing basic comfort, requires special professional adjustment. It now involves proficiency in managing life-extending technologies, such as dialysis, and respiratory and infusion therapies, which are creating high-tech, biomedical environments in patients' homes. Nurses will continue to dominate the coordination and delivery of home care and can expect a growing demand for high-quality home care with verifiable patient outcomes.

In recognition of nursing's pivotal role in the treatment and care of an aging society, the federal government has recently established a Center for Nursing Research within the National Institutes of Health. This center will support nursing research projects with an emphasis on promoting health and preventing disease and with a special focus on chronic health problems and terminal illness. Such research will

continue to validate the benefits of expert nursing care. With its sights on maintaining and restoring health, it can provide guidelines for preventing illness in our aging population. In clinical practice, it will help nurses keep up with new developments in nursing practice and health care technologies.

3

Technologic adjustments

Despite fiscal constraints, the development of new biomedical technology marches on. Undaunted by so many failures, medical scientists still struggle to develop a safer, more practical artificial heart. They extend transplantation technology to new applications, even though the cost of immunosuppressant drugs necessary to sustain the successful transplant is exorbitant and will probably continue to be so. And researchers work frantically to solve the mystery of AIDS, as the incidence of this disease reaches epidemic numbers. Meanwhile, an endless parade of new equipment, new diagnostic tests, new applications of computerized information, and new life support systems simultaneously simplifies, complicates, and extends the work of nurses.

We can expect the American health care system to continue its romance with technology in future years, even though financial realities and ethical questions concerning the fair distribution of resources will inevitably inhibit technology's growth. In the past, nurses have quickly accommodated and even taught new technology, though some of it was questionable and shortlived. But we can no longer accept new methods just because they are new. Nurses have always had good instincts about delivering quality care within limited resources. We now have to apply these instincts to becoming more discerning critics of new biomedical technology—evaluating new tools and new methods according to the cost-benefit ratio and promoting only those that work best in patient care.

4

Entrepreneurial advances

Not since pioneers like Lillian Wald and Lavinia Dock started the Henry Street Settlement to provide nursing services to immigrants in the New York tenements have so many nurses ventured out on their own. Enormous financial pressures on hospitals and a growing realization that high technology can't solve every clinical problem have created unique and exciting entrepreneurial opportunities for nurses. Last year, for example, the number of states with health insurance laws that mandate direct reimbursement for nurses' services has grown to 25. This signals growing recognition that nurses offer health care consumers high-quality service at cost-effective rates.

Not only are nurses venturing into individual and private practices, they are also developing unique health care businesses. Such businesses offer skilled nursing care, respite care services, health assessment and promotion services, and health education, research, and consultation services to industrial and individual consumers. A sense of professional autonomy, advanced education in business and professional practice, and a venturesome outlook have equipped nurse entrepreneurs to compete in the changing health care environment.

5

Future adjustments

More change will be the only thing we can count on in the year ahead, but we can expect some of it to bring exciting new options. The nursing profession is now geared to offer us the education and tools we will need to prepare for an uncertain future. A two-tiered level of licensure, finally differentiating technical from professional practice, may soon become a reality. And to encourage further professional advancement, more opportunities to acquire advanced degrees in a reasonable time and without sacrificing employment are becoming available. Declining enrollments in traditional nursing schools and an impending nursing shortage may soon give those who persevere greater opportunities to find in nursing an exciting career and a rewarding life's work.

Let's prepare to make the most of these opportunities by continuing to move nursing practice in positive new directions. Clearly, we must define nursing specialties in terms of promoting and maintaining health; emphasize issues that surround the care of the elderly; and push for more education in business practice and in the ethics of health care. Thus prepared, we can meet our future with confidence. Then no one can dare tell us to "know our place" since we will have so many different places to be.

We've weathered a lot of change and there's more to come. With the right attitude and the right preparation, we can do more than just meet it. We can welcome it.

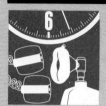

Emergency care

CPR update

Despite the initial success of many cardiopulmonary resuscitation (CPR) efforts, long-term survival statistics are discouraging. Only 10% to 20% of patients who have CPR in-hospital survive to discharge and, of the survivors, up to 20% die within 6 months after discharge. Obviously, improving these survival rates requires ongoing refinement of CPR techniques. To this end, the American Heart Association (AHA) has issued new guidelines for both basic and advanced cardiac life support. Here are some highlights of these latest AHA guidelines, as well as of recent important research into more effective CPR techniques.

Opening the airway

If a cardiac arrest victim loses consciousness, his lower jaw relaxes, possibly causing his tongue to fall back into and occlude his airway. Of the various techniques available to open the airway of an unconscious person with no evidence of neck or spinal cord injury, the AHA now recommends the head-tilt/chin-lift method. (The AHA still recommends the jaw-thrust without head-tilt method for a patient with suspected neck or spinal injury.) To use the head-tilt/chin-lift method, place one hand on the patient's forehead and tilt his head back slightly, hyperextending his neck (see the illustration at right). Then, being careful not to close his mouth completely, gently lift up his chin with the fingertips of your other hand to help move his tongue forward out of the airway.

To relieve airway obstruction from a foreign body in an adult or a child, the abdominal thrust technique (Heimlich maneuver) is now preferred over the previously recommended combination of back blows and abdominal thrusts. You can safely repeat the Heimlich maneuver an unlimited number of times in a choking victim.

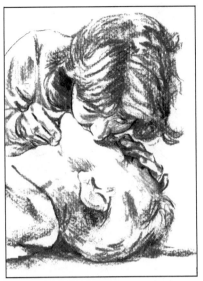

The head-tilt/chin-lift method for opening the airway in an unconscious patient

Ventilation and chest compression

The latest AHA guidelines also include changes in recommended ventilation and chest compression techniques. Previous recommendations were based on the assumption that ventilation is most effective when delivered rapidly and under high pressure. But continuing research has shown that rapid, high-pressure breaths during CPR often produce gastric distention that can actually interfere with adequate ventilation. Based on this discovery, the AHA now calls for initial ventilation with two breaths, each given over 1 to 1½ seconds, with partial lung deflation between the breaths, rather than the previously specified four rapid "staircase" breaths with no interposed lung deflation. For continuing CPR with a single rescuer, you should deliver these two breaths in the same manner between every 15 chest compressions. For two-rescuer CPR, the new standard is one breath, delivered over 1 to 1½ seconds, between every 5 compressions. Concurrently, the optimum number of

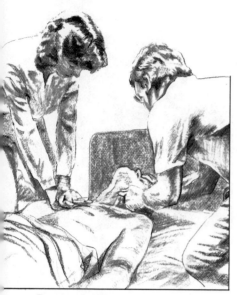

Two-rescuer CPR

chest compressions is now increased from the previously recommended rate of 60 compressions per minute (cpm) to between 80 and 100 cpm in adults and children, and at least 100 cpm in infants.

Although not included in the latest AHA guidelines, newer chest compression techniques that increase intrathoracic pressure show much promise. Increased intrathoracic pressure, not only the compression of the heart between the sternum and the vertebrae as previously believed, seems to be the reason why chest compressions may restore blood flow during CPR. Researchers have found that binding the abdomen or applying medical anti-shock trousers increases intrathoracic pressure, which improves blood flow during chest compressions. Alternating chest compressions with abdominal thrusts, a technique known as interposed abdominal compressions, achieves the same result. Some researchers have proposed that simultaneous compression-ventilation (SCV) CPR replace the current standard of one ventilation for every five compressions.

SCV–CPR, which involves simultaneous high-pressure ventilation and closed-chest compression, further increases intrathoracic pressure during CPR. But it can only be done on an intubated patient who's receiving high-pressure ventilation capable of overcoming the increased resistance caused by the compressions.

Defibrillation
The value of defibrillation in converting ventricular fibrillation or pulseless ventricular tachycardia to a more effective cardiac rhythm is unquestioned. But just how much electrical energy should be administered? The AHA now calls for an initial electrical charge of 200 joules, followed by (if necessary) a charge of 200 to 300 joules and then one of 360 joules. You should administer the three countershocks in rapid succession, without interruption for drug administration.

Drugs
Major changes have occurred in the area of recommended drug therapy during CPR, particularly in the use of calcium chloride, sodium bicarbonate, and bretylium tosylate.

Routine administration of calcium in the treatment of asystole and electromechanical dissociation is no longer recommended. The reason? When coupled with the endogenous calcium buildup that normally occurs during cardiac arrest, exogenous calcium administration may produce dangerously elevated serum calcium levels that can threaten vital organs. Consequently, the AHA now recommends calcium administration only in certain cases of cardiac arrest with concomitant hypocalcemia, calcium channel blocker toxicity, or hyperkalemia.

In the past, sodium bicarbonate was commonly given immediately after cardiac arrest. But the current thinking is that this isn't always necessary or advisable, especially if the patient is on a cardiac monitor and can be promptly converted to a sinus rhythm through

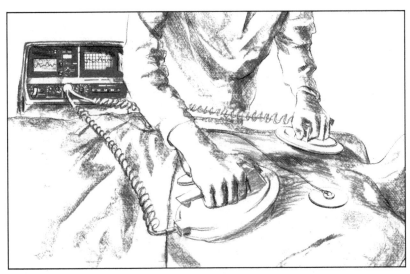

Defibrillation

defibrillation. Recent research shows that sodium bicarbonate actually can depress organ function by enhancing release of carbon dioxide, which can cross cellular membranes and induce hyperosmolality and hypernatremia, and by inhibiting intracellular oxygen release.

The new recommendations? In most code situations, sodium bicarbonate should be given strictly as needed, preferably based on arterial blood gas analyses and only after the use of more proven interventions—cardiac compression, ventilation with or without intubation, defibrillation, and administration of epinephrine and antiarrhythmic agents.

Controversy has surrounded the use of bretylium and lidocaine in treating and preventing ventricular dysrhythmias. Until recently, bretylium was the AHA's drug of choice for ventricular fibrillation. But based on new concerns about bretylium's potential hypotensive effects, the latest AHA guidelines call for lidocaine in this application.

Cerebral resuscitation
Recently, much attention has been fo-

cused on cerebral resuscitation to improve the neurologic prognosis of cardiac arrest victims. Research has focused on two areas in particular: improving blood oxygenation and cerebral blood flow during resuscitation and providing brain-oriented postresuscitation management.

Two classes of drugs—calcium channel blockers and iron-chelating agents—appear particularly promising for increasing cerebral blood flow and preventing postresuscitation brain cell damage. Calcium channel blockers, such as nimodipine and lidoflazine, dilate cerebral vessels, which theoretically improves cerebral blood flow during the delayed postischemic hypoperfusion state. Iron-chelating agents, such as deferoxamine, have a high affinity for extracellular iron ions; they may prevent free-radical reactions, which can cause widespread cerebral degeneration postarrest.

But drugs aren't the only means of preventing postresuscitation cerebral damage. Good nursing care, including prompt recognition of and intervention immediately after cardiac arrest and ongoing assessment for signs of cerebral involvement, can also play an important part. Nursing interventions that help prevent postresuscitation cerebral complications include measures to achieve hyperventilation, hyperoxygenation, adequate mean arterial pressure, and normal arterial pH and body temperature. This often requires careful balancing of interventions to ensure that a measure designed to improve one parameter doesn't disrupt another. For instance, maintenance of mean arterial pressure at the desired 90 to 100 mm Hg is commonly achieved through fluid volume loading. However, although volume loading may increase cardiac output, raising mean arterial pressure, it may also contribute to increased intracranial pressure, which can decrease cerebral blood flow. Thus, constant monitoring of the patient's total systemic response to all medical and nursing interventions is an essential part of postresuscitation care to prevent serious neurologic deficits.

MADELINE E. FASSLER, RN, BSN, CEN

Today's nursing triage

As you probably know, triage itself is nothing new—it's been part of nursing duties in many emergency departments (EDs) for over a decade now. But triage is becoming increasingly important, as current health care cost-containment trends force more efficient use of time, personnel, and equipment in every hospital. Many large EDs have one nurse per shift assigned to do triage on incoming patients. But whether or not you ever serve as triage nurse in your hospital's ED, you should familiarize yourself with triage basics.

What is triage?
Appropriately, the word triage comes from the French word for "sort out." For triage is a sorting process, originally developed to classify victims of war and other disasters according to

urgency of medical need and likelihood of survival if treated. In the ED, nursing triage involves deciding which patients should be treated before others and where the treatment should take place. This ensures that patients who need immediate care receive it, while also ensuring the best possible use of available emergency medical and nursing personnel and facilities. Nursing triage may also involve basic first aid and preliminary care (such as wound care) before a patient goes to a treatment area.

How are triage decisions made?
Triage activity consists of obtaining a focused history of the patient's chief complaint, performing a limited physical examination, and determining the urgency of the patient's problem, while at the same time reassuring him that he'll receive definitive medical care as soon as possible. Triage decision making is based on the data gathered from the history and examination, and follows the rule "when in doubt, triage up"—that is, if you're uncertain as to the seriousness of a patient's condition, treat it as more, rather than less, serious until you have solid evidence to the contrary.

The extent of your history taking and physical examination during triage depends on the nature of the patient's chief complaint and on his level of distress. Naturally, you'll ask the fewest questions and perform the briefest examination possible to provide you with the information you need to assign the patient to the appropriate triage category—you're not making a diagnosis, after all. For a patient who's clearly in distress, triage assessment may consist only of a quick inspection with no questioning necessary—or, of course, vice-versa.

Patient history in triage
Obtaining a focused patient history can be one of the greatest challenges in triage. Triage is typically done in the middle of a crowded, noisy ED with

little or no privacy and under strict time constraints. To be effective, you must be able to gather and interpret both subjective and objective data rapidly and accurately. Focus the history on the patient's chief complaint. Record this complaint on the triage record (in the patient's own words, if possible), making sure you understand what he really means by his descriptions. Have him qualify his complaint as precisely as he can, using the "P-Q-R-S-T" acronym or a similar device, if necessary (see *The "P-Q-R-S-T" Device*). Also record such information as the patient's age, current medications and the time of the last dose, allergies, date of last tetanus toxoid innoculation (if appropriate), and any other pertinent medical history. The patient's chief complaint may take on new meaning in light of some of this information.

Physical examination in triage
Apart from observing the patient's general appearance, the most important part of the physical examination during triage is assessing vital signs.
• Temperature. Take an oral or axillary temperature in all patients, as appropriate.
• Pulse. Check the apical pulse and, if appropriate, determine the apical-radial pulse deficit in all patients who complain of chest pains or palpitations. Note pulse rate, rhythm, and quality. While assessing pulse, also check skin temperature and capillary refill time. If warranted by the patient's history (for example, if he complains of dizziness or fainting), check both sitting and standing pulse rates.
• Blood pressure. During triage, check blood pressure as quickly and accurately as possible. If indicated by the patient's chief complaint or history, check orthostatic blood pressure as well. Check pressure in both arms for any patient with an unexpectedly high or low initial blood pressure reading.
• Respirations. Note the rate, depth, symmetry, and quality of respirations. Also note the patient's skin color and

---

THE "P-Q-R-S-T" DEVICE

When eliciting a patient's history of present illness, you can remember the questions that help him describe his problems fully by using the sequential letters PQRST:

P	**Provocative/palliative** What causes the problem? What makes it better? What makes it worse?
Q	**Quality/quantity** How does it feel, look, or sound, and how much of it is there?
R	**Region/radiation** Where is it? Does it spread?
S	**Severity** How does it rate on a severity scale of 1 to 10?
T	**Timing** When and how did it begin? How often does it occur? How long does it last?

---

turgor, facial expression, accessory muscle use, and any audible breath sounds. (Of course, you can easily identify a patient in respiratory distress without a detailed respiratory assessment.)

Only after obtaining a complete history and vital signs do you perform a more detailed physical examination—assuming you have the time and that such an examination is necessary.

The challenge of triage
Effective triage is often vital to the smooth operation of today's busy EDs. The triage nurse has a unique opportunity to exercise all her professional skills and judgment to ensure proper triage decisions and optimum patient care. Besides general nursing skills, expertise in such areas as crisis intervention and crowd control also comes into play. Performing effective triage isn't easy: learning to bring all the necessary elements to bear in the ED set-

TRIAGE CATEGORIES

Triage classifies emergency room patients into various categories that represent priority levels with specific time requirements for further assessment and treatment. This chart shows the popular three-category triage system.

EMERGENT

Patients with conditions classified as emergent are in critical condition and need immediate medical attention. Their illnesses or injuries are potentially threatening to life or function, and even a short delay in care can harm the patient. These conditions take the highest priority:
- Respiratory distress or arrest
- Cardiac arrest
- Severe chest pain with dyspnea or cyanosis
- Seizure states
- Severe hemorrhage
- Severe head injury
- Coma
- Poisoning or drug overdose
- Open chest or abdominal wounds
- Profound shock
- Multiple injuries
- Hyperpyrexia (over 105° F. or 40.5° C.)
- Emergency childbirth or complications of pregnancy

Start lifesaving measures; transfer to a treatment room; patient must be seen by a doctor immediately.

URGENT

These conditions are serious but generally not dangerous if medical support and treatment are briefly delayed. Patients with these conditions are your second priority:
- Chest pain associated with no respiratory symptoms
- Burns
- Major fractures
- Decreased level of consciousness or other acute neurologic deficits
- Back injuries
- Persistent nausea, vomiting, and/or diarrhea
- Severe abdominal pain
- Temperature of 102° to 105° F. (39° to 40.5° C.)
- Acute panic states
- Bleeding from any orifice

Transfer to a treatment room for more thorough assessment by a nurse or doctor; treatment should begin within 20 minutes to 2 hours.

NONEMERGENT

These conditions of lowest priority allow longer delay of medical attention without harming the patient. Such illnesses and injuries are nonacute or considered minor to moderately severe:
- Chronic backache or other chronic complaint
- Moderate headache
- Minor fractures, sprains, and strains
- Minor burns
- Vaginal/penile discharge
- Upper respiratory or urinary infections
- Dead on arrival

Patients with nonemergent conditions receive treatment after all emergent and urgent conditions have been treated; triage to other clinics if available.

ting takes time and practice. But the result, accurate triage, goes a long way in ensuring that patients who come to your ED receive timely and appropriate care.

SUSAN E. SHAPIRO, RN, MS, CEN

Continuous SvO₂ monitoring

For many patients in a critical care setting, rapid and accurate hemodynamic assessment may make the difference between life and death. Of the various hemodynamic monitoring techniques now available, few appear more promising than continuous monitoring of mixed venous oxygen saturation (SvO₂). Done through a fiberoptic flow-directed thermodilution pulmonary artery (PA) catheter, SvO₂ measurements perform several important functions. They provide an early warning of hemodynamic instability and cardiopulmonary problems; aid in assessing the patient's immediate response to medical and nursing interventions, including drug administration; and reduce the need for repeated measurement of routine parameters, such as arterial blood gases and cardiac output. In addition, the fiberoptic catheter helps detect and thus prevents certain complications associated with traditional PA catheters, such as clot formation at the catheter tip.

SvO₂ reflects the body's ability to meet tissue oxygen demands—the amount of oxygen needed by tissues for metabolic requirements. SvO₂ is influenced by two primary factors—oxygen transport and tissue oxygen consumption. Factors affecting oxygen transport include cardiac output, hemoglobin, and arterial oxygen saturation. A deficiency in any one of these factors can trigger compensation through a change in one or more of the other factors; for example, low hemoglobin results in increased

cardiac output. However, in a seriously compromised patient (such as a patient in shock, with severely reduced cardiac output), secondary compensation occurs by increasing oxygen tissue extraction from capillary blood to meet oxygen tissue demand. When primary compensation fails and secondary compensation takes over, the SvO₂ level invariably falls.

Tissue oxygen consumption refers to the amount of oxygen actually used by body tissues. When oxygen consumption rises (as in hyperthermia, for instance), cardiac output usually rises to meet tissue demands. However, compromised cardiac output inhibits tissue oxygen delivery and the SvO₂ level falls, indicating lactic acidosis.

Equipment and nursing considerations

The SvO₂ monitoring system consists of a flow-directed PA catheter with fiberoptic filaments and the CO-oximeter module (see the illustration on page 12). Catheter insertion follows the same technique as with any thermodilution flow-directed PA catheter. The distal lumen connects to an external PA pressure monitoring system; the proximal or central venous pressure lumen, to another monitoring system or to a continuous fluid administration unit; and the optical module, to the CO-oximeter unit.

The CO-oximeter consists of a digital display panel for continuous readout of SvO₂ values, a keyboard for data entry, and a strip recorder that marks SvO₂ levels (updated every 5 seconds) and the intensity of the signal received.

Nursing responsibilities for the SvO₂ monitoring system involve standard PA catheter care, equipment calibration, setting and adjustment of alarm parameters, maintenance of the strip recording system, and system troubleshooting. Calibration is necessary on initial catheter insertion, any time the catheter is disconnected from the CO-oximeter module, and routinely once a day. It's done by drawing a mixed ve-

THE SvO₂ MONITORING SYSTEM

The SvO_2 monitoring system includes a fiberoptic catheter, an optical module, and a CO-oximeter. On the CO-oximeter, a digital display panel displays a continuous digital SvO_2 value, and a strip recorder provides a permanent record of SvO_2 measurements.

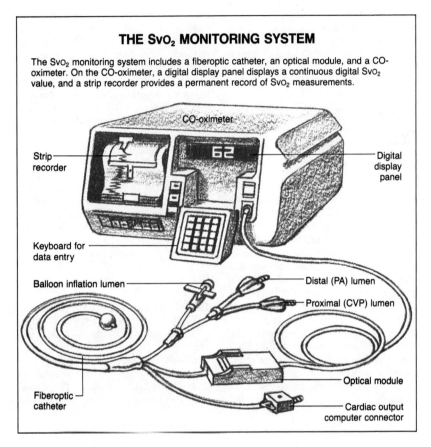

nous blood sample for laboratory analysis, then comparing the SvO_2 level of the sample to the SvO_2 reading on the CO-oximeter at the time of sampling. A difference greater than 4% between the two values necessitates recalibration according to the equipment manufacturer's instructions.

Alarm parameters are set, using the keyboard, usually at a range of 10% above and below the displayed SvO_2 level. These parameters must be updated with any change in SvO_2 greater than 5% and any time recalibration alters SvO_2 readings. The strip recorder, consisting of graph paper and marking pens, records the SvO_2 level every 5 seconds. At the lower edge of the graph paper, intensity bars measure the intensity of data transmission every 2 minutes. Inadequate signal intensity, as may result from a small clot at the catheter tip or from wedging of the tip against a vessel wall, causes the intensity bars to shorten and an alarm to sound. If the alarm sounds, SvO_2 readings are invalidated and system troubleshooting must begin. Troubleshooting involves checking catheter placement and patency, removing any air bubbles and kinks from the catheter and flushing it, and repositioning the patient.

Values and implications

In a healthy adult, an SvO_2 level between 60% and 80% usually indicates adequate tissue perfusion. However, normal values vary in critically ill patients, depending on the disorder; thus,

INTERPRETING SvO₂ MEASUREMENTS

High or low SvO_2 levels reflect problems with oxygen delivery and/or oxygen demand. This chart lists the physiologic problems that can alter SvO_2 levels, with their possible causes.

SvO₂ RANGE	PHYSIOLOGIC STATE	POSSIBLE CAUSES
High (80% to 95%)	• Increased oxygen delivery	• Increased FIO_2 from mechanical ventilation
	• Artifact	• Wedged catheter in pulmonary artery
	• Decreased oxygen uptake	• Hypothermia • Septic shock • Anesthesia • Left to right shunting
	• Increased cardiac output	• Inotropic drug administration
Normal (60% to 80%)	• Normal oxygen delivery and normal oxygen demand	• Adequate tissue perfusion
Low (below 60%)	• Increased oxygen demands	• Hyperthermia • Seizures • Severe pain and anxiety • Shivering
	• Decreased oxygen delivery resulting from: —Decreased hemoglobin	• Anemia • Hemorrhage
	—Decreased arterial oxygen saturation	• Disconnection from ventilator • Suctioning • Inadequate FIO_2 from mechanical ventilation
	—Decreased cardiac output	• Cardiogenic shock • Hypovolemia • Use of positive end-expiratory pressure (PEEP) • Discontinuation of intraaortic balloon pump

baseline SvO_2 values should be established for each individual patient. If the SvO_2 level falls below 60% or varies by more than 10% above or below the baseline value, you need to reassess the patient immediately and possibly troubleshoot the monitoring system as well. In general, an SvO_2 level below 60% is associated with cardiac decompensation; below 53%, with lactic acidosis; below 32%, with unconsciousness; and below 20%, with permanent cellular damage. High SvO_2 values—above 80%—occur in states of increased oxygen delivery, reduced oxygen demands, or decreased oxygen extraction by the tissues. See *Interpreting SvO₂ Measurements* for disorders associated with high and low SvO_2 levels. But, although this chart provides a guide for interpreting SvO_2 values, you also need to assess trends for a complete and accurate clinical picture—for example, a slowly diminishing SvO_2 reading can indicate bleeding, as hematocrit and hemoglobin levels decrease and impair tissue oxygen delivery.

JOAN M. BAUMANN, RN, BSN

Two new blood-filtering techniques to help treat renal failure

Diuretics and dialysis are the traditional methods of controlling fluid overload in patients with renal failure. But for patients with oliguria or anuria, diuretics often prove ineffective and may produce potentially serious adverse effects, such as hyperglycemia or electrolyte imbalance. And dialysis, which is both costly and time-consum-

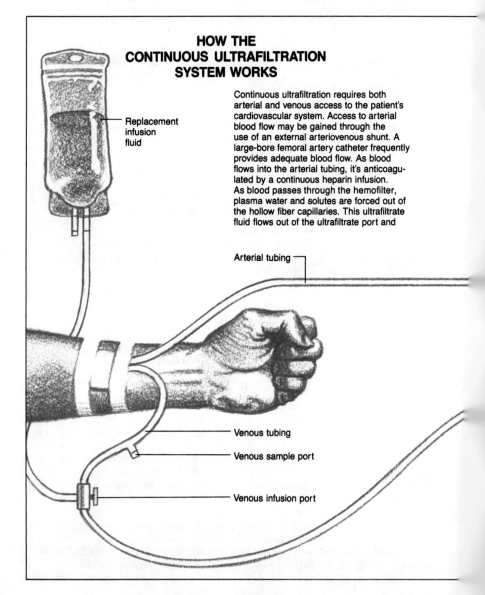

HOW THE CONTINUOUS ULTRAFILTRATION SYSTEM WORKS

Continuous ultrafiltration requires both arterial and venous access to the patient's cardiovascular system. Access to arterial blood flow may be gained through the use of an external arteriovenous shunt. A large-bore femoral artery catheter frequently provides adequate blood flow. As blood flows into the arterial tubing, it's anticoagulated by a continuous heparin infusion. As blood passes through the hemofilter, plasma water and solutes are forced out of the hollow fiber capillaries. This ultrafiltrate fluid flows out of the ultrafiltrate port and

Replacement infusion fluid

Arterial tubing

Venous tubing

Venous sample port

Venous infusion port

ing, may actually be contraindicated in hemodynamically unstable patients.

But two recently developed methods of controlling fluid balance—slow continuous ultrafiltration (SCUF) and continuous arteriovenous hemofiltration (CAVH)—offer safe, effective therapeutic alternatives. Both systems use a small-volume, low-resistance hemofil-

ter to slowly and continuously remove excess water and, in the case of CAVH, electrolytes and metabolic wastes from blood. Depending on the filter size, the SCUF system removes plasma water at a rate of 300 to 400 ml/hour; the CAVH system, at a rate of 400 to 800 ml/hour. Primarily used to treat patients with oliguric acute renal failure, they're par-

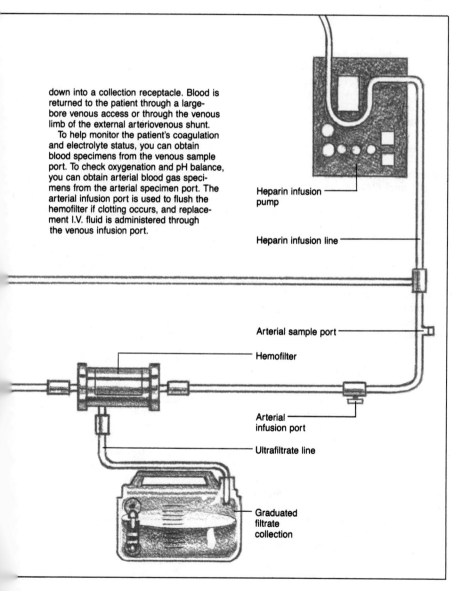

down into a collection receptacle. Blood is returned to the patient through a large-bore venous access or through the venous limb of the external arteriovenous shunt.

To help monitor the patient's coagulation and electrolyte status, you can obtain blood specimens from the venous sample port. To check oxygenation and pH balance, you can obtain arterial blood gas specimens from the arterial specimen port. The arterial infusion port is used to flush the hemofilter if clotting occurs, and replacement I.V. fluid is administered through the venous infusion port.

Heparin infusion pump

Heparin infusion line

Arterial sample port

Hemofilter

Arterial infusion port

Ultrafiltrate line

Graduated filtrate collection

ticularly valuable in controlling fluid balance in patients who can't tolerate dialysis and in those for whom diuretic therapy proves ineffective or contraindicated; in patients receiving dialysis, they can reduce the required frequency of treatments. And because CAVH removes solutes as well as water from plasma, it's also effective in controlling various electrolyte disturbances, such as hypernatremia and azotemia.

With SCUF and CAVH, the patient remains hemodynamically stable; equally important, he needn't restrict his fluid intake to prevent hypervolemia and pulmonary edema. He can take larger and safer dilutions of I.V. medications and, if necessary, receive hyperalimentation in full volume to meet his nutritional needs.

Nursing considerations for SCUF and CAVH

Basic nursing responsibilities for the patient undergoing either form of hemofiltration include assisting with system setup and maintenance; continually monitoring the patient's blood pressure and taking steps to help ensure normotension; checking his fluid and electrolyte status and providing replacements as needed; maintaining anticoagulation in the hemofilter; assessing composition and volume of the ultrafiltrated fluid; and monitoring for potential problems, particularly bleeding. System setup and maintenance follows the equipment manufacturer's instructions and your hospital's protocol; the other nursing responsibilities are discussed below.

• *Assessing the patient's fluid and electrolyte balance.* The rate of ultrafiltration necessary to remove the desired volume of fluid is determined primarily by the patient's blood pressure and is also influenced by plasma oncotic pressure (pressure exerted on vessel walls by plasma proteins). Decreased blood pressure or increased plasma oncotic pressure (as can result from dehydration or excessive colloid administra-

tion) can decrease or halt ultrafiltration, To prevent this problem, try to maintain the patient's mean arterial blood pressure at 60 mm Hg or greater by administering vasoactive agents, as ordered.

The rate of ultrafiltration is also influenced by the amount of negative hydrostatic pressure exerted by the column between the hemofilter and the collection bag. Raising the collection bag decreases column length and slows the ultrafiltration rate; conversely, increasing the column length by lowering the collection bag speeds ultrafiltration. A screw clamp installed on the ultrafiltrate tubing can also regulate the rate of fluid removal.

Fluid and electrolyte replacement requirements can vary widely among patients. Since the ultrafiltration rate in SCUF is usually less than 300 ml/hour, the patient's fluid replacement needs are usually covered by hyperalimentation and maintenance I.V. infusions. On the other hand, the patient on CAVH will probably need hourly I.V. fluid replacement, usually with normal saline or Ringer's lactate solution, of at least one half of his fluid output during the previous hour. You need to monitor the patient's serum electrolyte levels carefully during CAVH therapy; he may require additional calcium and potassium if his fluid replacement needs are great.

To prevent fluid volume depletion— a potential adverse effect of SCUF or CAVH therapy—you need to consider all sources of fluid loss and intake when calculating the patient's fluid replacement requirements. Carefully monitor his response to fluid removal for signs of volume depletion—hypotension, tachycardia, and decreasing central venous pressure or pulmonary capillary wedge pressure. If you note these signs, slow or stop the ultrafiltration rate by clamping the ultrafiltration line, then recalculate the patient's fluid replacement requirements.

• *Ensuring hemofilter anticoagulation.* Anticoagulation of the hemofilter and blood lines, done with continuous heparin infusion into the arterial blood line, is necessary to prevent clotting in the ultrafiltration system. You need to determine the optimum rate of heparin infusion to prevent clots while also avoiding bleeding problems in the patient. To do so, be sure to obtain baseline anticoagulation studies for the patient before beginning ultrafiltration therapy. Then, during therapy, draw clotting studies, such as partial thromboplastin time (PTT) or activated clotting time (ACT), every 4 hours to determine the patient's level of systemic anticoagulation, and adjust the heparin infusion as necessary to maintain PTT or ACT within the range specified by the doctor.

If the system begins to clot, decreasing the ultrafiltration rate, first check the patient's blood pressure to rule out a drop in blood pressure as the cause of the decreased rate, then check the hemofilter and tubing for signs of clotting. Normally, arterial blood appears bright red in the filter and tubing; dark streaks or separation of the blood indicates clotting. If you suspect clotting, flush the hemofilter by injecting a 50-ml heparinized saline bolus into the arterial port. After flushing, inspect the hemofilter for clots. If a large number of the hemofilter fibers are clotted, you need to change the filter and possibly reevaluate the entire anticoagulation system.

• *Assessing the patient for bleeding problems.* Although rare, bleeding during ultrafiltration therapy is a major concern. To minimize the risk of bleeding, make sure all blood lines are carefully positioned and securely bridge-taped to prevent accidental disconnection. Because rupture of the hollow fibers in the hemofilter can result in loss of blood into the ultrafiltrate, be sure to test the ultrafiltrate for occult blood regularly, and change the hemofilter when necessary. Further safety measures include inserting all necessary I.V. lines before beginning therapy and exercising caution during routine procedures, such as tracheal suctioning, to prevent injury to the patient.

The minimal level of systemic heparinization from the anticoagulation system rarely causes bleeding problems; however, you still need to assess the patient thoroughly for any evidence of bleeding, including occult bleeding from the gastrointestinal and urinary tracts. As an added precaution, obtain baseline coagulation studies from every patient before starting ultrafiltration therapy, and check his PTT and ACT values regularly during therapy.

ALICE A. WHITTAKER, RN, MS, CCRN

Nursing strategies for nonoliguric acute renal failure

One common and characteristic sign of acute renal failure (ARF) is oliguria, or urine output of less than 400 ml/day. But in fact, 20% to 50% of patients with ARF may have a urine output greater than 400 ml/day, a condition known as nonoliguric ARF. Incidence of nonoliguric ARF is rising, due in part to improved diagnostic techniques that enable detection of ARF at earlier, preoliguric stages; in part to increased use of nephrotoxic aminoglycoside antibiotics; and in part to current treatment regimens that use infusion of large volumes of intravenous fluids early to improve cardiac output, followed by administration of diuretics to increase urine output.

In general, nonoliguric ARF is less serious than oliguric ARF, with less associated morbidity and mortality. However, potentially fatal uremic complications—including anemia, metabolic acidosis, GI hemorrhage, and neurologic abnormalities—can still develop in nonoliguric ARF; and dialysis, while used less commonly than in oliguric ARF, may still be necessary.

DIFFERENTIATING BETWEEN OLIGURIC AND NONOLIGURIC A.R.F.

To help you differentiate between oliguric and nonoliguric ARF, here's a summary of important differences between the two conditions.

VARIABLE FEATURES	OLIGURIC A.R.F.	NONOLIGURIC A.R.F.
Urine output	Less than 400 ml/day	400 to 2,000 ml/day
Solute excretion	Minimal excretion of daily solute load	Excretion of solute load up to 350 mOsm/1,000 ml/day
Creatinine clearance	Low (about 1ml/min)	Considerably higher (2 to 15 ml/min)
Electrolyte balance	High sodium excretion and water overload, resulting in hyponatremia; low potassium excretion, resulting in hyperkalemia	Hyperkalemia is the only significant electrolyte problem.
Morbidity	Longer average length of hospitalization; greater frequency of dialysis	Shorter average length of hospitalization; reduced frequency of dialysis
Mortality	Approximately 50%	Approximately 26%

While nonoliguric and classic oliguric ARF share many clinical features, certain crucial differences influence patient management.

Nursing management of nonoliguric ARF

Nursing care of the patient with nonoliguric ARF involves careful assessment of all body systems, with special consideration given to maintaining fluid balance, replacing electrolyte losses, and providing nutritional support.

• *Maintaining fluid balance.* Even with a normal urine output, the patient with nonoliguric ARF may experience fluid volume overload if his fluid intake exceeds output. Your assessment of the patient's extracellular fluid volume involves careful consideration of all sources of fluid loss as well as all possible means of fluid replacement. Although intake and output records provide information on fluid volume

trends, the patient's body weight is the most reliable indicator of fluid balance. Based on the fact that 1 liter of water weighs approximately 1 kg, you can quickly and accurately estimate any fluid loss or gain through daily body weights.

Typically, initial treatment for nonoliguric ARF consists of fluid therapy, based on the patient's individual needs. This may involve fluid restriction. Usual daily fluid orders include replacement of urine volume plus a variable allowance for insensible water loss.

You can assess the patient's response to fluid therapy by observing him for signs of fluid volume overload, including increased body weight and evidence of peripheral edema. Auscultate the patient's lungs for rales, which may point to pulmonary edema. Also check such parameters as central venous pressure, pulmonary capillary wedge pressure, cardiac output, and systemic blood pressure—elevated values may indicate fluid volume overload.

If you detect any signs of fluid volume overload, notify the doctor immediately. Expect to administer a loop diuretic, such as furosemide, which enhances diuresis by blocking reabsorption of sodium and water in the renal tubules and increases glomerular filtration through its vasodilating effect on the renal vasculature.

For most patients with nonoliguric ARF, fluid balance is achieved by fluid therapy and administration of diuretics. But if these measures prove ineffective, the patient may need dialysis therapy.

Although less common than fluid overload, fluid volume deficit can also occur in nonoliguric ARF when total fluid loss exceeds fluid replacement. If untreated, this fluid volume deficit can result in hypovolemia, hypotension, and hypoperfusion of the kidneys, which could cause permanent renal damage. So, besides monitoring the patient for fluid overload, you also need to be alert for early signs of fluid volume deficit: poor skin turgor, sticky mucous membranes, flat neck veins, and orthostatic pulse and blood pressure changes.

• *Ensuring electrolyte balance.* Maintaining electrolyte balance involves accurate assessment of electrolyte loss and appropriate replacement therapy. Probably the most significant electrolyte problem in nonoliguric ARF is hyperkalemia, which can develop despite near-normal urine output. An elevated serum potassium level results from decreased renal excretion as well as from the metabolic acidosis that almost invariably accompanies ARF. Hyperkalemia can seriously affect the cardiac conduction system, often producing potentially fatal dysrhythmias. Thus, you need to monitor the patient's serum potassium level carefully, remaining alert for signs of cardiac dysrhythmias. In nonoliguric ARF, hyperkalemia is most effectively treated by administering an ion-exchanging agent, such as Kayexalate, which removes a milliequivalent of potassium for every milliequivalent of sodium absorbed. The longer the ion-exchanging agent remains in the GI tract, the more potassium is exchanged. Administered by mouth or as a retention enema, ion-exchanging agents should be given with an osmotic agent, such as sorbitol. Sorbitol creates an osmotic diarrhea, which helps remove potassium and prevents constipation.

• *Providing nutritional support.* The primary goals of nutritional management in nonoliguric ARF include decreasing protein catabolism and limiting the accumulation of nitrogenous waste products and potassium in extracellular fluid. Secondary goals include preventing malnutrition, promoting recovery, and enhancing resistance to infection. Most patients with ARF, either oliguric or nonoliguric, are in a catabolic state and require increased calorie and protein intake. A high-carbohydrate diet usually supplies the required calories. Of course, individual protein requirements vary, but recent studies suggest that patients with nonoliguric ARF have higher creatinine clearance than those with oliguric ARF, and thus may better tolerate the increased solute load that results from a higher protein intake. Carefully assess such a patient for any rapid rise in blood urea nitrogen level and for any other signs or symptoms of developing uremia. If these occur, dialysis will be necessary to maintain a positive nitrogen balance while minimizing uremic complications.

If oral feeding is inappropriate for your patient, intravenous hyperalimentation (IVH) can ensure that he receives proper intake of calories, protein, and other nutrients to promote rapid recovery. However, a patient on IVH may require daily dialysis to maintain fluid and electrolyte balance, which makes IVH an unattractive alternative for many patients.

ALICE A. WHITTAKER, RN, MS, CCRN

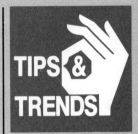

TIPS & TRENDS

New burn dressing

If you take care of burn patients, you may be interested in a new burn-care product: a one-step burn dressing designed for emergency use on many types of thermal and chemical burns. Called Water-Jel, the new dressing is made of 100% new wool combined with a bactericidal, biodegradable, water-soluble gel containing natural oils. The dressing, which comes in sizes ranging from 2″ × 2″ to 18″ × 8″, can be applied at the accident scene or in the emergency department and can be left in place for up to several hours, if necessary, before secondary burn care begins. Water-Jel decreases pain, reduces swelling, cools and soothes the skin, and lessens the progression of burns by absorbing excess heat.

Another Water-Jel product for burns is a fire blanket that extinguishes flames while at the same time providing primary burn therapy. The blanket can withstand temperatures up to 2,800° F. (1,538° C.).

Central pontine myelinolysis

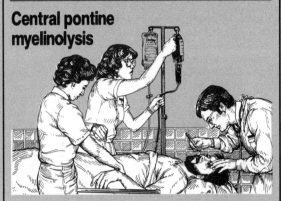

Rapid infusion of intravenous saline solutions to correct fluid volume deficiencies, long a standard practice in emergency departments, has been linked to the development of central pontine myelinolysis (CPM) in some patients. Marked by destruction of the pontine myelin and disruption of the pyramidal tract, CPM causes severe, often fatal, neurologic impairment. Patients with a severe electrolyte disturbance, particularly hyponatremia (a serum sodium level less than 130 mEq/liter) are especially susceptible. The primary predisposing factors are malnutrition and alcoholism; others include chronic renal failure, hepatic disease, advanced cancer, acute hemorrhagic pancreatitis, and severe bacterial infections.

Typical clinical features of CPM include nystagmus and palsies of cranial nerve VI, which restrict lateral eye movement; altered level of consciousness, sometimes with pseudocoma or "locked in" syndrome; pseudobulbar palsy, as evidenced by dysarthria and dysphagia; and quadriparesis. Many of these mental and ocular changes are similar to those found in acute thiamine (vitamin B_1) deficiency or Wernicke's encephalopathy; in fact, CPM and Wernicke's encephalopathy often coexist in the same patient.

If any patient—especially one suffering from malnutrition and/or alcoholism—develops these signs and symptoms, suspect CPM and notify the doctor immediately. Expect to administer thiamine (50 to 100 mg either I.V. or I.M.). Perform frequent neurologic checks, as ordered, and monitor trends in serum sodium level. The doctor may order diagnostic studies, such as computed tomography scanning, magnetic resonance imaging, and brain stem and somatosensory evoked potentials.

To help prevent CPM, provide fluid and electrolyte replacement judiciously to volume-depleted patients, and avoid hypertonic saline solutions unless absolutely necessary.

The THI heat stress index

Heat emergencies—heat cramps, heat exhaustion, and, most importantly, heat stroke—are preventable. But prevention requires knowledge of the mechanisms and the risks of such emergencies. Athletes, laborers in non–air-conditioned environments, persons taking diuretic or anticholinergic drugs, and the elderly are particularly susceptible; these people need an easy, reliable way to assess the risk of heat emergencies for any given environmental condition. In response to this need, a simple formula known as the temperature-humidity index (THI) has been developed. This formula requires only the day's high temperature, expressed in degrees Fahrenheit (°F.), and relative humidity, both of which are readily obtained from media sources or a weather service.

The THI formula is as follows:

$$(\text{temperature [°F.]} + \text{relative humidity}) \times 0.4 + 15 = \text{THI}$$

So, on a day with a high temperature of 85° F. and a relative humidity of 80, the THI is calculated as follows:

$$(85 + 80) \times 0.4 + 15 = 81$$

After calculating the THI for a given day, the value is compared to these standards to estimate the risk on that day:

THI below 65	No significant risk
THI between 65 and 80	Moderate risk; discretion advised
THI over 80	High risk; extreme caution advised

Warn your patients in high-risk groups about the dangers of heat emergencies, and take the time to explain this simple formula.

Computerized burn estimation

For a seriously burned patient, fluid volume replacement is especially important in the first 72 hours of treatment. Accurate initial estimation of the patient's total burn surface area (TBSA) determines optimum fluid replacement therapy. However, whether they use the "rule of nines" or the Lund and Browder chart, health care professionals tend to overestimate TBSA, which can result in overhydration of the patient.

A new method of calculating TBSA—computer-assisted burn surface area estimation—may help ensure more accurate TBSA estimates. Consisting of a personal desktop computer and a special grid-pattern tracing easel, the computer-assisted system calculates TBSA quickly (on average, within 5 minutes), easily, and with little significant variation between users. A recent study at the University of Virginia Medical Center compared doctors' estimates to computer-generated calculations of TBSA on a diagram of a burned adult male. The results? The doctors' estimates ranged from 38.3% to 44.2% TBSA, compared to the computer-assisted calculation of 29.6% TBSA—a significant discrepancy that could have serious clinical implications.

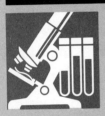

Diagnostic tests

Fetal-maternal erythrocyte distribution

Some transfer of red blood cells from fetal to maternal circulation occurs during most spontaneous or elective abortions or most normal deliveries. Usually, the amount of blood transferred is minimal and of no clinical significance. But transfer of significant amounts of blood from an Rh-positive fetus to an Rh-negative mother can result in maternal immunization to the Rh_o (D) antigen and the development of anti–Rh-positive antibodies in maternal circulation. During subsequent pregnancy, this maternal immunization subjects an Rh-positive fetus to potentially fatal hemolysis and erythroblastosis.

To prevent maternal Rh_o (D) immunization, Rh_o immune globulin (anti-D) is given to an unsensitized Rh-negative mother shortly after the birth of an Rh-positive infant or after an abortion. The amount of Rh_o immune globulin needed depends on the volume of fetal blood transferred; thus, this test measures the number of fetal red blood cells in maternal circulation to allow calculation of the Rh_o (D) immune globulin dosage needed for protection.

This test usually employs a modification of the Kleihauer technique, using a maternal blood smear fixed with ethanol. The adult hemoglobin is eluted from the red blood cells by a buffer at an acid pH of 3.2. Removal of hemoglobin does not destroy the red blood cells and therefore permits the counting of these adult cells and the normally stained fetal red blood cells. (A counterstain, such as aniline blue, may aid visualization of the eluted adult red cells by giving them a very light gray-blue color.) After counting, the percentage of fetal red blood cells is used to calculate the approximate fetal-maternal erythrocyte volume, based on average total red cell volume.

Purpose
• To detect and quantify fetal-maternal blood transfer
• To determine the amount of Rh_o (D) immune globulin needed to prevent maternal immunization to the Rh_o (D) antigen.

Patient preparation
Explain to the patient that this test determines the amount of Rh_o immune globulin she needs to protect future infants from complications resulting from Rh incompatibility. Review how Rh isoimmunization occurs (see *Pathogenesis of Rh Isoimmunization,* page 24). Tell her that she needn't restrict foods or fluids before the test, that the test requires a blood sample, who will perform the venipuncture and where, and that she may experience transient discomfort from the needle puncture and the pressure of the tourniquet. Reassure her that sample collection takes less than 3 minutes.

Procedure
Perform a venipuncture, and collect at least 1 ml of blood in a *lavender-top* tube.

Precautions
• To prevent hemolysis, handle the sample gently and keep it at room temperature—*do not freeze.*
• If possible, arrange for sample analysis within 24 hours of collection—72 hours at the latest.

Values
Normal maternal whole blood contains no fetal red blood cells.

Implications of results
An elevated fetal red blood cell volume in maternal circulation necessitates administration of Rh_o (D) immune globulin. The number of vials needed is based on multiples of 15 ml of fetal red blood cells in maternal circulation.

PATHOGENESIS OF RH ISOIMMUNIZATION

Rh-negative woman prepregnancy.

Pregnancy with Rh-positive fetus.

Placental separation.

Postdelivery, mother becomes sensitized to Rh-positive blood and develops anti–Rh-positive antibodies (squares).

Administration of Rh_o (D) immune globulin to an unsensitized Rh-negative mother as soon as possible (no later than 72 hours) after the birth of an Rh-positive infant or after a spontaneous or elective abortion prevents complications in subsequent pregnancies. Some doctors are now administering Rh_o (D) immune globulin prophylactically at 28 weeks' gestation to Rh-negative women who have no detectable Rh antibodies.

The following patients should be screened for Rh isoimmunization or irregular antibodies:
• all Rh-negative mothers during their first prenatal visit, and at 24, 28, 32, and 36 weeks' gestation
• all Rh-positive mothers with histories of transfusion, a jaundiced baby, stillbirth, cesarean birth, or induced or spontaneous abortion.

Post-test care
If a hematoma develops at the venipuncture site, apply ice.

Interfering factors
• Hemolysis caused by improper temperature control or rough handling of the sample may interfere with accurate determination of test results.
• Sample analysis done after 72 hours of collection may yield inaccurate results.
• Improper test ordering, such as ordering a "Kleihauer test," may result in performance of the wrong test. (The Kleihauer method is also used to detect abnormal hemoglobin with hereditary persistence of high fetal hemoglobin.)

DENNIS E. LEAVELLE, MD

Immunofixation of cerebrospinal fluid

This test, which uses immunoelectrophoresis to analyze cerebrospinal fluid (CSF) and serum samples for immu-

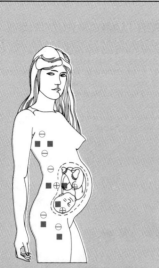

During the next pregnancy with Rh-positive fetus, maternal anti–Rh-positive antibodies enter fetal circulation and attach to Rh-positive red blood cells, subjecting them to hemolysis.

noglobulins, helps confirm diagnosis of multiple sclerosis (MS). Increased total protein content of CSF, primarily due to increased CSF immunoglobulin synthesis, is characteristic of MS and certain other degenerative neurologic disorders. The CSF immunoglobulins in MS electrophorese as discrete populations, known as oligoclonal bands, rather than as the broad, homogeneous polyclonal bands characteristic of normal, polyclonal immunoglobulin. These discrete immunoglobulins presumably come from restricted clones of immune cells in the CSF of MS patients. Although establishing the presence of oligoclonal bands in CSF through electrophoresis may give sufficient diagnostic information in most cases (see "Multiple sclerosis screening panel," page 31), immunofixation provides confirmation by ruling out rare bands that aren't composed of immunoglobulin.

In this test, a sample of CSF is concentrated to approximately 200 mg/dl

of the IgG concentration, then analyzed through an agarose gel electrophoresis technique. Specific antibodies to IgG, IgM, IgA, and other immunoglobulins are added to the electrophoresed proteins; these react to form insoluble precipitates in the agarose. After unreacted protein (nonimmunoglobulin) is removed by washing, the precipitates are visualized by staining with amido black. In the final evaluation, the oligoclonal band pattern of the CSF sample is compared to the stained immunofixation pattern, and the immunoglobulin and light chain classes of the oligoclonal bands are recorded. As a cross-check, a serum sample is also analyzed for oligoclonal bands. (The bands aren't clinically significant if the same bands occur in both CSF and serum.)

Purpose
To help confirm diagnosis of MS.

Patient preparation
Explain to the patient that this test helps determine whether his symptoms are caused by MS. Advise him that he needn't restrict food or fluids before the test. Tell him that the test requires both blood and CSF samples, and who will collect the samples. Warn that he may experience transient discomfort from the needle puncture and the pressure of the tourniquet during blood sample collection, and that he may feel some stinging from injection of the anesthetic and local pain from insertion of the spinal needle during lumbar puncture for CSF sampling. Advise the patient that he may experience headache during the lumbar puncture, but that his cooperation during the procedure will minimize this and other possible side effects.

Before the test, make sure the patient or a responsible member of his family has signed a consent form. If the patient seems unusually anxious, tell the doctor; he may order a mild sedative to help the patient relax before lumbar puncture.

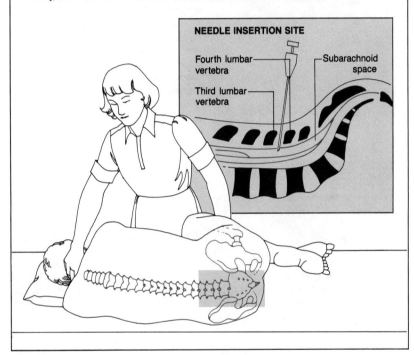

POSITIONING THE PATIENT FOR LUMBAR PUNCTURE

Position the patient on his side at the edge of the bed, with his knees drawn up as far as possible. Place a small pillow under his head, and bend his head forward, so that his chin touches his chest. Support the patient during the procedure by standing in front of him and placing one of your arms around his neck and your other arm around his knees. Usually, the needle is inserted between the third and fourth lumbar vertebrae.

NEEDLE INSERTION SITE

Fourth lumbar vertebra

Third lumbar vertebra

Subarachnoid space

Procedure

Perform a venipuncture, and collect a blood sample in a 7-ml *red-top* tube. Then, within 2 hours of blood sampling, assist the doctor in performing a lumbar puncture, and collect at least 3 ml of CSF in a sterile tube that contains no additives. Label the samples properly and send them to the laboratory promptly.

Precautions

• Send the samples to the laboratory immediately after collection. If the test can't be performed on the day of collection, refrigerate, but don't freeze, the samples.

• During the lumbar puncture, observe the patient for any signs of adverse reaction, such as elevated pulse rate, pallor, or cool, clammy skin. Alert the doctor immediately of any significant changes.

Findings

Normally, CSF contains no oligoclonal bands or only one band of any immunoglobulin class and light chain.

Implications of results

Positive test results (two or more oligoclonal bands found in CSF but not in the concomitant serum sample) support a diagnosis of MS *only* in conjunction with characteristic clinical findings. This test may also be positive in a variety of central nervous system disorders, including cryptococcal meningitis, idiopathic polyneuritis, neurosyphilis, chronic rubella panencephalitis, and subacute sclerosing panencephalitis.

Post-test care
• If a hematoma develops at the venipuncture site, apply ice.
• Have the patient remain supine for at least 8 hours after lumbar puncture, and encourage the patient to increase fluid intake.
• If the doctor orders slight head elevation, raise the head of the patient's bed 20 degrees.
• Monitor vital signs and neurologic status frequently, and check the lumbar puncture site for redness, swelling, and drainage.

Interfering factors
• Freezing and thawing of specimens can cause false-negative results.
• Delay between collection time and laboratory testing can invalidate results.

JERRY A. KATZMANN, PhD
RAYNELL J. CLARK, BA, MT

Autoimmune liver disease test panel

This panel evaluates patients with a suspected immune-mediated liver disease, including chronic active hepatitis (CAH) and primary biliary cirrhosis (PBC). The panel includes tests for

_____NEW TEST_____

AUTOIMMUNE LIVER DISEASE TEST PANEL: FINDINGS AND IMPLICATIONS

TEST	NORMAL VALUES	IMPLICATIONS OF ABNORMAL RESULTS
Antinuclear antibodies	Negative	Antinuclear antibodies are present in some patients with CAH and in other immune-mediated liver diseases.
Serum protein electrophoresis	• Total protein: 6.3 to 7.9 g/dl • Albumin: 3.1 to 4.3 g/dl Alpha₁ globulin: 0.1 to 0.3 g/dl • Alpha₂ globulin: 0.6 to 1.0 g/dl • Beta globulin: 0.7 to 1.4 g/dl • Gamma₁ globulin: 0.7 to 1.6 g/dl	Patients with hepatic cirrhosis or CAH often have elevated globulins and decreased albumin.
Antimitochondrial antibodies	Negative	Antimitochondrial antibodies have been reported in 79% to 94% of patients with PBC.
Anti–smooth muscle antibodies	Negative	Anti–smooth muscle antibodies are present in sera from up to 85% of patients with CAH and less than 50% of patients with PBC.

serum protein electrophoresis, which is often abnormal in patients with cirrhosis; antinuclear antibodies, which are often detected in both CAH and PBC; antimitochondrial antibodies, often found in PBC; and anti–smooth muscle antibodies, common in CAH.

Purpose
To screen for immune-mediated liver disease.

Patient preparation
Explain to the patient that this test panel helps determine whether his symptoms are caused by an immune-mediated liver disease. Inform him that he needn't restrict food or fluids before the tests. Tell him that the tests require a blood sample, and that he may feel transient discomfort from the needle puncture and the pressure of the tourniquet. Reassure him that sample collection takes less than 3 minutes.

Procedure
Perform a venipuncture, and collect the sample in a 10-ml *red-top* tube.

Precautions
Send the specimen to the lab immediately, or freeze it at −4° F. (−20° C.) if prolonged storage is necessary.

Post-test care
If a hematoma develops at the venipuncture site, apply ice.

Interfering factors
None known at this time.

HENRY A. HOMBURGER, MD
RAYNELL J. CLARK, BA, MT

Connective tissue disease test panel

These three test series aid the differential diagnosis of a variety of immune-mediated connective tissue diseases, including systemic lupus erythematosus, rheumatoid arthritis, Sjögren's syndrome, and mixed connective tissue disease.

The *connective tissue disease screen,* which includes a test for antinuclear antibodies (ANA) and rheumatoid factor (RF) screen and titer, is useful in the initial evaluation of patients with suspected immune-mediated inflammatory disease. The *connective tissue disease autoantibody panel* identifies the specific autoantibodies detected by the ANA test. IgG antibodies to double-stranded DNA (ds-DNA) occur in lupus erythematosus; antibodies to extractable nuclear antigens (ENA) are found in lupus erythematosus and other connective tissue diseases. The *connective tissue disease activity assessment* monitors exacerbations of lupus erythematosus.

Purpose
To aid differential diagnosis of immune-mediated connective tissue disease and help monitor disease activity.

Patient preparation
Explain to the patient that this test panel helps diagnose and evaluate his disease. Instruct him to fast for 12 hours before the tests. Tell him the tests require one or more blood samples, who will perform the venipuncture and where, and that he may experience transient discomfort from the needle puncture and the pressure of the tourniquet. Reassure him that sample collection takes less than 3 minutes.

Procedure
Perform a venipuncture, and collect each sample in a 3-ml *red-top* tube.

Precautions
Send the samples to the laboratory immediately. If the disease activity assessment assay can't be performed within 4 hours of collection, the serum must be separated from the clot and frozen at −94° F. (−70° C.) until it can be done.

NEW TEST

CONNECTIVE TISSUE DISEASE TEST PANEL: FINDINGS AND IMPLICATIONS

TEST	NORMAL VALUES	IMPLICATIONS OF ABNORMAL RESULTS
Connective tissue disease screen		
ANA (antinuclear antibodies)	Negative	60% to 90% of lupus erythematosus patients test positive.
RF (rheumatoid factor screen)	Nonreactive	> 75% of patients with rheumatoid arthritis test positive.
Connective tissue disease autoantibody panel		
ENA (extractable nuclear antigens):		
RNP (ribonucleoprotein antigens)	Negative	Found in mixed connective tissue disease.
Sm (Smith antigens)	Negative	Found in lupus erythematosus.
SSB	Negative	Found in Sjögren's syndrome and lupus erythematosus.
SSA	Negative	Found in lupus erythematosus, Sjögren's syndrome, and congenital complete heart block.
ds-DNA (double-stranded DNA)	< 70 units	60% of lupus erythematosus patients test positive during active disease.
Connective tissue disease activity assessment		
ds-DNA	< 70 units	A rise in titer may indicate an increase in disease activity.
CH_{50} (total complement)	25 to 70 units	Depressed levels of complement occur during active inflammation in lupus erythematosus.

Post-test care
If a hematoma develops at the venipuncture site, apply ice.

Interfering factors
• Falsely low total complement (CH_{50}) values can result from a delay in testing or from improper storage of specimens.

• The following drugs can cause false-positive results for ANA: chlorpromazine, phenytoin, ethosuximide, hydralazine, methyldopa, oral contraceptives, isoniazid, procainamide, and trimethadione.

HENRY A. HOMBURGER, MD
RAYNELL J. CLARK, BA, MT

Hereditary angioedema test panel

The most common genetic abnormality associated with complement, hereditary angioedema (HAE) is characterized by episodes of acute edema in subcutaneous tissue, the gastrointestinal tract, or the upper respiratory tract. Acute respiratory involvement may be life-threatening. The disorder, inherited as an autosomal dominant trait, can result from a low concentration of C1 esterase inhibitor or from the presence of an abnormal, nonfunctional inhibitor protein; either condition disrupts normal regulation of the classical complement pathway, causing excessive breakdown of C4 and C2 and generation of a kinin-like fragment of C2.

In this test panel, designed to confirm diagnosis of HAE, the concentration of C1 esterase inhibitor is determined through a nephelometric assay, in which a specific antiserum is reacted with the patient's serum sample, with the resultant turbidity compared to a known standard. The functional assay for C1 esterase inhibitor, the second part of the panel, detects the presence of abnormal inhibitor protein. In this assay, patient serum is activated with aggregated human immunoglobulin, then monitored in a radial immunodiffusion plate. Absence of reaction indicates presence of a normal functional inhibitor protein; reaction indicates abnormal inhibitor protein.

Purpose
To confirm diagnosis of HAE.

Patient preparation
Explain to the patient that this test panel can confirm whether his symptoms are caused by HAE. Instruct him to fast for 12 hours before the tests; he needn't restrict fluids. Tell him that the panel requires a blood sample, who will perform the venipuncture and where, and that he may experience transient discomfort from the needle puncture and the pressure of the tourniquet. Reassure him that sample collection takes less than 3 minutes.

NEW TEST

H.A.E. TEST PANEL: FINDINGS AND IMPLICATIONS

TEST	NORMAL VALUES	IMPLICATIONS OF ABNORMAL RESULTS
C1 esterase	8 to 24 mg/dl	Values below 8 mg/dl point to HAE.
C1 esterase inhibitor, functional assay	Functional	Nonfunctional result indicates HAE.
C4	• White males: 12 to 72 mg/dl • White females: 13 to 75 mg/dl • Black males: 11 to 75 mg/dl • Black females: 12 to 67 mg/dl	Lower-than-normal values indicate complement consumption and require further investigation.

Procedure

Perform a venipuncture, and collect the sample in a 7-ml *red-top* tube.

Precautions

- Be sure the patient fasts for at least 12 hours before collecting the blood sample.
- Send the sample to the lab at once. Serum must be separated from the clot and tested within 8 hours of sample collection, or the sample must be frozen at $-94°$ F. ($-70°$ C.) until testing.

Post-test care

If a hematoma develops at the venipuncture site, apply ice.

Interfering factors

Improper specimen handling or delay in testing can cause falsely low readings for C4 and C1 esterase inhibitor.

HENRY A. HOMBURGER, MD
RAYNELL J. CLARK, BA, MT

Multiple sclerosis screening panel

The unpredictable nature of multiple sclerosis (MS), with its periodic exacerbations and remissions and variable progression, often makes early diagnosis difficult. This test panel, consisting of two tests performed on cerebrospinal fluid (CSF) samples, helps screen patients for MS and also for certain other demyelinating diseases. Certain abnormalities in CSF— increased total protein (which occurs primarily from increased IgG synthesis) and detectable IgG proteins that appear as discrete populations (known as oligoclonal bands) rather than as a broad homogeneous band on electrophoresis—point to MS or possibly other demyelinating disease. The first test in the screening panel, the CSF IgG index test, detects IgG synthesis in the central nervous system. The index is determined by calculating and then comparing the ratio of IgG to albumin in both CSF and serum samples. A CSF ratio greater than the serum ratio suggests IgG synthesis in central nervous system tissues. The second test in the panel, the oligoclonal band test, uses electrophoresis to inspect and compare the immunoglobulin region of both CSF and serum samples.

Purpose

To aid diagnosis of MS.

Patient preparation

Explain to the patient that these tests help determine whether his symptoms are caused by MS. Inform him that he needn't restrict food or fluids before the tests. Tell him the tests require samples of blood and CSF. Explain who will collect the samples and when. Warn that he may experience transient discomfort from the needle puncture and the pressure of the tourniquet during blood sample collection and will probably feel some burning from injection of local anesthetic and local pain from insertion of the spinal needle during CSF collection. Advise him that headache may occur during lumbar puncture, but that his cooperation during the test will minimize this and any other possible side effects. Make sure the patient or a responsible family member has signed a consent form. If the patient seems unusually anxious, notify the doctor, who may order a mild sedative before the procedure.

Procedure

First, perform a venipuncture and collect the blood samples in 7-ml *red-top* tubes. Then, within 2 hours of blood sample collection, assist the doctor in performing a lumbar puncture, and collect at least 3 ml of CSF in a sterile tube that contains no additives.

Precautions

- During lumbar puncture, observe the patient closely for signs of adverse reactions, such as elevated pulse rate,

M.S. SCREENING PANEL: FINDINGS AND IMPLICATIONS

TEST	NORMAL VALUES	IMPLICATIONS OF ABNORMAL RESULTS
Cerebrospinal fluid (CSF) IgG index	• CSF IgG: ≤ 8.4 mg/dl • CSF albumin: ≤ 26.0 mg/dl • Serum IgG: 640 to 1,430 mg/dl • Serum albumin: 2,584 to 4,792 mg/dl • CSF IgG index: ≤ 0.77 • CSF IgG/albumin ratio: 0.15 to 0.38 • Serum IgG/albumin ratio: 0.15 to 0.41	Greater-than-normal ratios are consistent with MS, as well as with other demyelinating diseases such as neurosyphilis, acute inflammatory polyradiculopathy, and subacute sclerosing panencephalitis.
Oligoclonal banding	0 to 1 band in both serum and CSF	Multiple bands seen in CSF but not in serum are consistent with MS but also may occur in other diseases, including neurosyphilis, subacute sclerosing panencephalitis, cryptococcal meningitis, idiopathic polyneuritis, and chronic rubella panencephalitis.

pallor, or clammy skin. Be sure to alert the doctor immediately to any significant changes.
• Record the CSF collection time on the test request form. Send properly labeled specimens to the laboratory immediately. Take care never to freeze CSF samples.

Post-test care
• Have the patient remain supine for at least 8 hours after lumbar puncture, and instruct him to increase his fluid intake.
• Monitor vital signs and neurologic status frequently.
• If a hematoma develops at the venipuncture site, apply ice.

Interfering factors
Improper handling of blood or CSF samples or excessive delay before CSF testing may cause false-negative results

for oligoclonal banding.

HENRY A. HOMBURGER, MD
RAYNELL J. CLARK, BA, MT

Lyme disease serology

Lyme disease is a multisystem disorder characterized by dermatologic, neurologic, cardiac, and rheumatic manifestations in various stages. Epidemiologic and serologic studies implicate a recently discovered, commonly tickborne spirochete, *Borrelia burgdorferi*, as the causative agent. Serologic tests, both indirect immunofluorescent and enzyme-linked immunosorbent assays, measure antibody response to this spirochete and indicate current infection or past exposure. These assays identify 50% of patients with early-stage Lyme disease; essentially 100% of patients with later complications of carditis, neuritis, and arthritis; and 100% of patients in remission.

In an indirect immunofluorescent assay, *B. burgdorferi* is grown in culture, fixed to a microscope slide, and then incubated with a human serum sample. A fluorescein-labeled antiglobulin is then introduced into the antigen-antibody complex. Any human antibody that binds to the spirochete is detected by viewing (under an ultraviolet microscope) the fluorescent antiglobulin that attaches to it.

Purpose

To confirm diagnosis of Lyme disease.

IMMUNOFLUORESCENCE AND ENZYME-LINKED IMMUNOSORBENT ASSAY

In **Immunofluorescence,** a histochemical technique, fluorescent dyes are attached to antibody molecules. When complexed with antigen, the antibody appears as a colored fluorescence when viewed under an ultraviolet microscope. Both direct and indirect immunofluorescence allow precise detection and demonstration of human tissue antigens and of bacterial, viral, and protozoan antigens. In the *direct* method, the fluorescein-labeled antibody reacts with an antigen specific to it. In the *indirect* method, a fluorescein-labeled antiglobulin reacts with an unlabeled antigen-antibody complex; the antiglobulin then binds to the unlabeled antibody. Both methods are widely used to detect autoantibodies, immunoglobulins of cell surfaces, components of complement, T and B lymphocytes, tumor-specific antigens, and microorganisms.

Enzyme-linked immunosorbent assay (ELISA) can identify antibody or antigen, and is replacing or supplementing radioimmunoassay and immunofluorescence. This method is safe, sensitive, and simple to perform, and provides reproducible results at a low cost. To measure a specific antibody, antigen is fixed to a solid-phase medium, incubated with a serum sample, and then incubated with an antiimmuno-globulin-tagged enzyme. Excess unbound enzyme is washed from the system and a substrate is added. To measure a specific antigen, antibody instead of antigen is fixed to a solid-phase medium. Hydrolysis of the substrate produces a color change, quantified by a spectrophotometer. The amount of substrate hydrolyzed is directly proportional to the amount of antigen or antibody in the serum sample.

ULTRAVIOLET (FLUORESCENCE) MICROSCOPE

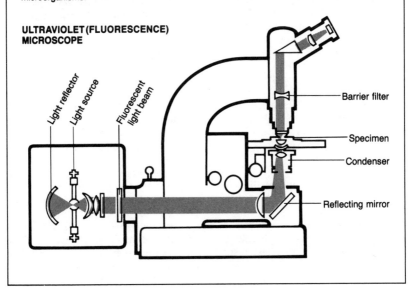

Light reflector

Light source

Fluorescent light beam

Barrier filter

Specimen

Condenser

Reflecting mirror

Patient preparation

Explain to the patient that this test helps determine whether his symptoms are caused by Lyme disease. Instruct him to fast for 12 hours before the blood sample is drawn; he needn't restrict fluids. Tell him that the test requires a blood sample, who will perform the venipuncture and where, and that he may experience transient discomfort from the needle puncture and the pressure of the tourniquet. Reassure him that sample collection takes less than 3 minutes.

Procedure

Perform a venipuncture, and collect the sample in a 7-ml *red-top* tube.

Precautions

Handle the specimen carefully to prevent hemolysis.

Values

Normal serum values are nonreactive or a serum titer of <1:256. A serum titer of 1:128 is considered borderline, and calls for repeat testing in 4 to 6 weeks.

Implications of results

A positive Lyme serology can help confirm diagnosis but is not definitive. Other treponemal diseases and high rheumatoid factor titers can cause false-positive results. Patients with other treponemal diseases demonstrate considerable cross-reactivity, and, although rheumatoid factor isn't normally associated with Lyme disease, up to 20% of patients with high rheumatoid factor titers may have positive Lyme disease serologies.

Post-test care

If a hematoma develops at the venipuncture site, apply ice.

Interfering factors

• Analysis of serum with high lipid levels may cause inaccurate test results and requires repetition of the test after a period of restricted fat intake.

• Blood samples contaminated with other bacteria can cause false-positive results.

• Hemolysis caused by rough handling of the sample can interfere with accurate determination of test results.

JERRY A. KATZMANN, PhD
RAYNELL J. CLARK, BA, MT

Protein C

In contrast to other vitamin K–dependent enzymes, activated (converted from a zymogen to an active enzyme) protein C is a potent and specific anticoagulant, which acts to suppress the procoagulant activity of activated platelets. Protein C is not activated during the blood coagulation process, but becomes activated as a result of interactions of products of the clotting system (thrombin) with the capillary endothelium. Thus far, only congenital deficiencies of protein C have been identified.

Exceedingly rare, *homozygous* deficiency (usually the result of consanguinity) is characterized by rapidly fatal thrombosis in the perinatal period, a syndrome known as *purpura fulminans*. The more common *heterozygous* deficiency occurs in about 10% of patients with familial venous thrombosis. In members of families carrying the deficiency, susceptibility to venous thromboembolism begins at puberty and continues throughout life.

The test for protein C remains largely experimental. Most measurements entail immunochemical assay of protein C antigen. Any of the standard immunochemical methods—immunoelectrophoresis, radioimmunoassay, or enzyme-linked immunosorbent assay (ELISA)—is used; each method requires a monospecific antibody to protein C. The assay is standardized by plasma pooled from a large group of normal donors.

In a different approach, done only in

research laboratories, protein C is isolated from the patient's plasma, activated, and then assayed for enzymatic activity either as an anticoagulant or with cologenic peptide substrates. Again, the test is standardized by comparison with plasma pooled from normal donors.

Whatever the methodology, the test is used to investigate the cause of otherwise unexplained thrombosis and to establish patterns of inheritance. It's rarely positive even when the level of suspicion is high. A positive finding for heterozygous deficiency is used for informational purposes only, as the clinical significance of the deficiency isn't fully understood, and interventions are still largely experimental. Prothrombin concentrate, which contains protein C, and plasma have been given to one homozygous newborn, with some success.

Purpose

To investigate the mechanism of idiopathic venous thrombosis.

Patient preparation

Explain to the patient that the test is part of an attempt to understand the underlying cause of his disease. Advise the patient that he needn't restrict food, fluids, or activity before the test. Tell him that the test requires a blood sample, who will perform the venipuncture and when, and that he may feel transient discomfort from the needle puncture and the pressure of the tourniquet. Assure him that these procedures take less than 3 minutes.

Check patient history for coumadin-type anticoagulants, which will affect test results.

Procedure

Perform a venipuncture, and collect the sample using a 3-ml *blue-top* vacutainer tube or a special syringe and anticoagulant provided by the coagulation laboratory. (At most centers, sample collection is done by laboratory personnel.)

Precautions

Send the sample to the laboratory immediately.

Values

Normal range is 50% to 150% of population mean, which is standardized by each laboratory.

Implications of results

Identification of the role of the deficiency of protein C in idiopathic venous thrombosis may lead to prevention of some cases of thromboembolism in the future.

Post-test care

If a hematoma develops at the venipuncture site, apply ice.

Interfering factors

Anticoagulant therapy may alter test results.

WHYTE G. OWEN, PhD

Urine tetrahydrocannabinol

Δ-9 Tetrahydrocannabinol, commonly referred to as THC, is the major psychologically active constituent of the marijuana plant *(Cannabis sativa)*. Ingestion of THC results in intoxication, the degree of which depends on the dose and frequency of use. Of the several THC metabolites identified in human urine, the major one is 11-nor-Δ_9-tetrahydrocannabinol-9-carboxylic acid (THC-COOH), which exists in urine in the free or conjugated state as a glucuronide.

Most analytic techniques for THC metabolites in urine are directed toward THC-COOH, to determine marijuana use. The length of time THC metabolites remain in the body varies, depending on individual metabolism rate, frequency and amount of drug use, and time of last ingestion. Generally, analysis can detect drug ingestion up to 6 weeks after last ingestion in a chronic user and up to 3 days after last ingestion in an occasional user.

The analysis is usually carried out in two stages, screening and confirmation testing. Immunoassays (radioimmunoassays or enzyme immunoassays) are the most commonly used methods for screening urine specimens for THC metabolites. Confirmation of immunoassay results requires any of several chromatographic techniques, however. Gas chromatography with mass selective detector (GC/MS) is the most accurate, specific, and dependable method known today and the one most recommended for confirmation, particularly when the test results are to be used for forensic purposes.

Purpose

To determine the presence and level of THC metabolite (THC-COOH) in the body.

Patient preparation

Explain to the patient or a family member, if appropriate, that this test determines recent use of marijuana or hashish. Inform him that he needn't restrict food or fluids before the test. Tell him the test requires a urine sample, and explain the proper collection techniques. Make sure that the patient or a responsible family member signs an appropriate consent form. Thoroughly check the patient's recent drug history, noting time and route of administration of all drugs.

Procedure

Collect a random urine specimen. The first morning void usually contains higher levels than later specimens.

Precautions

Send the specimen to the laboratory immediately. If the specimen will be sent to an outside laboratory for analysis or if testing will be delayed for more than 72 hours, freeze the specimen to minimize decomposition.

Values

Normally, no THC metabolites are found in urine.

Implications of results

A positive test for THC metabolites confirmed by GC/MS indicates ingestion of marijuana or hashish or passive exposure through inhalation. (However, a THC-COOH level higher than 20 ng/dl usually indicates drug ingestion rather than passive exposure.)

Post-test care

None.

Interfering factors

Delayed analysis of an unfrozen specimen may result in misleading test results.

MAHMOUD A. ELSOHLY, PhD

Serum tocainide

This quantitative analysis, done by high-performance liquid chromatography, measures serum levels of tocainide hydrochloride (Tonocard) to identify subtherapeutic, therapeutic, and potentially toxic doses during initial dose titration and maintenance therapy. A new oral antiarrhythmic used for suppression of premature ventricular contractions, tocainide has Class 1B antiarrhythmic properties similar to those of lidocaine and, like lidocaine, is indicated for the treatment of ventricular dysrhythmias. But although tocainide's electrophysiologic properties are very similar to those of lidocaine (in fact, tocainide is commonly known as "oral lidocaine"), tocainide levels must be monitored via this tocainide-specific assay.

Purpose

• To monitor therapeutic levels of tocainide
• To detect drug toxicity and monitor its treatment.

Patient preparation

Explain to the patient that this test helps determine the safest and most effective dosage of tocainide. Inform him that he needn't restrict foods or fluids before the test. Tell him the test requires a blood sample, who will perform the venipuncture and where, and that he may experience transient discomfort from the needle puncture and the pressure of the tourniquet. Reassure him that sample collection takes only a few minutes, and that test results should be available within 2 to 3 days. Before sample collection, check the patient's history for use of other drugs.

Procedure

Perform a venipuncture, and collect a trough-level or peak-level sample, as ordered, in a *red-, green-,* or *lavender-top* tube, as directed by the testing laboratory. Record the date and time of the last drug dose and the time of sample collection on the laboratory slip.

Precautions

Handle the sample gently to prevent hemolysis, and send it to the laboratory immediately.

Values

The therapeutic range for serum tocainide is 4 to 10 µg/ml. The toxic level is over 10 µg/ml.

Implications of results

Trough levels guide the adjustment of therapeutic dosage; peak levels can detect toxicity and monitor its treatment. Because side effects of tocainide (commonly gastrointestinal disturbances, vertigo, dizziness, blurred vision, paresthesias, tremor) increase with drug concentration, even in the therapeutic range, the lowest effective dose should be prescribed for long-term therapy. At therapeutic serum concentrations, 24-hour continuous EKG tracings help determine the optimum dose.

Therapeutic effects of tocainide are more likely when serum concentrations are within the therapeutic range. If a patient demonstrates serum concentrations in the upper end of the therapeutic range but doesn't receive therapeutic benefit, administration of another antiarrhythmic drug should be considered.

Patients with concentrations in the toxic range require immediate assessment for severe central nervous system and cardiovascular effects. Serious toxic effects can be minimized by reducing the dose immediately when serum concentrations fall in the toxic range.

Post-test care

If a hematoma develops at the venipuncture site, apply ice.

Interfering factors

Hemolysis caused by rough handling of the sample can interfere with accurate determination of test results.

HARRY G. McCOY, PharmD
JEANANNE KREJCI, RN, BA

Antibody tests in diabetes mellitus

These tests detect various antibodies in the blood of patients with known or suspected diabetes mellitus. Antibody formation in diabetes mellitus can take three forms. The most common is formation of anti-insulin antibodies from exogenous insulin sources—beef, pork, or human insulin preparations. Detection of insulin antibodies confirms this process as the cause of insulin resistance and suggests the necessity for alternate therapy to control hyperglycemia.

Another type of antibody formed in diabetes mellitus, the anti–beta cell antibody, is directed against the insulin-producing cells of the pancreas. Research continues on the possible link between these antibodies, on diabetes mellitus with distinct HLA typing, and on using these tests for these antibodies as a predictor of diabetes. Still basically a research tool, however, the test for anti–beta cell antibodies isn't commercially available at present.

A third type of antibody identified in diabetes, the anti–insulin receptor antibody, plays a role in the development of insulin resistance. Still largely experimental, measurement of these antibodies may help determine the cause of insulin resistance. Like the anti–beta cell antibody test, the test for anti–insulin receptor antibodies is also a research tool, not yet available for widespread clinical use.

Purpose
• To aid diagnosis of insulin resistance
• To assist in insulin management for control of hyperglycemia
• To aid diabetes research.

Patient preparation
Explain to the patient that the test for anti–insulin antibodies evaluates his diabetes and helps guide insulin therapy. If the patient's scheduled for the anti–beta cell antibody or anti–insulin receptor antibody test, explain that these experimental tests help researchers learn more about the nature of diabetes mellitus and its management.

Advise the patient to follow the doctor's instructions for preparations for this test. Tell him the test requires a blood sample, who will perform the venipuncture and where, and that he may feel slight discomfort from the needle puncture and the tourniquet.

Procedure
Perform a venipuncture, and collect the sample in a 7-ml *red-top* tube, or as directed by the testing laboratory.

Precautions
None.

Values
Normally, no anti-insulin, anti–beta cell, or anti–insulin receptor antibodies are present in blood.

Implications of results
The presence of anti-insulin antibodies in a diabetic patient may indicate the need for an alternative type of insulin or for increased insulin dosage to achieve euglycemia. Both pork and beef insulin set up an antigen-antibody response by the human body. Pure pork insulin produces less anti-insulin antibodies than either beef/pork combinations or pure beef insulin. Human insulin was theoretically produced to eliminate antibody formation; however, formation still occurs, although antibody levels are less than with pure pork insulin. The clinical difference between human and pure pork insulin remains to be determined. As of now, either type is recommended for patients starting on insulin therapy.

Positive anti–beta cell antibodies may indicate that the patient is at increased risk of diabetes mellitus, if it hasn't already developed. This finding may also indicate a greater risk of ketoacidosis, hypoglycemic reactions, and possibly long-term complications of diabetes.

The presence of anti–insulin receptor antibodies indicates a decreased ability of endogenous or exogenous insulin to exert an appropriate metabolic effect. In research studies, a positive test result usually confirms a diagnosis of insulin resistance of unknown etiology (as opposed to the more common diagnosis of insulin resistance due to down-regulation of insulin receptors that occurs in obese Type II diabetic patients).

Post-test care
If a hematoma develops at the venipuncture site, apply ice.

Interfering factors
None.

BARBARA L. SOLOMON, RN, DNSc, CCNS

The opinion or assertions contained herein are the private views of the author and are not to be construed as official or as reflecting the views of the Department of the Army or the Department of Defense.

Diagnostic protocols for complications of diabetes

Although advances in the therapeutic management of diabetes mellitus have significantly reduced mortality directly related to insulin deficiency, certain long-term complications continue to plague diabetics. In particular, metabolic changes associated with progressive thickening of the muscle capillary basement membrane cause a variety of microvascular complications, most significantly diabetic retinopathy and nephropathy. Other, less well-understood changes produce a third major complication, diabetic neuropathy.

Traditionally, assessment and treatment of diabetes complications occurred only after such complications were well-established, with clearly recognizable signs and symptoms. But recently developed protocols adopted by the National Diabetes Advisory Board promote three basic changes in this approach:
• Improved treatment of diabetes before complications develop
• Early detection of physical changes that point to complications
• Prompt initiation of treatment once complications are detected.

Crucial to such a philosophy, however, is a knowledgeable patient who understands the relationship between diabetes, its complications, and his health and who is capable of performing recommended self-care protocols. This requires comprehensive patient teaching on the principles of day-to-day management that can help prevent complications. It also requires that health care providers themselves understand the baseline physical assessment protocols that enable early detection of complications and prompt treatment or prevention.

DIABETIC RETINOPATHY

Of the 5,000 annual cases of diabetes-related blindness in the U.S., most result from retinopathy—either the non-proliferative (background) or proliferative form. About half of all diabetic patients develop some form of retinopathy within 10 years after diagnosis of diabetes; this number increases to 80% of diabetic patients by 15 years after diagnosis. Characterized by slight retinal vein dilation and aneurysms, background retinopathy eventually results in retinal hemorrhage and leakage from vessel deterioration, which leads to macular edema. Symptoms usually develop only after significant pathologic changes have occurred. In proliferative retinopathy, the advanced form of background retinopathy, diminished circulation to retinal vessels results in hypoxia and infarction. New vessel growth is fragile and prone to hemorrhage into the vitreous. Without treatment, hemorrhage or retinal detachment can cause blindness.

Diagnostic protocols

The National Diabetes Advisory Board recommends close monitoring of diabetic retinopathy for all diabetic patients. All examinations should be performed by an ophthalmologist or another doctor skilled in the detection of retinopathy. Recommended measures include:
• An annual visual acuity examination and complete visual history
• Ophthalmoscopic examination with dilated pupils for patients with Type I diabetes of more than 5 years' duration and for all patients with Type II diabetes regardless of duration
• For diabetic patients planning a pregnancy, an ophthalmoscopic examination 6 months before conception; for pregnant diabetic patients, ophthalmoscopic examination during both the first and third trimesters
• Fluorescein angiography, when appropriate, as a supplementary method of detecting sensitive diabetic changes within the eye.

Patient education

Comprehensive patient teaching about diabetic retinopathy can encourage compliance with recommended treatment and improve prognosis. Teach all diabetic patients:

• How diabetic retinopathy causes vision loss

• The potential relationship of poor metabolic control to the development or exacerbation of retinopathy

• The importance of self-care procedures, such as blood glucose monitoring, in achieving metabolic control

• The connection between hypertension and retinopathy, and the need for control of hypertension

• The importance of regular visual acuity and ophthalmoscopic examinations even when the patient has no visual symptoms

• The need to immediately report any blurred vision or visual halos not related to low blood glucose levels—possibly early signs of retinopathy

• How laser photocoagulation therapy is used to treat retinopathy, with the optimum time for such treatment being before vision problems develop

• The availability of vocational rehabilitation programs and other social services for the visually impaired.

DIABETIC NEPHROPATHY

Diabetes-related renal disease occurs in 50% of patients with diabetes of more than 20 years' duration that was diagnosed before age 20. A much lower

DIAGNOSTIC TESTS FOR DIABETES COMPLICATIONS

TEST	PURPOSE	PROCEDURE
Ophthalmoscopic examination	Inspection of the interior structures of the eye and/or the ocular fundus to reveal signs of retinopathy, including: • hard yellow exudates • soft white exudates • intraretinal microvascular abnormalities • hemorrhage • neovascularization • lens opacity	• Follows complete visual history and acuity examination. • Pupils are dilated with 1 to 2 drops of 1% tropicamide (Mydriacyl). • In a darkened room, the examiner views the optic disk, the physiologic cup, the retinal vessels and background, and the macula and fovea centralis.
Fluorescein angiography	Documentation of subtle changes not apparent on ophthalmoscopic examination; associated with interior structures of the eye and/or the ocular fundus to aid early detection of retinopathy	• After his pupils are dilated, the patient is situated in front of a camera that takes funduscopic pictures. • The patient receives I.V. infusion of fluorescein dye. • Photographs are taken immediately before, during, and after dye injection.
Nerve conduction tests	Evaluation of nerve functions by assessing velocity of nerve impulses and pathways used; allows early detection of abnormalities that indicate neuropathy	• Small conducting pads are placed over the skin at selected body areas to deliver charges of electric current.

incidence (2% to 4%) of nephropathy occurs in those diagnosed after age 40. Diabetic nephropathy develops as a result of basement membrane thickening, which leads to inadequate glomerular filtration of waste products from the blood. Important contributing factors to diabetic nephropathy include hypertension and neurogenic bladder, which predispose the diabetic patient to chronic urinary tract infections. Administration of a nephrotoxic contrast medium for radiographic studies can also contribute to nephropathy.

Diabetic nephropathy progresses in three stages. The first stage, the progression of subclinical disease, can last up to 20 years. During this stage, treatment focuses on prevention of irreversible damage while the kidney is still functioning. Evidence of kidney damage marks the onset of the second stage—a period of worsening proteinemia that typically lasts from 3 to 5 years. In the third and final stage, renal failure progresses rapidly and usually proves fatal.

Diagnostic protocols

Although recommended protocols for assessing renal function in diabetic patients vary, depending on the individual, general guidelines include:
- Routine and complete urinalysis at diagnosis
- Complete urinalysis for patients over age 40 or those with diabetes of 10 or more years' duration
- A thorough history of any symptoms related to renal function, such as frequent urinary tract infections or hypertension
- Frequent routine blood pressure screenings.

If urinalysis detects proteinuria, additional protocols include:
- A 24-hour urine collection to confirm abnormal protein levels
- Serum or plasma blood tests for albumin, creatinine, and blood urea nitrogen
- Collection of a clean-catch urine specimen for culture to check for infection, and appropriate treatment for any infection detected
- Consultation with a nephrologist or a diabetes specialist if serum creatinine is elevated (serum creatinine level greater than 5 mg/dl may point to the need for kidney transplantation).

Patient education

All diabetic patients need to know:
- The relationship of poor metabolic control and the development of diabetic nephropathy
- The importance of self-care methods in achieving metabolic control
- The need to avoid frequent episodes of diabetic ketoacidosis
- The relationship of hypertension to the progression of nephropathy; the

PATIENT TEACHING

- Advise the patient that the procedure takes approximately 1 hour.
- Warn him that he'll experience some blurring of vision for 6 to 12 hours, due to pupil dilation.
- Advise him to reduce light sensitivity post–pupil dilation by wearing sunglasses.
- Instruct him not to drive until his vision returns to normal.

- Advise the patient that the actual procedure takes approximately 30 minutes.
- Tell him that he'll be observed for 1 hour postprocedure for any adverse effects of dye injection.
- Warn him that injection of fluorescein dye may cause nausea, vomiting, or local allergic reactions.
- Warn him that he'll experience some blurring of vision and light sensitivity for 6 to 12 hours, due to pupil dilation.
- Instruct him not to drive until his vision returns to normal.

- Advise the patient that the procedure takes approximately 1 hour.
- Warn him that the electric current may produce a mild electric shock or tingling sensation to the area, but that discomfort should be minimal.

need for frequent blood pressure monitoring and the importance of compliance with hypertension treatment; and the need to achieve and maintain ideal body weight to help decrease high blood pressure
• The importance of recognizing and seeking early treatment for symptoms of urinary tract infections.

DIABETIC NEUROPATHY

Another common complication of diabetes, neuropathy is directly correlated to age, occurring in only 5% of diabetic patients before age 30 and in 70% of diabetic patients over age 50. Although the exact pathophysiology of diabetic neuropathy is unclear, many researchers believe that it develops as a direct result of ischemia or as an effect of a metabolic lesion. Neuropathies fall into various classifications, depending on the involved nerve segment. These classes include peripheral neuropathies, which typically lead to foot problems, and autonomic neuropathies, which disrupt cardiovascular and gastrointestinal reflexes. Because symptoms vary with the area of nerve involvement, they serve as the major diagnostic aid.

Diagnostic protocols

Although specific diagnostic measures depend on the type and extent of neuropathic involvement, certain general protocols provide important baseline information on neuropathic changes and encourage preventive measures. These recommended protocols apply to all newly diagnosed diabetic patients; patients with diabetes of more than 10 years' duration; diabetic patients over age 40; and all patients with a history of neuropathy or related diabetic complications, including peripheral vascular disease (PVD) and foot problems.

Patients in these groups require at least annual examinations according to the following protocols:
• A thorough history of any symptoms that suggest neuropathy or PVD, such as intermittent claudication

• A complete physical examination, including evaluation of these pulses—femoral, tibial, popliteal, and dorsalis pedis
• Evaluation of sensory function in the toes and feet
• A complete foot examination, including careful inspection for poor hygiene or ulcers
• A nerve conduction evaluation to serve as a baseline indicator of nerve function.

Patient education

Patient education for diabetic neuropathy involves increasing the patient's awareness of the importance of:
• Promptly reporting symptoms of altered sensation, such as temperature changes, burning, tingling, or numbness
• Maintaining as near-normal a metabolic state as possible, and the role of self-care in achieving this goal
• Prevention or correction of risk factors, such as smoking and hypertension
• Proper foot care
• Prompt referral and treatment for symptoms of neuropathy.

DEBRA HAIRE-JOSHU, RN, MSN, MSEd

Electrophysiologic study

Electrophysiologic study (EPS) is a valuable new diagnostic tool that traces and graphically records the location and pathway of recurrent dysrhythmias in the conduction system of the heart. EPS is most commonly used for patients with recurrent dysrhythmias, particularly ventricular tachycardia. It's also used to evaluate congenital anomalies that affect conduction for possible surgical correction. Two basic forms of EPS are currently in use; the most frequently performed type, endocardial catheter mapping, is discussed here.

Purpose

• To evaluate the heart's conduction system by characterizing the electrophysiologic properties of various heart tissues
• To define the mechanism, origin, conduction pathway, and severity of a recurrent cardiac dysrhythmia
• To uncover latent dysrhythmias following cardiac ischemia or infarction
• To help plan and evaluate different therapeutic regimens (surgery or drug therapy).

Patient preparation

Explain to the patient that this procedure helps evaluate his heart's function by recording its electrical activity. Instruct him to avoid food and fluids for at least 6 hours before the test. Also instruct him to discontinue medications, as ordered, unless EPS is being done to evaluate the effectiveness of an antiarrhythmic drug. Tell him who will perform the test and where, and that it takes 2 to 3 hours. Explain that he'll receive a mild sedative but will remain conscious throughout the procedure.

Supplement the doctor's explanation of EPS, answering any questions the patient may have about the procedure and its potential risks. If appropriate, arrange for the patient and his family to visit the catheterization laboratory to familiarize themselves with the equipment and decrease their anxiety about the procedure. Point out that, although the laboratory isn't an operating room, sterile technique is observed; members of the catheterization team wear gowns, gloves, and masks to protect the patient from infection. Explain to the patient that at least two electrode-tipped catheters are inserted into arteries or veins in his arm or leg and threaded through the vessels to his heart. Tell him the skin over the catheter insertion sites will be shaved, if necessary, and cleansed with an antiseptic solution. Warn that he'll feel a transient stinging sensation from the local anesthetic injected to numb the insertion sites and he may feel pressure as the catheters are advanced through the blood vessels; assure him that these sensations are normal, but tell him to report any other adverse sensations.

Inform the patient that he'll have an I.V. line inserted to allow administration of medications during the procedure. Obtain a complete drug history at this time, and make sure the patient or a responsible family member has signed a consent form.

Procedure

The patient is placed in a supine position on the table, and EKG leads are applied for continuous cardiac monitoring. An I.V. line is started with heparin solution to prevent thrombus formation. An arterial line also may be inserted for blood pressure monitoring. After local anesthetic is injected at the selected catheter insertion sites, small incisions or percutaneous punctures are made into the arteries or veins and the catheters are passed through the needles into the vessels. Generally, right-sided heart studies involve catheter insertion through the antecubital, internal jugular, or femoral vein; left-sided studies, through the femoral or antecubital artery. Under fluoroscopy, the catheters are then guided to place the electrode tips at the desired locations in the heart.

The number and location of electrodes varies with the complexity of the study. For example, EPS for sinus node function requires two electrodes placed in the high right atrium and the His bundle; ventricular mapping may require electrodes in the coronary sinus, right atrium, His bundle region, and the right and left ventricles.

Once the electrodes are in place, mapping begins. Each section of the endocardium under an electrode is activated by an electrical impulse, producing an electrogram of that area. This enables mapping of several areas during sinus rhythm, including any existing aneurysm sites and ischemic areas. If mapping is being done to evaluate a dysrhythmia or for antiarrhyth-

ANTIARRHYTHMIC DRUG RESPONSE IN E.P.S.

In antiarrhythmic drug testing in EPS, the drug is administered intravenously or orally, followed by programmed electrical stimulation to test the drug's effectiveness in suppressing the dysrhythmia. The results are indicated on continuous EKG tracings. A typical set of drug responses, obtained during drug testing for a patient with recurrent ventricular tachycardia (VT), is presented below.

CONTROL   Sustained VT (285 beats/minute)

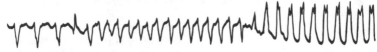

PROCAINAMIDE   Sustained VT (160 beats/minute)

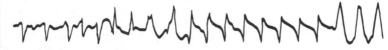

QUINIDINE   Sustained VT (180 beats/minute)

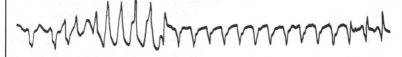

DISOPYRAMIDE   Sustained VT (200 beats/minute)

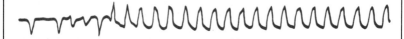

MEXILETINE   Sustained VT (170 beats/minute)

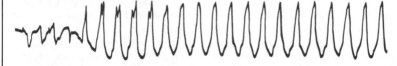

APRINDINE   No inducible VT

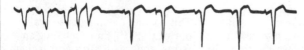

Adapted with permission from *Critical Care Quarterly*, 7(2), September 1984.

mic drug testing, the doctor attempts to induce a specific dysrhythmia, most commonly ventricular tachycardia, through electrical stimulation. When he confirms the dysrhythmia (as shown on the continuous EKG tracing), and it's recorded by the electrodes placed throughout the heart, antiarrhythmic drug testing can begin. In this procedure, the test drug is administered through the I.V. line, and the doctor attempts to induce the dysrhythmia again. If he cannot, the drug is considered successful in preventing the dysrhythmia.

Once the necessary data are obtained, the catheters are removed and pressure dressings are applied to the insertion sites. Heparinization may be reversed with protamine sulfate. The patient is then transferred to his room, where he's monitored closely. Depending on EPS results, he may remain hospitalized for several days for evaluation of treatment options.

Precautions
EPS is contraindicated in patients who are hemodynamically unstable.

Findings
Normal individuals will not have easily inducible dysrhythmias.

Implications of results
Identification of the origin and conduction pathway of a dysrhythmia guides the choice of medical or surgical intervention. Testing of various antiarrhythmic drugs determines the most effective form of drug therapy.

Post-test care
• Monitor vital signs carefully, and watch for any signs or symptoms of dysrhythmia, such as chest pain, dizziness, dyspnea, erratic pulse, or drop in blood pressure. Keep emergency resuscitation equipment handy.
• Observe the catheter insertion sites for hematoma or blood loss; replace pressure dressings as needed. Also check color, skin temperature, and pe-

ripheral pulse below the insertion sites.
• Check with the doctor on resuming medications. Provide analgesics if needed.

Interfering factors
Current antiarrhythmic therapy may alter results.

TERRI C. MURRELL, RN, MSN

Neonatal screening test for cystic fibrosis

This test, still largely investigational, measures serum immunoreactive trypsinogen (IRT) in the neonate to screen for cystic fibrosis (CF). The most common fatal genetic disease, CF strikes about 1 in every 2,000 neonates in the United States. It causes generalized exocrine gland dysfunction, affecting sweat gland, respiratory, and gastrointestinal function. The median life expectancy for CF patients is only about 21 years. Although no cure yet exists for CF, identification of affected neonates soon after birth and before the development of significant respiratory involvement may help extend survival.

Unlike most neonatal screening tests that detect inborn errors of metabolism, the IRT test is directed at pancreatic manifestations of the disease. But because about 15% of CF patients show no pancreatic involvement, this screening test may not detect all affected neonates. Nevertheless, experimental results are encouraging. In studies of the IRT test's effectiveness, repeat testing was done on infants who tested positive on initial screening. Those that tested positive on the second screening were then referred for diagnostic sweat testing for CF. Based on those results, the predictive value of a positive IRT test (specificity) with two-tiered screening is estimated at 75%; specificity based only on initial screening is between 15% and 22%. The predictive value of a negative test result (sensitivity) hasn't yet been determined.

At present, no other reliable CF screening methods exist. Although the CF gene is reportedly located on chromosome 7, the specific gene hasn't been identified, and available genetic markers presently cannot be used for widescale screening of any type.

Purpose
To screen neonates for CF.

Patient preparation
Explain to the infant's parents that this test helps detect CF. Tell them that the test requires a blood sample obtained through a heel prick. Because of the relatively high rate of false-positive results on initial screening, be sure to discuss the nature and limitations of this test with the parents. Also be sure they sign a consent form before the test begins.

Equipment
Alcohol or povidone-iodine swabs/ sterile lancet/specially marked filter paper/2″ by 2″ sterile gauze pads/small adhesive bandage strip/labels for the infant's and mother's name, doctor's name, room number, and date of sample collection.

Procedure
After assembling the necessary equipment and washing your hands thoroughly, wipe the infant's heel with an alcohol or povidone-iodine swab and dry it with a gauze pad. Then perform a heel stick. Squeezing the infant's heel gently, fill the circles on the filter paper with blood. Make sure the blood saturates the paper. Then apply gentle pressure with a gauze pad to ensure hemostasis at the puncture site. When the filter paper is dry, label it appropriately and send it to the laboratory promptly.

Precautions
None.

Values
Normal and suspect IRT levels are based on percentiles derived from reference neonate populations. To date, the 99.8th percentile, IRT concentration of 140 ng/dl, is considered positive on the first screening. The 99.5th percentile, or 120 ng/dl, is considered positive for the second screening.

Implications of results
Positive results, even after two-tier screening, aren't sufficient for definitive diagnosis of CF, but do indicate the need for further diagnostic evaluation. The sweat test, which detects the presence of elevated sodium and chloride concentrations in sweat, is necessary for confirmation.

Post-test care
• Heel sticks heal quickly and require no special care.
• If results are positive, tell the parents that additional testing is needed to confirm diagnosis.

Interfering factors
The following factors may interfere with accurate determination of test results:
• failure to allow the filter paper to dry completely
• failure to follow proper procedures for sample collection.

SHERRY L. KERAMIDAS, PhD

Protocols for prenatal detection of neural tube defects

All high-risk pregnant women should undergo prenatal testing for fetal neural tube defects (NTD), such as spina bifida and anencephaly. Such women include those who previously had a child with an NTD; those with a family history of NTD or related disorders; and those with elevated maternal serum alpha-fetoprotein (MSAFP) levels, detected on routine prenatal screening. High MSAFP levels at 16 to 18 weeks' gestation may suggest fetal NTD. But positive confirmation requires ultrasonography and/or amniocentesis for measurement of alpha-fetoprotein (AFP) and acetylcholinesterase (AChE) in amniotic fluid. These tests are typically performed concomitantly and in various combinations to confirm diagnosis.

Ultrasonography

Level I ultrasonography detects the presence of fetal heart motion, gestational date based on the measurement of fetal biparietal diameter, the presence of multiple fetuses, and the amount of amniotic fluid present. Level I ultrasonography is always performed on any patient with an elevated MSAFP level. Because it can visually confirm anencephaly, Level I ultrasonography usually precludes the need for amniocentesis in suspected anencephaly.

Most neural tube defects observed in the second trimester of pregnancy are open, not covered with skin or bulging membrane as usually occurs in affected term infants. For this reason, Level II ultrasonographic diagnosis of fetal spina bifida may require cross-sectional views of the spinal column from the cervical spine to the sacrum to detect abnormally formed vertebrae and associated soft-tissue defects. But ultrasonographic examination of the fetus at risk shouldn't be limited to the spine. Measurement of the lateral ventricles can be helpful, because spina bifida is frequently associated with secondary hydrocephalus resulting from ventricular enlargement.

In experienced hands, Level II ultrasonography is better than 95% accurate in the diagnosis of fetal spina bifida. Level II ultrasonography is also important for the diagnosis of certain easily visualized defects of the fetal abdominal wall (such as omphalocele and

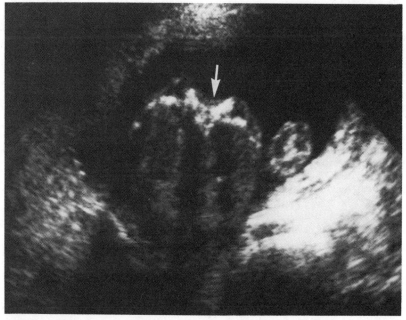

Horizontal cross-section ultrasonography of open spina bifida in a second-trimester fetus. Arrow points to V-shaped lumbar vertebra.

gastroschisis) and sacrum (such as sacrococcygeal teratoma), which can produce false-positive results for spina bifida on amniotic fluid analysis.

Amniotic fluid analysis

If MSAFP screening or ultrasonography suggests a fetal defect, amniocentesis for the measurement of AFP and possibly AChE is performed to help confirm diagnosis. In fetal spina bifida, blood and cerebrospinal fluid leak out of the open defect into the amniotic fluid. Thus, detection of AFP, the major fetal serum protein in amniotic fluid, suggests the presence of fetal spina bifida; detection of AChE, an enzyme present in neural tissue, including the spinal cord, helps confirm it. Contamination of an amniotic fluid sample with fetal blood can falsely elevate AFP levels; therefore, testing for AChE (which isn't found in fetal serum) is important to rule out such false-positive results. When combined, these two tests diagnose fetal spina bifida with better than 99% accuracy. However, because elevated AChE also occurs in open gut defects that expose the mesenteric plexus, Level II ultrasonography is also required to positively differentiate between fetal defects of the spine and of the abdomen. If ultrasonography doesn't show a fetal defect (and especially if the amniotic fluid specimen shows blood contamination), amniocentesis must be repeated to confirm abnormal test results. Timing is also significant; amniotic fluid drawn during the third trimester may yield false-negative results for AFP, since hydramnios associated with NTD may cause an apparent reduction of AFP levels. Thus, in the third trimester, both AChE testing and ultrasonography are necessary.

Testing procedure

For convenience, most high-risk patients undergo amniocentesis and ultrasonography during the same visit. Ultrasonography requires a full bladder for proper uterine visualization; if the patient's bladder is empty, she should drink three to five glasses of water within 45 minutes to fill it. The procedure carries no risk to the mother or fetus.

Amniocentesis is performed on an outpatient basis under ultrasonographic guidance. The procedure rarely produces maternal or fetal complications. Before needle insertion, the nurse prepares the patient by cleansing the abdominal skin with an iodine-containing preparation; the doctor may inject a local anesthetic to numb the aspiration needle insertion site. After inserting the needle, the doctor aspirates about 1 ml of amniotic fluid. Both amniotic fluid AFP and AChE are stable for several days at room temperature, but require freezing for longer storage before testing.

Because AFP levels decrease with each week of gestation from the second trimester to term, accurate determination of date of conception is essential for accurate interpretation of test results. AFP levels, determined by radioimmunoassay, are reported by week of gestation in terms of multiples of the normal median (MOM), or the normal mean plus the number of standard deviations. Values above 2.5 MOM or the mean plus 3 to 5 standard deviations are considered abnormal.

AChE isoenzymes are measured by gel electrophoresis, to separate the enzyme pseudocholinesterase from the specific AChE isoenzyme. Electrophoresis testing performed first with and then without an AChE inhibitor added more clearly identifies this isoenzyme. Normally, amniotic fluid contains no AChE; any detectable level is considered abnormal.

F. SUSAN COWCHOCK, MD

Serum flecainide

This quantitative analysis uses either capillary gas chromatography with electron capture detection or liquid chromatography with fluorescent detection to measure serum levels of flecainide acetate (Tambocor). A new oral antiarrhythmic drug used for suppression of premature ventricular contractions, flecainide is classified as a Class 1C antiarrhythmic, with properties including increased refractory time; slowed atrial, nodal, and ventricular conduction; and prolonged PR interval and QRS complex on electrocardiography. Measurement of serum flecainide concentration detects subtherapeutic, therapeutic, and potentially toxic doses during initial dose titration and ongoing therapy.

Purpose

• To monitor therapeutic levels of flecainide
• To detect flecainide toxicity and monitor its treatment.

Patient preparation

Explain to the patient that this test helps determine the safest and most effective dosage of flecainide. Tell him he needn't restrict food or fluids before the test. Tell him the test requires a blood sample, who will perform the venipuncture and where, and that he may experience transient discomfort from the needle puncture and the pressure of the tourniquet. Reassure him that collecting the sample takes less than 3 minutes, and that test results are usually available within 2 to 3 days. Before sample collection, take a complete drug history.

Procedure

Perform a venipuncture, and collect a trough-level or peak-level sample, as ordered, in a *red-, green-,* or *lavender-top* tube, as directed by the testing laboratory. Record the date and time of the last dose of flecainide and the time of sample collection on the laboratory slip.

Precautions

Handle the specimen gently to prevent hemolysis, and send it to the laboratory immediately.

Values

The therapeutic range for serum flecainide is 0.2 to 1.0 µg/ml (200 to 1,000 ng/dl), reported as flecainide acetate. The toxic level is over 1 µg/ml.

Implications of results

Trough levels guide adjustment of therapeutic dosage; peak levels detect toxicity and monitor its treatment. Therapeutic effectiveness of flecainide is more likely when serum concentration is within the therapeutic range; if control of dysrhythmia isn't achieved by therapeutic dosage, another antiarrhythmic agent should be considered. Serum concentration at the upper end of the therapeutic range is more likely to produce side effects such as cardiac conduction disturbances and reduction of left ventricular function; thus, the lowest effective dose should be prescribed for long-term therapy.

Because serum flecainide concentration correlates well with electrocardiographic interval prolongation, both baseline and 24-hour continuous EKGs are useful in guiding drug therapy.

A patient with serum flecainide concentration in the toxic range requires immediate assessment for dangerous EKG interval prolongation and slowed conduction, evaluation of left ventricular function (especially in the presence of congestive heart failure), and neurologic assessment for characteristic side effects such as dizziness, paresthesias, and tremor. Serious toxic effects can be minimized by immediately reducing the dose when concentration reaches the lower limit of the toxic range.

Post-test care

If a hematoma develops at the venipuncture site, apply ice.

Interfering factors

Hemolysis caused by rough handling of the sample can interfere with accurate determination of test results.

HARRY G. McCOY, PharmD
JEANANNE KREJCI, RN, BA

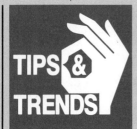

TIPS & TRENDS

MONITORING DIABETES

Glycosylated hemoglobin test

A relatively new diagnostic tool for monitoring diabetes mellitus therapy, the glycosylated hemoglobin test uses chromatographic or chemical techniques to measure levels of hemoglobin A variant HbA_{1c}. Unlike blood and urine glucose tests, which require repeated samplings and reflect glucose metabolism only at the time of collection, measuring glycosylated hemoglobin requires only one venipuncture every 6 to 8 weeks and reflects diabetes control over this period.

Research work continues on a related test that measures glycosylation of albumin molecules introduced into the blood of diabetes patients. This test, not yet available for clinical use, reflects metabolic glucose control over a 2- to 3-week period, providing an intermediate indicator between traditional blood and urine glucose tests and glycosylated hemoglobin testing.

FOR DIAGNOSIS AND TREATMENT

Sleep disorder centers

An estimated 12% to 15% of the population of industrialized nations suffers from some type of sleep disorder, generally involving either deficient or excessive sleep. Besides interfering with a person's quality of life, such a disorder can also lead to severe emotional and physical problems. Until recently, sufferers had nowhere to turn; most hospitals and medical centers simply don't have the equipment and specialists necessary for proper diagnosis and treatment.

But now, in response to this pervasive problem, sleep disorder centers are opening across the country. In such a center, a sleep disorders specialist reviews the patient's history for medical problems, family history of sleep disorders, and use of prescription and recreational drugs, including alcohol and caffeine. He then

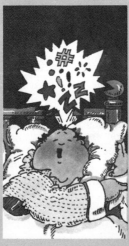

analyzes the patient's sleep habits and performs a comprehensive physical examination.

Later, while the patient sleeps (or attempts to sleep) in a specially equipped laboratory, a battery of tests known collectively as polysomnography is performed to help evaluate the nature and severity of the patient's sleep disorder. Polysomnography typically consists of continuous electroencephalography (EEG) to detect the various stages of sleep; electrooculography (EOG) to detect rapid eye movement (REM) sleep, the deepest sleep stage; electromyography (EMG) to detect muscle activity during the different sleep stages; electrocardiography (EKG) to monitor heart rate and rhythm during sleep; respiratory monitoring to detect periods of apnea; oximetry to measure tissue oxygen saturation levels; and continuous audiovisual recording to observe sound and movement throughout the sleep cycle. This battery of tests, modified to meet the individual patient's needs, may be repeated for several nights to gather sufficient data. Analysis of the multiple tracings and other information obtained from polysomnography enables diagnosis of the particular sleep disorder—such as sleep apnea or narcolepsy—and, consequently, development of an effective treatment plan.

Brain scans in psychological disorders

Two frequently used neurologic tests—computed tomography (CT) and positron emission tomography (PET)—may enhance understanding of certain psychological disturbances and lead to more effective prevention and treatment. Many studies using CT scans have shown dilated cerebral ventricles in patients diagnosed as schizophrenic, particularly chronic schizophrenics. Some studies have reported widened brain sulci, suggesting atrophy of the cerebral cortex, and mild to moderate cerebellar atrophy. Based on these studies, two subtypes of schizophrenia may exist: one type (with good prognosis) that has few visible signs on CT scan, and another

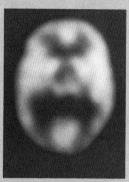

Normal positron emission tomogram of the brain (cross-sectional image)

type (with poor prognosis) with structural abnormalities visible on CT scan.

CT studies of patients with other psychological disorders, such as dementia, alcoholism, anorexia nervosa, and autism, have

turned up abnormalities similar to those found in schizophrenics. Abnormal findings in these disorders, while of unclear significance in treatment or prevention, do strongly support arguments for an organic basis of certain psychological disorders.

PET scans show the diffusion of arterial blood glucose in the brain by visualizing an injected radioactive glucose marker. Initial studies suggested diminished blood flow in the frontal lobes of schizophrenics, a finding unsupported by later research. However, recent investigations point to abnormalities of both cortical and subcortical levels of neural activity in schizophrenia. Research into this possibility continues.

Preoperative testing—no longer routine

Every hospital nurse knows the standard preoperative testing routine, which commonly includes urinalysis, complete blood count, chemistry profile, and coagulation studies for every patient, regardless of the surgery he's scheduled for. Apart from the time these tests take, their annual aggregate cost is in the billions—money that could be better spent in other areas of health care.

But a recent study may help change this situation. Researchers from the University of California,

San Francisco, have completed a study exploring the actual usefulness of routine preoperative laboratory screening tests. The results? In the 2,000 patients studied, 60% of tests ordered were not indicated by even the most conservative medical criteria, and less than 1% of all tests done revealed abnormalities that might influence surgical management. The conclusion? Routine preoperative

screening can be safely eliminated and replaced by tests for specific indications only, such as coagulation disorders, anemia, fluid and electrolyte imbalances, and diabetes. Besides saving billions of health care dollars, such a policy would free nurses from the time-consuming routine of ordering tests, obtaining samples, checking results, and notifying the doctor—and allow more time for patient teaching, emotional support, and other more important nursing duties.

Colorectal cancer screening at home

Until recently, a thermometer was the only practical tool most people had for self-health monitoring. But today, the average person has access to a multitude of home-testing equipment, including blood pressure monitors, pregnancy tests, and now even tests to detect hidden blood in stool. The latter test is particularly valuable, since the American Cancer Society estimates that 75% of colorectal cancer cases could be cured if detected and treated early—and occult blood in stool is an important early sign.

Several home-screening tests for occult blood in stool are available. They yield quick results with no discomfort and can be done in the privacy of the home, at an average cost of under $2.00 per test. Testing procedures vary with the individual product, but all the tests provide early indication of possible colorectal cancer.

When advising a patient on the use of these home tests, stress the following points:
• For accurate results, test three consecutive bowel movements.

• A positive result doesn't necessarily indicate cancer; such diverse factors as diet, medication, bleeding gums, ulcers, hemorrhoids, polyps, and even long-distance running could cause such a reading. But it should be reported immediately nonetheless.
• Conversely, negative test results don't guarantee the absence of colorectal cancer. All persons over age 40 still need an annual physical examination to ensure they remain cancer-free.

RECOMMENDATIONS FOR COLORECTAL CANCER SCREENING

RISK CATEGORY	TYPE OF SCREENING	FREQUENCY OF SCREENING
High-risk Patients with Gardner's syndrome or with chronic ulcerative colitis (over 10 years' duration)	• Colonoscopy with cytology (Frequent false-positive findings for occult blood in stool contraindicates home screening for this risk group.)	• Every 4 to 6 months
Moderate-risk Patients with prior resected colon carcinoma or with a history of polyps	• Colonoscopy or sigmoidoscopy • Occult blood in stool	• Colonoscopy or sigmoidoscopy once a year • Occult blood every 6 to 12 months
Low-risk Patients age 40 or older with no history of colorectal disease	• Digital rectal examination • Occult blood in stool	• Once a year for both screens

The dexamethasone suppression test and depression

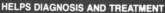

The dexamethasone suppression test (DST), a standard diagnostic tool for adrenocortical disorders, also appears useful in diagnosing major depression and monitoring its treatment. This use is based on the finding that certain patients with major depression have high levels of circulating adrenal steroid hormones. Administration of a synthetic oral steroid, such as dexamethasone, to such patients fails to suppress these levels but does lower them in nondepressed subjects.

In the DST, a patient is given 1 mg of dexamethasone at 11 p.m.; then, blood samples are drawn at 4 p.m. and 11 p.m. the next day. (More frequent sampling may increase the likelihood of measuring a nonsuppressed cortisol peak.) A cortisol level of 5 ng/dl or greater indicates failure of dexamethasone suppression.

False-positive results can occur in a variety of medical conditions, such as diabetes mellitus; pregnancy; and situations of severe bodily stress (such as trauma, severe weight loss, dehydration, and acute alcohol withdrawal). False-positives can also follow use of certain drugs, particularly barbiturates, within 3 weeks before the test.

Although not indicated as a screening test for depression, the DST aids diagnosis of major depression as the EEG aids diagnosis of epilepsy: a normal test result doesn't rule out the diagnosis, but an abnormal test result strengthens a clinically based diagnosis. The DST has proven disappointing in differentiating dysthymic disorder (neurotic depression) from major affective illness (psychotic depression), but may have use in patients with other psychological diagnoses (such as schizoaffective disorder, for example) to establish the need for treatment of coexisting depression.

Multimineral hair analysis

Numerous commercial laboratories advertise multimineral hair analysis in professional journals and other health industry publications and, until a recent FTC ruling discouraged the practice, directly to the public.

Based solely on the data obtained from the analysis, many of these laboratories prescribe vitamin and mineral supplements (which they often sell) and sometimes even provide diagnostic suggestions. But while hair analysis has established value in forensic pathology and as a screening test for heavy metal exposure, it can't accurately detect individual mineral deficiencies and is certainly unreliable in indicating specific disease states. So many factors affect the mineral content of hair—including use of shampoos and dyes, environmental conditions, age and gender, and even color, diameter, and growth rate—that hair can't possibly reflect current body conditions. Warn your patients about this unscientific and expensive scam.

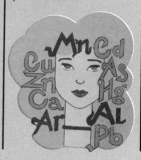

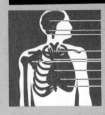

Diseases

CLINICAL UPDATES

AIDS update

Acquired immune deficiency syndrome (AIDS), a most frightening and serious disease, continues to spread and poses a challenge to nurses and other health care workers as well as to those who have the disease. AIDS is characterized by a deficiency in cell-mediated immunity (T cell immunity) that causes susceptibility to a wide range of opportunistic infections and unusual cancers. This defect in cell-mediated immunity is caused by infection with retrovirus HTLV-III (human T cell lymphotrophic virus III). The virus is transmitted through sexual contact, through inoculation with blood or blood products, and transplacentally.

The incubation period for AIDS appears to be anywhere from 2 to 5 years, possibly longer. However, a person infected with the HTLV-III virus usually develops an antibody to this virus within 6 weeks to 6 months.

Patient population

Since it was first identified in the United States, AIDS has occurred predominantly among certain groups of people, including homosexual and bisexual men (73%), intravenous drug abusers (17%), hemophiliacs (1%), persons who received contaminated blood transfusions (2%), heterosexual partners of infected persons (1%), and children born to infected mothers (1%). Although the AIDS virus is transmitted more efficiently from male to female, it can also be transmitted from female to male through sexual contact.

The Centers for Disease Control (CDC) defines AIDS for surveillance purposes as the presence of an illness, such as an opportunistic infection or Kaposi's sarcoma (KS), that indicates a deficiency in cell-mediated immunity in a person without a known source of immunosuppression other than infection with HTLV-III.

The CDC has also described a related syndrome called AIDS-related complex (ARC). ARC is characterized by two or more of the following symptoms, which persist for 3 months or longer: fever, weight loss (of 15 lb [6.8 kg] or 10% of normal body weight), diarrhea, night sweats, fatigue, lymphadenopathy (in two or more extrainguinal sites), and laboratory values that indicate abnormal cell-mediated immunity. The syndrome can range from mild to severe. Patients with ARC may die of other causes without ever developing the opportunistic infections or cancers that are diagnostic of AIDS. Other patients with ARC eventually develop AIDS.

The number of people in the United States with ARC is unknown. An estimated 1,000,000 people in the United States have been infected with HTLV-III, and are, therefore, antibody-positive but may be asymptomatic. Epidemiologic predictions estimate that between 5% and 30% of these people will eventually develop AIDS.

AIDS has been reported in every state in the United States and in most other countries as well. This infection generally (about 90% of the time) affects men between the ages of 20 and 49. Mortality is high: 50% overall but up to 80% within 2 to 3 years after diagnosis. According to some forecasts, at least tens of thousands more people will require nursing care for AIDS.

Causes

AIDS results from an infection with the HTLV-III virus. This virus has a particular predilection for the helper T, or T_4, cell but has also been shown to directly infect other cells, including B cells, macrophages, and central nervous system cells. HTLV-III is a retrovirus, a type of ribonucleic acid (RNA)

COMMON CLINICAL SYNDROMES SEEN IN A.I.D.S.

RESPIRATORY

- *Pneumocystis carinii* pneumonia
- Cytomegalovirus (CMV) pneumonitis
- Pulmonary Kaposi's sarcoma
- *Mycobacterium avium intracellulare*
- *Mycobacterium tuberculosis*

GASTROINTESTINAL

- CMV colitis
- Cryptosporidiosis
- *Giardia lamblia* infection
- *Candida albicans* esophagitis/stomatitis
- Kaposi's sarcoma
- *Mycobacterium avium intracellulare*

NEUROLOGIC

- *Toxoplasma gondii* encephalitis
- *Cryptococcus neoformans* meningitis
- CMV encephalitis
- HTLV-III infection

SKIN

- Kaposi's sarcoma lesions
- Herpes simplex virus abscesses
- Varicella zoster infection

virus. Once inside a T_4 cell, the virus replicates with the help of a viral enzyme called reverse transcriptase. HTLV-III then integrates itself into the cell's genetic machinery (the deoxyribonucleic acid). The result is an abnormally functioning T_4 cell. When activated, it produces more virus, which, in turn, infects other cells. Over time, the number of normally functioning T_4 cells decreases and the individual becomes more susceptible to the types of intracellular organisms and tumors that the T_4 cell usually protects him against (for example, viruses, fungi, parasites, and mycobacteria). Because the T_4 cell normally induces many other immune functions, the HTLV-III virus damages other parts of the immune system as well. Thus, the HTLV-III virus impairs natural killer-cell function, macrophage function, and the B cell's ability to respond to new antigens.

Signs and symptoms

Typically, the person with AIDS seeks medical help because of an infection or malignancy that indicates deficient cell-mediated immunity. Many patients report a recent history of mild to severe nonspecific symptoms, such as fever, weight loss, fatigue, lymphadenopathy, or night sweats. However, some patients are asymptomatic, then abruptly develop a KS lesion or symptoms of an opportunistic infection. For most persons with AIDS, the clinical course is one of peaks and valleys. After successful treatment of an opportunistic infection, the patient may feel healthy for several months until he develops another opportunistic infection or lesion. Although the course is variable, most patients continue this pattern of recurring infection for 8 months to 2 years or longer. Finally, they succumb to an opportunistic infection.

About 30% of patients with AIDS develop KS, which usually presents as a purplish, palpable, discrete skin lesion anywhere on the body. The lesions generally aren't painful or pruritic, except in certain places such as the foot. Over time, the patient may develop multiple and diffuse KS lesions. The incidence of extracutaneous KS is high, with lesions commonly found in the mucous membranes of the GI tract, in the lymph nodes, and in the lungs.

The most common opportunistic infection found among AIDS patients is *Pneumocystis carinii* pneumonia. Its presenting symptoms include an insidious or acute onset of shortness of breath, chest tightness or discomfort, cough, and fever. Other common opportunistic infections include:
- *Candida albicans* stomatitis or esophagitis, which is characterized by white patchy spots, an altered sense of taste, difficulty swallowing, and retrosternal burning or pain
- *Toxoplasma gondii* encephalitis,

which is marked by headaches, confusion, subtle central nervous system (CNS) changes, or full-blown seizures
• Cryptosporidiosis, cytomegalovirus (CMV) infection, or parasitic infestation, which causes voluminous diarrhea and abdominal discomfort.

In children, the clinical course of AIDS varies slightly from that of adults. The incubation period appears to be shorter, approximately 5 to 11 months. Children develop KS and most of the same opportunistic infections. In addition, children often have a chronic diffuse interstitial pneumonitis of unknown etiology and chronically enlarged parotid glands.

Diagnosis

A firm diagnosis of AIDS requires one of the clinical manifestations described above (an opportunistic infection or unusual cancer) as well as a positive test result for antibody to HTLV-III.

Antibody to HTLV-III is measured by an enzyme-linked immunosorbent assay (ELISA) test. A positive ELISA test is always repeated. Results are confirmed by a more specific antibody test called the western blot analysis. A person who has antibody to HTLV-III doesn't necessarily have AIDS but has been infected with the virus. For this reason, a person who is positive for antibody to HTLV-III must be considered capable of transmitting the virus through sexual activity or blood. The ELISA test is currently being used in blood banks in the United States and in many other parts of the world to screen blood and blood products for AIDS contamination. Blood that tests positive for antibody to HTLV-III is discarded.

The HTLV-III virus can also be cultured from an infected person's cells. This is a long and difficult test that is not widely available but is useful in evaluating the effectiveness of experimental antiviral therapy. Generally, it takes 4 to 6 weeks to culture the virus from cells.

Several diagnostic tests are crucial to the clinical evaluation of the patient with AIDS. A complete blood count with differential can reveal lymphocytopenia. An immune profile, consisting of absolute numbers of T_4 and T_8 cells and a T_4:T_8 ratio, can reveal a low T_4 cell count and a low T_4:T_8 ratio. Skin testing with common antigens is often used to evaluate in vivo cell-mediated immunity. However, most AIDS patients are anergic and don't respond to skin testing.

Additional diagnostic tests are necessary to diagnose the opportunistic infections or malignancies associated with AIDS. For example, KS lesions are diagnosed by biopsy; *Pneumocystis carinii* pneumonia is diagnosed via the bronchial washings or transbronchial biopsy obtained during bronchoscopy; *Candida albicans* and herpes simplex are diagnosed via culture.

Patients need support and teaching during these diagnostic procedures. They are told that the diagnosis of *Pneumocystis carinii* pneumonia or KS confirms the diagnosis of AIDS, and they worry about its implications. At this difficult time, the patient needs nonjudgmental nursing support.

Treatment

Currently, no treatment exists for the retroviral infection that causes AIDS or for the resulting immunodeficiency. Researchers continue to search for an effective antiviral agent to combat the HTLV-III virus and to restore or augment the impaired immune system. Several different antiretroviral agents with good activity against HTLV-III in vitro are currently being studied in Phase I and II clinical trials. Methods of enhancing or restoring immune function continue to be investigated, including therapy with biological response modifiers, such as interleukin-2, the interferons, and thymosin (see "Cancer update: Interleukin-2 [IL-2] therapy," pages 60 to 62); lymphocyte transfusions; and bone marrow transplantation. Most researchers believe that a combination of antiretroviral therapy and immune system enhancement will be necessary to cure AIDS.

Treatment is available for the secondary opportunistic infections and malignancies associated with AIDS. KS can be treated with single-agent or combination chemotherapy, radiation therapy, or alpha-interferon. The most commonly employed chemotherapeutic agents are vinblastine and etoposide (VP-16). Both are bone marrow suppressants that can further suppress im-

mune function. Combination chemotherapy is usually reserved for life-threatening KS because its side effects can be lethal. Radiation therapy has been used successfully for cosmetic or palliative reasons but is not a viable systemic therapy. Alpha-interferon induces partial or complete remission of KS lesions in approximately 30% of patients studied. In general, alpha-interferon appears to work better in patients with stronger immune profiles. Some clinicians recommend no therapy for KS unless associated morbidity exists.

Although some agents can effectively fight many of the opportunistic infections, the incidence of adverse and often dose-limiting side effects in AIDS patients is extraordinarily high. In addition, many of the infections recur when therapy is stopped. The drug of choice for *Pneumocystis carinii* pneumonia is oral or I.V. co-trimoxazole (Bactrim, Septra). Its common side effects are hypersensitivity, rash, and leukopenia. If treatment fails or toxicity occurs, I.M. or I.V. pentamidine may be substituted. Pentamidine can be toxic to the kidneys or liver and can cause hyperglycemia or hypoglycemia and hypotension.

Toxoplasma gondii encephalitis can usually be treated with a combination of pyrimethamine and silver sulfadiazine. Side effects include hypersensitivity reactions and bone marrow suppression. Patients with toxoplasmosis usually require long-term therapy.

Candida albicans can be treated with nystatin or clotrimazole; in severe cases with ketoconazole or amphotericin B. *Cryptococcus neoformans* meningitis is treated with I.V. amphotericin B, usually in combination with flucytosine. Amphotericin B is highly toxic, especially to renal function. Herpes simplex lesions are treated with I.V. or P.O. acyclovir, which is often needed chronically.

Currently, no standard treatment is available for infections with *Cryptosporidium*, *Mycobacterium avium intracellulare*, or CMV. However, a new

PROMISING ANTI-A.I.D.S. AGENTS

A new family of drugs, designed to inhibit the AIDS virus' ability to reproduce, may offer hope of survival to victims of AIDS. One of these drugs is azidothymidine (AZT, also called Compound S).

At a recent meeting of the Interscience Conference on Antimicrobial Agents and Chemotherapy (ICAAC), investigators reported that AZT has been shown to limit multiplication of the human T cell lymphotrophic virus III (HTLV-III) in laboratory tests. AZT appears to work by inhibiting reverse transcriptase, an enzyme essential for multiplication of HTLV-III. The HTLV-III virus multiplies by imposing reverse transcriptase over the genetic code of the human host cell, transforming it into a producer of the virus. AZT so closely resembles this enzyme that the virus can't distinguish between them, but, by using the AZT molecule, the virus loses its ability to reproduce.

Early reports from Phase I trials suggest that AZT arrests the virus with milder side effects than any agent tested so far. And it has the advantage of being effective with oral administration. Moreover, preliminary data indicate that AZT can reach the cerebrospinal fluid; thus, it can even attack the virus that has spread to neurologic sites. Encouraged by these preliminary data, some investigators suggest that preventing uncontrolled reproduction of this virus may stabilize the patient's condition, allowing his immune system to regenerate and recover normal function, possibly effecting an indefinite remission.

Several other drugs also receiving clinical trials in patients with AIDS are suramin, ribavirin, interferon A, and the French agent HPA-23.

agent called DHPG has shown some promise in treating CMV infections.

Complications

Complications can occur in almost any organ system as a result of an opportunistic infection, multiple infections, malignancy, or drug toxicity. The systems most frequently involved are respiratory, GI, neurologic, and skin. The most common cause of death in AIDS patients is respiratory failure either from CMV pneumonitis, *Pneumocystis carinii* pneumonia, or pulmonary KS. Neurologic complications can follow direct infection of nervous system cells with the HTLV-III virus.

Nursing intervention

Comprehensive, careful, and continuous assessment of AIDS patients is an essential aspect of nursing care. Symptoms of many of the characteristic clinical syndromes are subtle. Yet, early detection and intervention can make a significant difference in outcome. Take special care to monitor the patient's respiratory, neurologic, nutritional, eliminatory, and skin status. Give AIDS patients detailed information on self-care, how to avoid infection, and how to avoid transmission of the virus to others.

• For respiratory problems, position the patient properly, provide oxygen therapy, and pace activities to prevent overexertion. Give antimicrobials promptly according to dosage schedule.

• Regularly assess neurologic and mental status. Patients with CNS infections may need reality orientation as well as safety precautions. Seizure precautions and anticonvulsants may be needed.

• Closely monitor nutritional and electrolyte status, especially in a patient with diarrhea. Such patients often require supplemental, high-calorie feedings; some may require intravenous hyperalimentation. Antidiarrheals such as Lomotil or tincture of opium are often helpful. Meticulous mouth care is important. Rinses with normal saline solution plus hydrogen peroxide or sodium bicarbonate help maintain hygiene and comfort.

• Monitor KS lesions and encourage or provide good skin care. Herpes simplex lesions are often painful and may require analgesic drug treatment as well as a careful regimen for wound healing.

• Encourage healthy behaviors, for example, good nutrition, rest, exercise as

GUIDELINES FOR INFECTION CONTROL IN THE CARE OF PATIENTS WITH A.I.D.S.

When caring for a hospitalized AIDS patient, impose blood and body fluid precautions for infection control.

Wash hands before and after contact with the patient or with any soiled items.

Wear gloves to avoid contact with blood or body fluids, or with objects and materials soiled with them.

Wear a gown if a chance exists that your clothing will be soiled with the patient's blood or body fluid.

Wear a mask only if a possibility exists that blood or other secretions will splash in your face, for example, when suctioning a patient or while assisting with an endoscopy.

Dispose of needles in an accessible, impervious container as soon as possible after use. Needles should not be bent, cut, or resheathed.

Label laboratory specimens "Blood and Body Fluid Precautions" and place in a plastic bag for transport.

Label and bag linen according to hospital policy for infection control precautions.

Clean blood spills with a 1:10 solution of sodium hypochlorite 5.25% (household bleach).

Visitors don't need to take precautions unless they might come into contact with the patient's blood or body fluids.

tolerated, good hygiene, and avoidance of infection.

• Teach patients the signs and symptoms of infection and what to do if symptoms appear.

• Provide patients with information about safe sexual practices.

• Instruct them not to donate blood, organs, or semen; not to share razors, toothbrushes, or other items that might be contaminated with blood; and to avoid pregnancy.

• Advise patients to inform their doctors, dentists, and sexual partners of their diagnosis.

• Be prepared to deal with the AIDS patient's numerous psychosocial concerns. Besides having to deal with the prognosis of a terminal illness and the isolation of social disapproval, AIDS patients must face rapid and severe changes in body image that can crush self-esteem. Some patients lose their jobs, financial security, and health insurance. Many lose the support of their families due to geographic distance, emotional separation, or fears of family members for their own health. Other family members may simply not know what to do. Nurses can help by offering support to AIDS patients, helping them to maintain hope, teaching them what they need to know to cope with their disease, and referring AIDS patients and the people close to them for appropriate counseling.

CHRISTINE GRADY, RN, MSN, CS

Cancer update: Interleukin-2 (IL-2) therapy

Traditionally, three standard types of cancer treatment have been available: surgery, radiation, and chemotherapy. Currently, a group of substances is being studied that, if shown to be useful, will likely become the fourth type

of cancer treatment. These substances are called biological response modifiers (BRMs).

BRMs have been defined as agents or approaches to cancer treatment that change the relationship between tumor and host by changing the host's biological response to tumor cells and thereby producing a therapeutic effect. Such agents include interferon, thymic factors, monoclonal antibodies, and interleukin-2 (IL-2), among others. IL-2 is a substance that alters the host's immune system in response to the growth of cancer cells.

Biological theories

The concept that the immune system helps to prevent or control cancer through such mechanisms as immune surveillance, whereby cells of the immune system scan for and eliminate early malignant cells from the body, has been under consideration for some time. The immune system's primary function is to recognize and destroy anything foreign to the host. Cancer cells are, in a sense, foreign and can therefore serve as antigens, stimulating an immune response.

Researchers have discovered complex mechanisms of immune response. The challenge now is to learn how to stimulate or modify these mechanisms to potentiate the body's natural defense against cancer. In this area, IL-2 appears promising.

Origin of IL-2

Lymphocytes, which constitute about 22% to 25% of the white blood cell population, produce cell products called lymphokines. IL-2 (originally called T-cell growth factor) is a naturally occurring lymphokine secreted by T lymphocytes (a specific type of lymphocyte that matures in the thymus gland) and is thought capable of altering the immune response associated with tumor-related antigens.

When lymphocytes are exposed to a specific antigen, they secrete IL-2 into the surrounding tissue. The released

IL-2 then acts as a powerful signal, causing cell division and proliferation of other T lymphocytes. IL-2 also induces lymphocytes to become activated killer cells that have been shown to destroy a wide variety of tumor cells.

Since the supply of natural human IL-2 is limited, the technique of gene splicing has been developed for producing this substance in large amounts. Recombinant IL-2 is produced by inserting the gene for human IL-2 into *Escherichia coli* bacteria, which provide the environment for synthesizing IL-2 molecules. The bacteria are then killed, thus making possible the recovery of a highly purified form of IL-2 in sufficient quantity for use in research and clinical trials.

Phase I clinical trials

Currently, IL-2 studies are being conducted in both laboratory and specialized clinical settings, using small numbers of patients with various types of refractory cancers. Phase I clinical trials will identify IL-2–related side effects, toxicities, and any biological effects occurring with various doses.

Phase I trials of BRMs differ from Phase I trials of chemotherapy. With BRMs, the largest tolerated dose isn't necessarily the most effective dose. A lower dose may actually be more effective as an immunomodulator. As a result, Phase I trials of BRMs test different doses for their effect on biological and immune function as well as for side effects and toxicity.

At one institution, IL-2 was administered intravenously in escalating single doses during a Phase I trial. The 14 patients who participated in the trial had histologically documented advanced cancer that resisted conventional cancer therapy. The patients were screened for adequate performance status and kidney, liver, and hematologic function. Before hospitalization, patients signed a consent form for the four weekly treatments.

IL-2 with normal saline solution was given through a peripheral I.V. line, and the infusion rate was monitored by an infusion control device. Essential, frequent nursing assessments included vital signs, observation for systemic reaction, and inspection of the I.V. insertion site for local reaction. In addition, serum and urine samples were obtained at frequent intervals before, during, and after the infusion to measure IL-2 levels.

The effectiveness of IL-2's antitumor activity was evaluated in various ways. Microscopic observations were made of the effects of IL-2 on the lymphocyte population after each IL-2 infusion as well as the effect of foreign antigens on the lymphocytes. In addition, the patient's malignancy was measured for response appropriate for the type of cancer (for example, chest X-ray for lung metastasis, cancer antigen 125 serum level for ovarian cancer). A 50% reduction in tumor size was required as a prerequisite for continued treatment with IL-2.

Side effects appeared to be dose related, since four patients at the low-dosage range had only mild chills, fever of 99.5° F. to 102.2° F. (37.5° C. to 39° C.), and mild aching. Three of five patients who received the higher dosage experienced nausea with vomiting, severe chills, fever, and mild aching. All symptoms resolved shortly after the infusion ended. When complete, the results of this and other studies will determine the next phase of clinical trials for IL-2.

Nursing intervention

Nurses play an important role in caring for patients who are participating in a Phase I clinical trial of a BRM agent. The informed consent document each patient must sign outlines the purposes of the study, the expected outcomes, and the expected side effects. Use this document as a teaching aid to measure each patient's level of understanding. Be prepared to reinforce and reexplain areas of misunderstanding.

Since the nature and severity of any agent's side effects are not fully known when Phase I trials begin, carefully observe and document any subjective or objective signs. The fact that little is known about the agent and its effects can frighten the patient. Allay his fears by assuring him that he will be closely monitored. Remember that a patient who's accepted for such a study has already undergone aggressive therapy; now he is being asked to participate in an experimental treatment that may do little good but may cause side effects. The patient's anxiety is understandable. Offer your reassurance and support.

Be aware of the frequency and volume of blood samples required in such a study. A large volume of blood drawn for study often results in a declining hematocrit level. Observe significant complete blood count results. Watch for and report signs and symptoms of anemia to the doctor.

Document the time at which side effects occurred in relation to dosage and infusion rate. This can be important in planning future treatments. For example, if chills or fever is significant at an initial dose, be prepared to premedicate the patient for subsequent treatments. (In one study, I.V. meperidine and diphenhydramine were found to reduce severity of chills.) To prepare the patient for discharge, instruct him about potential symptoms to minimize fears.

Indications for the future

IL-2 therapy has shown exciting promise in other studies. In 1985, the National Cancer Institute conducted a study involving leukapheresis in combination with IL-2. A patient's blood was withdrawn, and the lymphocytes were separated and exposed to IL-2. This facilitated proliferation of a type of lymphocyte termed lymphokine activated killer (LAK) cell. Then the combination of IL-2 and LAK cells was infused intravenously.

IL-2 was administered in high doses up to three times a day. In this study, 40% of patients whose tumors failed to respond to all preceding conventional treatment showed measurable tumor regression. These patients developed various side effects that included weight gain due to profound fluid retention, pulmonary edema, respiratory distress, and a generalized erythematous rash.

In the treatment of malignant glioma, a type of brain cancer, and in another study of bladder cancer, IL-2 or LAK cells were injected intratumorally. Injecting IL-2 directly into the tumor elicited an antitumor effect without systemic toxicity.

The future direction of IL-2 will depend on the analysis and development of data from several levels of research. To date, research findings as discussed above are preliminary and not all toxicities are known. More clinical trials are necessary. Consequently, the availability of these treatments at community hospitals seems unlikely in the near future. However, IL-2 may be used as an adjunct therapy after surgical excision of tumors as well as a primary form of treatment when infused with LAK cells. In some cancers, the best use of IL-2 may be in combination with standard therapy; in others, it may be effective when used alone. As IL-2's effectiveness is determined, nursing input will be essential for developing standards of nursing care specific to BRM therapy.

DEBORAH C. FOISIE, RN, BS
BEVERLY VINCENT, RN, MSN

Cancer update: Laser therapy

Photodynamic therapy (PDT) is a new and experimental treatment for nonoperable bronchogenic cancer. Malignant cells saturated with hematoporphyrin derivative (HPD) are destroyed by the photochemical reaction that occurs when the cells are exposed to a specific spectrum of red light delivered by an argon laser–pumped tunable-dye laser.

HPD is injected intravenously and absorbed by all cells within 12 to 24 hours, but only malignant cells retain the chemical. The nonthermal laser beam selectively targets only HPD-saturated malignant cells that may or may not be visible. The healthy tissue is unaffected.

To date, PDT has been used mainly as a palliative treatment for obstructive endobronchial tumors. Although PDT appears to have eliminated tumors permanently in some patients, the current goal of PDT is to improve the quality of life for patients with endobronchial tumors that haven't responded to conventional treatment. New protocols are being developed for similar treatment of bladder and skin cancer.

Preparation for PDT

An assessment bronchoscopy establishes the extent of obstruction by the tumor and its exact location. A computed tomography scan determines if the tumor has invaded the bronchial wall or extended into the pleural space. An invasive tumor can't be treated by PDT because the treatment would destroy the bronchus.

Preoperative care of the patient about to undergo PDT is similar to that of any patient with a compromised airway. Adequate nutrition is essential, since these patients, usually debilitated and exhausted, have probably been unable to eat a regular diet.

The patient receives HPD intravenously (dose calculated at 2 mg/kg of body weight) 24 to 72 hours before treatment. Timing of the injection depends upon the type and size of the tumor. After the injection, the patient must be protected from sunlight, which would cause severe skin burns as a result of photosensitivity. Keep drapes and bedside curtains drawn in the patient's room. Room lights may be left on, however, since artificial light doesn't react with HPD.

The patient is visited by the operating room (OR) nurse, who assesses his physical and mental status as well as his anxiety level. Since most patients are over age 55, the OR nurse should communicate all the patient's medical problems, such as cardiovascular disease, concurrent respiratory problems, or liver disease, to other members of the operating team in case the patient's status becomes compromised in any way during PDT. The OR nurse should be prepared to answer any questions the patient might ask and to inform the patient and his family about the sequence of events that precedes the treatment.

PDT procedure

On admission to the operating room, the patient's vital signs are taken and cardiac monitoring is begun. The patient is then sedated with I.V. morphine and diazepam and asked to gargle with a flavored oral lidocaine solution to anesthetize the throat and vocal cords. When the patient is sufficiently anesthetized, the OR nurse assists the doctor or respiratory therapist in intubating the patient and instituting mechanical ventilation. (Arterial blood gases may be drawn at this time.)

Next, a flexible bronchoscope is inserted and the tumor is visualized. Additional lidocaine solution is injected down the bronchoscope, allowed to pass over the tumor site, and then suctioned out.

Close monitoring of the patient's cardiac status is necessary throughout the procedure since lidocaine and bronchoscopy can cause dysrhythmias. Maintaining adequate topical anesthesia is important to ensure the patient's comfort and cooperation during the procedure, which may last 1½ hours or more. Since the patient remains conscious during the procedure, additional sedation is given as needed to relieve discomfort and lessen anxiety. Psychological support is also important since the patient may be frightened.

The laser quartz fiber is passed through the bronchoscope and is directed close to or into the tumor. The laser operator activates the laser, stopping and starting on the doctor's instructions. The laser light is interrupted frequently to inject lidocaine, to suction tumor debris away from the airway, to relocate the laser fiber, and to check the laser fiber's tip. Treatment time varies with the size and type of tumor. Upon completion of PDT, the laser fiber and bronchoscope are removed. When lidocaine's anesthetic effects have worn off sufficiently to allow the patient to maintain a patent airway, the endotracheal tube is removed.

Postoperative care
The patient is monitored closely in the recovery room. Moist oxygen is administered to prevent airway drying and irritation, and the patient is encouraged to breathe deeply and to cough up any accumulated exudate. Vital signs are monitored carefully until the patient is no longer drowsy and shows no new or unusual dysrhythmias. Stay alert for signs of respiratory distress, since tumor debris from dead malignant cells may obstruct the airway. After treatment of a large tumor, such obstruction may occur approximately 6 hours after treatment. An emergency bronchoscopy may be necessary to clear the airway.

Damaged malignant cells continue to die for 6 to 7 days after PDT. Up to three bronchoscopies may be performed to remove exudate and to assess tumor size. Large endobronchial tumors may require additional laser treatments. Since sufficient HPD remains in the malignant cells for several days, supplementary laser treatments can be performed during the cleanup bronchoscopies.

The outcome of the treatment is a clear airway. Most patients can breathe freely again and drink and eat as tolerated when the gag reflex returns.

The patient must avoid exposure to sunlight for 30 days, but he may go outside after sunset. If he must go out during the day, he should cover all skin and wear a hat that completely covers his head and shades his face. After 30 days, the patient may test for photosensitivity by exposing a small area of skin to filtered sunlight. If the exposed area develops redness, burning, or tingling, the patient must continue to avoid sunlight for 7 more days and then repeat the test.

KATHIE THOMPSON, RN, BBA

Cancer update: Monoclonal antibody therapy

Monoclonal antibody therapy is a promising new treatment for a variety of cancers, including lymphocytic leukemia and ovarian cancer. This treatment became possible only recently as a result of new understanding of immune mechanisms. However, it was first suggested in the 1890s by Paul Ehrlich, who postulated that antibody molecules could selectively target toxic substances to cancer cells and kill them. This combination of an antibody covalently linked to a modified toxin (see *How Immunotoxins Kill Tumor Cells*) is called an immunotoxin, designed to inactivate protein synthesis of cancer cells.

Mechanism of action
The antibody portion of an immunotoxin guides the immunotoxin to the antigen-specific tumor cell. The toxin portion is derived from certain plants or bacteria and contains an A chain and a B chain. The A chain, an enzymatically active peptide, inactivates protein synthesis. The B chain, a cell-binding peptide, must be modified by partial or complete removal from the toxin to allow the antibody to bind with antigen on the tumor cell surface. After binding, the antigen-immunotoxin moves inside the cell in an endosomal

HOW IMMUNOTOXINS KILL TUMOR CELLS

An immunotoxin, consisting of an antibody linked to a modified toxin, kills a tumor cell by antigen binding, inclusion into the cell, and release of toxin to inactivate protein synthesis at the ribosomes.

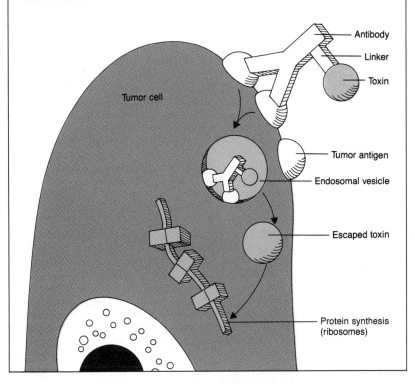

vesicle. The toxin portion eventually escapes from this vesicle into the cytosol. Here it interacts with ribosomes and inactivates them. Immunotoxins are extremely potent and can kill tumor cells at very low concentrations.

Developmental and clinical research

Early studies on animals with small tumors showed that radionuclides and cytotoxic drugs linked to antibodies have significant antitumor effects. In these studies, the antibody was injected directly into the tumor site.

Later biological research in the 1970s was responsible for the development of hybridoma monoclonal antibodies. The discovery of hybridoma technology enabled the fusion of two cell lines to form a hybrid cell that shared the genetic information of both cells. This event led to the development of monoclonal antibodies (mabs). Mabs are antibodies that are produced by a single clone of cells. The mab is specific for a single antigenic determinant.

In 1975, Köhler and Milstein developed a method to produce pure mabs from the cloned cells of mice. Antibody production occurs when a mouse is immunized with a desired antigen. Mouse spleen cells are then removed and fused with rapidly dividing mouse myeloma cells, producing the hybrid cells. Each hybrid cell, in turn, produces a single, or monoclonal, antibody. Selected hybrid cells can be grown in a special medium and cloned for specific antibody production. The clones may be frozen for future use, grown in mass culture, or injected into a mouse. After injection, the mouse develops a tumor, producing the desired antibody.

Human tumor cells have been found to carry specific antigens. When introduced into the body, mabs target these specific antigens. Mabs can be tagged with radionuclides or joined with certain drugs or toxins. Recently, mabs have been conjugated with ricin toxin, ricin toxin A chain, and *Pseudomonas* exotoxin A to enhance their ability to kill tumor cells.

Since the 1970s, a large number of immunotoxins have been identified; some are now being studied for their clinical effectiveness. At the University of California at San Francisco, patients with melanoma have been treated with an antibody to melanoma cells linked to ricin toxin A chain. At the National Institutes of Health, patients with T cell acute lymphoblastic leukemia (HTLV-I positive) have been treated with an antibody to the interleukin-2 receptor linked to *Pseudomonas* toxin. At the University of Toulouse in France, patients with chronic lymphocytic leukemia have received an antibody to these cells linked to ricin toxin A chain.

At the Fred Hutchinson Cancer Center and at the University of Minnesota, immunotoxins have been used to treat the bone marrow grafts of patients after allogeneic and autologous bone marrow transplantation. These grafts have been treated before transplantation with antibodies to T cells linked to ricin toxin A chain or to whole ricin to prevent graft-versus-host disease.

Duke University's Comprehensive Cancer Center has begun one new clinical trial, using I.V. immunotoxin therapy in patients with refractory chronic lymphocytic leukemia; and one new trial is anticipated, using intraperitoneal immunotoxin therapy in patients with Stage III ovarian cancer.

Adverse effects

To date, 4 patients at Duke have been treated with I.V. immunotoxin with no adverse effects. Twenty-six patients at the University of California at San Francisco have been treated with I.V. immunotoxin, and most had minimal adverse effects. Three developed mild allergic reactions that responded to antihistamines, fluid replacement, and steroids; 17 developed fluid retention and decreased serum albumin levels; and 1 showed moderate but reversible liver toxicity. One patient developed a fatal myocardial infarction; however, researchers didn't associate the immunotoxin with the infarction.

Complications

Several complications may follow immunotoxin therapy. Antigen shedding, antigen modulation, or antigen heterogeneity may prevent tumor cells from binding to the immunotoxin. This problem could possibly be circumvented by plasmapheresis or a combination of immunotoxins.

Another potential problem is the chance that immunotoxins might bind to normal tissue, increasing their potential toxicity. Also tumor cells may lack target antigen and resist internalization of immunotoxin after binding. The use of multiple toxins may prevent development of resistant tumor cells.

Finally, a human antibody response could inactivate the immunotoxin in the plasma. This may be prevented by altering the antibody or toxin or by using immunosuppressive agents to block the immune response.

Protocols for clinical trials

New clinical trials for immunotoxin therapy are beginning. Each phase of these trials depends on meticulous nursing documentation for data collection, timely and accurate specimen collections, and careful observation for unknown side effects, which may include life-threatening situations.

Nurses also participate in clinical trials by helping the patient and his family understand the new therapy and by providing support throughout the treatment regimen. Many patients selected for such clinical trials have undergone prior aggressive cancer therapy and may view this experimental treatment as their final hope. They also may experience fear and anxiety about the investigational drug's unknown side effects.

Specific protocols are now available for clinical trials of immunotoxin in patients with leukemia, and one is anticipated in patients with ovarian cancer.

CHRONIC LYMPHOCYTIC LEUKEMIA

Chronic lymphocytic leukemia (CLL) is the most common type of leukemia in Western countries and affects more men than women. Most cases of CLL involve B lymphocytes. Early symptoms of the disease include chronic fatigue and exercise intolerance. Advanced disease is marked by fever, weight loss, diaphoresis, severe fatigue, and anemia. Chemotherapy is the treatment of choice for CLL, with additional chemotherapy and radiotherapy after relapse. Patients who eventually have no further response develop resistance to the chemotherapeutic agents. For these patients, prolonged survival has seemed unlikely. The use of interferon and monoclonal antibodies has demonstrated little success; however, the use of I.V. immunotoxin may offer more effective treatment.

I.V. administration allows high circulating concentrations of the immunotoxin to interact directly with the high CLL-tumor antigen level and to bind in the circulating CLL cells. Patients selected for this protocol must be refractory to conventional therapy. Both pharmacokinetic and immunologic studies are performed.

Nursing intervention

Specific nursing interventions for the CLL protocol include the following:
• Monitor and observe for side effects

of circulating systemic immunotoxins, which may include rash, fever, chills, and bronchospasms. Keep emergency resuscitative equipment readily available at the bedside.
• Monitor laboratory chemistries for early signs of renal or hepatic damage. How easily the immunotoxin will be metabolized by humans is unknown.
• Monitor blood counts, particularly hematocrit, white blood cell count and differential, and platelets.
• Observe changes in weakness, fatigue, fever, and diaphoresis.

OVARIAN CANCER

Ovarian cancer is among the most lethal of all gynecologic cancers. This intraabdominal malignancy develops in the pelvis and spreads to surrounding structures and to serosal surfaces of the peritoneal cavity. Ovarian cancer usually doesn't spread beyond the abdominal cavity because the diaphragm, pelvic floor, and abdominal wall serve as barriers. Patients with Stage III ovarian adenocarcinoma are usually treated with surgery and combination chemotherapy. Currently, 40% to 50% of these patients have residual disease after surgery. Further chemotherapy and radiotherapy don't significantly change prognosis.

Intraperitoneal chemotherapy using peritoneal dialysis has been developed and administered (with few side effects) to patients with ovarian cancer. This method of therapy delivers a high concentration of antitumor drug to the tumor site and avoids systemic chemotherapy, which exposes normal tissue to chemotherapy toxicity.

A new clinical trial will test the effects of intraperitoneal immunotoxin therapy in patients with refractory Stage III epithelial ovarian adenocarcinoma. The immunotoxin is delivered by intraperitoneal dialysis via Tenckhoff catheters using 2 liters of dialysate solution. This large fluid volume enables total bathing of the abdominal cavity. Dose escalation of the immunotoxin is determined by evidence of toxicity. Pharmacokinetic and immunologic studies are performed throughout therapy.

Nursing intervention

Nursing care for patients receiving intraperitoneal immunotoxin therapy includes the following:

• Manage dialysis treatments, including accurate recording of fluid exchanges. The most common complication experienced with dialysis is abdominal pain or discomfort, which may result from inadequate warming of the dialysate solution, irritation from catheter placement, potential peritonitis from the immunotoxin, or bacterial peritonitis.

• Monitor and observe for signs and symptoms of bacterial peritonitis (fever, abdominal spasms, changes in respirations).

• Maintain Tenckhoff catheter sterility.

• Teach patients self-care techniques for their catheters.

• Provide emotional support to foster coping strategies for dealing with changes in body image and life-style related to dialysis.

SCARLOTT K. MUELLER, RN, BSN, MPH

Cancer update: Radiation therapy

Improvements in radiation therapy have made possible treatment of deeply embedded and superficial cancerous lesions without damaging skin and surrounding normal tissue. Radiation therapy targets high-energy beams of radiation directly to destroy cancer cells and stop their rampant proliferation.

How radiation combats cancer

Radiation therapy does the most damage to a cell while it is synthesizing deoxyribonucleic acid (DNA) and dividing. With damaged DNA, the cell is unable to divide further and eventually dies.

Because cellular growth and proliferation require oxygen and an adequate blood supply, small, well-oxygenated, and well-vascularized cells are more radiosensitive than large, less vascularized tumors. In addition, tumors made up of rapidly dividing cells (such as lymphatic and hematopoietic tissue, germ cells, and intestinal epithelium) are more sensitive to radiation than tumors made up of cells and tissue with low mitotic activity.

Radiation sources

In the last decade, great technical strides have improved radiation therapy. Formerly delivered by a machine that offered only a single energy, new machines (such as the 25 MeV linear accelerator) offer greater flexibility in treatments. For example, unlike the standard 4 MeV linear accelerator or cobalt 60 unit, the 25 MeV provides radiation treatments with two different modalities: high-energy X-ray beams and electron beams.

High-energy X-ray beams deliver radiation doses at great depths (the higher the energy, the deeper the penetration), thus sparing injury to the skin and surrounding normal tissue. High-energy beams are especially useful in obese patients whose tumors lie deep under the skin's surface.

In contrast, the finite penetration of the electron beam can treat superficial lesions more effectively, while sparing healthy tissue in the surrounding area of radiation damage. The electron beam is especially useful in treating recurrent chest wall lesions, such as those found in metastatic breast cancer, since it doesn't damage underlying tissue.

Intraoperative radiotherapy

The most innovative and still investigational application of the 25 MeV linear accelerator is intraoperative radiotherapy. Several national research protocols have recently been designed

DELIVERING HIGH-ENERGY RADIATION

High-energy linear accelerators deliver two types of radiation to cancer cells: X-ray beam and electron beam. X-ray beams, generating up to 25 million electron volts (MeV), direct radiation to deep tumors, sparing injury to the skin and surrounding tissue. Electron beams, with energy up to 22 MeV, deliver highly focused radiation to superficial tumors.

The high-energy linear accelerator shown here is the Clinac 2500. In operation, the electron gun of the Clinac 2500 shoots high energy electrons into the accelerator, a specially engineered metal tube. At the same time, a powerful microwave source supplies the accelerator with electromagnetic energy waves. Absorbing this added energy, the electrons are accelerated to nearly the speed of light. The electrons are used directly for treatment or, when X-rays are required, they're aimed at a metallic target. When the electrons strike the target, they're slowed or stopped and high energy X-rays are released.

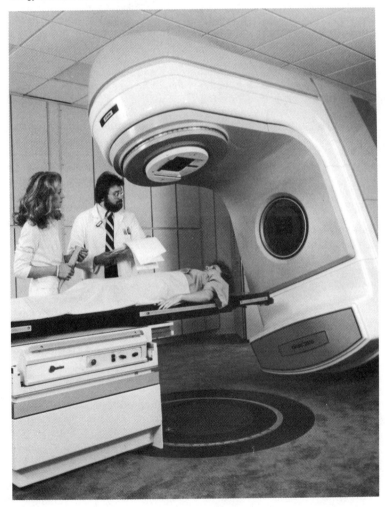

to study the efficacy of this treatment.

Intraoperative radiotherapy delivers a specific radiation dose (usually 6 to 10 times that of standard external beam radiation) to a tumor during surgery. After the surgeon has resected as much tumor as possible, radiation is delivered to the tumor bed using the electron beam. The surgical site is then closed, and further treatment, if necessary, is planned.

The advantage of intraoperative therapy is that it delivers a large dose of radiation directly to the tumor bed. No skin is present in the treatment field, and the surgeon can retract critical structures in the tumor area, thus preventing radiation damage to healthy tissue. The disadvantage is that in many hospitals, the patient must be transported from the operating room to the radiation therapy department during the surgical procedure, thus increasing the surgical risk and the risk of infection.

Some institutions overcome this disadvantage by performing intraoperative radiation in a special operating suite located near the 25 MeV linear accelerator.

Adverse effects

Since radiotherapy is a localized treatment, effects of therapy are specific to the area being treated. One of the most common adverse effects is skin irritation, ranging from slight redness to moist desquamation with skin breakdown. This is especially prevalent in patients treated with electron beams. To minimize such skin reactions, patients should be instructed to wash gently with a mild soap and to pat the area dry; to avoid use of perfumes, lotions, and powders; to avoid wearing tight, constricting clothing over the irradiated area; and to avoid exposing the treated area to the sun. If blistering or skin breakdown occurs, the patient should notify the doctor immediately so he can take appropriate action to prevent infection.

Other common adverse effects of radiation therapy are specific to the organ system(s) involved in the treatment field. When the head and neck area is treated, mucositis can be a severe problem. The patient should be encouraged to see his dentist before treatment and to maintain good oral hygiene. Diet modifications should be advised. The patient may also experience mouth dryness and loss of taste. Hypothyroidism may also occur.

If the esophagus or lung is treated, the patient may develop esophagitis. He should be instructed to avoid spicy and acidic foods as well as very hot and very cold foods. A topical anesthetic such as Xylocaine 2% Viscous Solution may be ordered to relieve mouth discomfort. If the patient is having difficulty eating, nutritional supplements should be recommended.

Nutritional supplements are also recommended for the patient who has undergone radiotherapy of the stomach or small intestine. Such a patient will most likely experience nausea and vomiting; he requires small, frequent meals and may be given antiemetics if necessary.

After radiation to the pelvis, the patient is likely to experience diarrhea. Antidiarrheal medications such as Lomotil are commonly ordered, and the patient is instructed to eat a low-fiber diet. A long-term adverse effect of pelvic radiation therapy is sterility.

If the treatment field includes the bladder, the patient may develop cystitis. In that case, he should be encouraged to increase his fluid intake to several quarts daily. He may receive treatment with bladder analgesics and/or antibiotics.

Nursing intervention

● Thoroughly educate the patient about radiation treatment. Explain procedures in detail. Arrange for the patient to tour the radiation therapy department before treatment.
● Include family members in your teaching. They may share the patient's questions and fears. Understanding the

treatment will help them support the patient more effectively.

• Reassure the patient that he won't become radioactive from the treatment. Many patients worry about this, so be sure to address this worry before treatment.

• Thoroughly explain anticipated side effects of radiation therapy and how they can be managed.

PATRICIA A. McLAUGHLIN, RN, BSN

Cancer update: Radioactive antibodies

Early results of studies of a new cancer treatment indicate that antibodies labeled with radioactive isotopes may help overcome hepatoma, an aggressive primary liver cancer. This experimental treatment was pioneered in 1978 by Dr. Stanley Order of Johns Hopkins Hospital, Baltimore. Since then, several protocols have been sponsored by the Radiation Oncology Group for radioactive antibody treatment of hepatomas, Hodgkin's disease, and non–small cell lung cancer. To date, such treatment is available only at Johns Hopkins Hospital; Albert Einstein Medical Center, Philadelphia; and the University of California Medical Center at San Francisco.

Treatment
Certain types of tumors secrete antigens (proteins) in high concentrations. Two such antigens are ferritin, associated primarily with hepatomas, lung cancer, and Hodgkin's disease; and carcinoembryonic antigen (CEA), associated primarily with lung and colon cancer. (Although these antigens can be found in healthy tissue, the concentration is small and the structure is slightly different.)

When ferritin or CEA is injected into a rabbit, pig, or monkey, the animal makes antibodies to the antigen, thus producing anti-ferritin or anti-CEA. The antibodies can then be tagged with the radioactive isotope iodine-131 (^{131}I). After purification, the radioactive antibody is then injected into a patient. The antibody is expected to travel to the tumor site, where it combines with the antigen, forming an antigen-antibody complex. While the antibody is at the tumor site, the tumor receives a high dose of radiation, much higher than can be delivered with external beam radiation therapy. Thus, the radiation and an immunologic response work together to destroy tumor cells to which the antibody is attached.

Adverse effects
Several adverse effects are associated with radioactive antibody treatment, including a rare allergic reaction with anaphylactic shock. To prevent severe allergic reactions, sensitivity tests of the skin and eyes precede this type of treatment.

Bone marrow suppression is common after radioactive antibody treatment because the antibody is administered I.V. and circulates through the bloodstream, irradiating bone marrow. Depending on the reduction in white blood cell and platelet counts, the patient may risk infection or bleeding. Another important risk with this treatment is the potential for destruction of the tumor-bearing organ(s) due to the high radiation dose and the antigen-antibody complex.

Because ^{131}I emits gamma rays that can pass through the body, the patient who has received radioactive antibodies must be isolated for 7 to 10 days to protect others from radiation exposure.

Nursing intervention
• Become familiar with all treatment procedures so you can perform or assist with them as needed.

• Assess the patient's ability for self-care before the infusion, since contact with him will be limited after treatment renders him radioactive. Be sure

NEW DRUG DEVELOPMENT: CLINICAL TRIALS

Clinical trials protect consumers from unsafe drugs and false and misleading drug labeling. They are the result of the 1962 Kefauver-Harris Amendments.

EARLY DRUG LAWS

The Kefauver-Harris Amendments followed two unsuccessful attempts to regulate the marketing of drugs. Unfortunately, in each case, inadequate legislation led to human tragedy. In 1906, Congress passed the Pure Food and Drug Act (Copeland Act) to protect false and misleading drug labeling. This weak legislation allowed seizure of drugs only after they had been marketed. In 1937 when sulfanilamide elixir appeared in drug stores across the country, the weakness became evident. The drug, which hadn't been tested for toxicity, killed 107 people.

As a result, Congress amended the Copeland Act in 1938 to require proof of a drug's safety before it was marketed. But the thalidomide tragedy in the early 1960s showed a need for stricter regulations.

In 1962, the Kefauver-Harris Amendments required that all new drugs must undergo premarketing clinical trials for proof of safety and efficacy. Drugs marketed between 1938 and 1962 were checked for efficacy by the Drug Efficacy Study Group of the National Academy of Sciences–National Research Council. Each drug was identified as either (1) meeting standards of the Kefauver-Harris Amendments; (2) showing insufficient effectiveness and thus requiring proof of efficacy within a certain time (failure would lead the Food and Drug Administration [FDA] to pull the drug off the market); or (3) ineffective and thus immediately withdrawn from the market by the FDA.

Unless new information indicates that they are unsafe or ineffective, old drugs that meet these requirements are exempt from clinical review.

ORIGIN OF NEW DRUGS

New drugs originate in the laboratory, where chemists and pharmacologists concoct new chemical compounds to produce various pharmacologic effects. Each new compound undergoes numerous tests to identify its pharmacologic properties (absorption, distribution, excretion, metabolism, mechanism of action, dose-response relationships, duration of action, effective dosage range, and potential toxicity). Results then guide decisions about clinical trials. Before clinical trials can begin, the drug's sponsor must submit an Investigational New Drug application to the FDA, which has 30 days to review the application. After 30 days, if the FDA has not told the sponsor to withhold or restrict the drug's use, clinical trials can begin.

PHASES OF CLINICAL TRIALS

Clinical trials for a new drug involve three phases and possibly a fourth after the drug has received FDA approval.
• *Phase I (clinical pharmacology)* to determine safety and confirm pharmacologic activity in humans. These studies determine dose ranges, toxicity, drug dynamics, and metabolism. Except for cancer chemotherapeutic agents, Phase I studies are performed on a few healthy volunteers. The initial drug dose is a fraction of the predicted therapeutic dose.

If Phase I trials show an acceptable margin of safety, Phase II trials may begin.
• *Phase II (clinical investigation)* to evaluate or define potential efficacy; the dose-response relationship; mechanism of action, physiologic effects; and pharmacokinetics; and safety and toxicity. These studies usually involve a limited number of hospitalized patients. If Phase II trials confirm efficacy and if the FDA agrees that the drug's potential benefits outweigh its risks, Phase III trials may begin.
• *Phase III (clinical trials)* to define the best regimen and to prove long-term safety and efficacy. These well-controlled trials involve large numbers of patients. If results show reasonable safety and efficacy, the drug's sponsor submits a New Drug Application to the FDA. If this application is approved, the drug can be marketed, but the FDA may require Phase IV trials.
• *Phase IV (postmarketing trials/similar to Phase III)* to monitor clinical experience, particularly in regard to rare effects.

to teach the patient how to take his vital signs.

• Encourage family members to visit the patient for a short time daily.

• Provide emotional support, especially during isolation. If questions arise concerning radiation exposure, consult the hospital's radiation safety officer.

PATRICIA A. McLAUGHLIN, RN, BSN

Infertility update

Currently, one in six couples either can't conceive or can't carry a pregnancy to term. Most of them can now find help in specialized medical techniques. As recently as 20 years ago, fewer than 30% of infertile couples were treated successfully. But today, comprehensive evaluation and treatment offer an infertile couple a 96.4% chance of conceiving a child. This dramatically improved success rate is due to technical advances and to a new understanding of endocrinology and genetics that have allowed researchers to develop more effective methods for aiding conception and supporting a pregnancy to term.

To the couple desiring a pregnancy, these advances in fertility management are not without emotional and financial sacrifice. Why, then, the increased demand for fertility assistance? First, the subject of infertility is no longer taboo. Second, the social milieu has changed. Couples are waiting longer to marry and to begin their families. Thus, they have less time to have genetically healthy children or to be eligible for adoption. In addition, multiple social and environmental factors actually cause infertility. Prolonged use of contraceptives has been associated with anovulation. Abortion and intra-uterine devices have been associated with infections and scarring that can interfere with conception. And finally, excessive environmental pollutants and the prevalence of sexually transmitted diseases, especially chlamydial infection, have also impaired normal reproductive functions.

Today's nurse has a responsibility to understand the basics of fertility and infertility, to know the various tests and treatments for infertility, and to teach fertile couples to value, rather than take for granted, their fertility.

Reproductive requirements

For pregnancy to occur, a female must ovulate, her fallopian tubes must be unobstructed and undamaged, and her uterine lining must allow an embryo to implant, grow, and develop. In addition, her cervical mucus must be receptive to sperm. The male must have sufficient sperm of normal form and mobility that are capable of fertilizing an egg.

Diagnostic methods

Specialized diagnostic tests now reliably identify the cause(s) of infertility.

Sperm tests. The sperm penetration assay (SPA) (or zona-free hamster egg test) is a new evaluation tool that measures the capacity of human sperm to penetrate a specially prepared hamster egg. This test confirms the characteristics necessary to fertilize a human egg. It offers much more information than the traditional semen analysis, which simply grades sperm on motility, count, and morphology.

The SPA can be used to diagnose unexplained infertility; to screen for in vitro fertilization, gamete intrafallopian transfer, and varicocele repair; and to screen sperm donors for artificial insemination. The SPA can also help identify appropriate treatment for oligospermia. However, its validity in assessing fertilization potential is controversial as a result of inherent variables, such as how sperm preincubation time affects results. Also controversial is SPA's interpretation of results and its determination of a cutoff point to distinguish infertile from fertile males. Generally, hamster egg penetration by 10% to 20% and more of

THE SPERM PENETRATION ASSAY

The sperm penetration assay is carried out in the laboratory using collected sperm and hamster-derived eggs to determine the ability of sperm to fertilize human eggs.

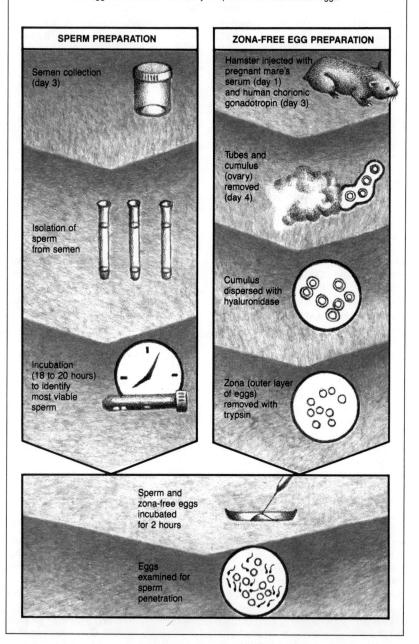

SPERM PREPARATION

Semen collection (day 3)

Isolation of sperm from semen

Incubation (18 to 20 hours) to identify most viable sperm

ZONA-FREE EGG PREPARATION

Hamster injected with pregnant mare's serum (day 1) and human chorionic gonadotropin (day 3)

Tubes and cumulus (ovary) removed (day 4)

Cumulus dispersed with hyaluronidase

Zona (outer layer of eggs) removed with trypsin

Sperm and zona-free eggs incubated for 2 hours

Eggs examined for sperm penetration

the sperm sample indicates positive fertility potential. Sperm that function below this range are considered infertile. Recently, however, a method has been developed to assist these infertile males. Their sperm is placed within a special egg yolk buffer prior to the test. Although the numbers are small, an increase in penetration rate has been noted.

Ovulation tests. The home ovulation prediction kit measures the level of luteinizing hormone (LH) in the urine to determine ovulation time more precisely. LH aids in the release of the mature egg from the ovarian follicle. The onset of this LH surge begins about 24 to 36 hours before ovulation.

Identifying a woman's fertile period can then be used to time intercourse for the greatest chance of conception. Predicting ovulation is also necessary for certain tests and for certain treatments associated with infertility.

The ovulation prediction kit (several brands are available) is a simple, rapid, noninvasive test that can be done in the privacy of one's home. It is less expensive than radioimmunoassay tests and ultrasound monitoring. However, results of this test may be ambiguous, and certain drugs can alter its results. In addition, the best time of day to perform the test and optimum frequency are still unknown.

Treatment methods

In vitro fertilization (IVF). Since 1981, IVF has helped couples conceive babies in the laboratory. With IVF, male sperm and female eggs are placed together for fertilization outside the body. The fertilized egg is then transferred to the uterus. IVF was initially used to treat women whose fallopian tubes were damaged or absent. Today, IVF is an option for couples with unexplained infertility and is viewed as the ultimate test for male infertility.

Gamete intrafallopian transfer (GIFT). This abbreviated IVF procedure places sperm and eggs immediately into the woman's fallopian tube(s) instead of growing them first in culture media.

A disadvantage of GIFT is that fertilization cannot be documented unless pregnancy occurs. The GIFT procedure is about 2 days shorter than IVF and thus less expensive.

Cryopreservation. This is a process of preparing and freezing fertilized eggs for future implantation. Its advantages include the freedom to postpone the transfer until the most optimal uterine environment exists; to use a limited number of fertilized eggs for transfer at a single time, saving some for future use; and to decrease the risk of multiple pregnancy by limiting the number of fertilized eggs transferred.

A future use for cryopreservation might be embryo adoption by infertile couples for whom the regular adoption channel isn't an option.

Laparoscopy. This technique allows visualization of the ovaries, fallopian tubes, uterus, and pelvis through the insertion of a special instrument through the umbilicus. In just over a decade, it has become the most frequently performed procedure for women. Laparoscopy can diagnose pelvic problems such as infertility and can provide access for procedures such as tubal ligations, for draining or removing cysts from the ovary or fallopian tubes, and for repairing damaged tubes via microsurgery. When used with the laser, the laparoscope can replace laparotomy in treating endometriosis and adhesions; it's also being used increasingly to monitor results of therapy and to evaluate and treat fetal problems in utero, a process known as fetoscopy.

Laparoscopy can usually be done as an outpatient procedure with shorter hospitalization time, quicker recovery, and potentially reduced risk of postoperative adhesion formation. It is, of course, less costly than laparotomy.

The cervical cup. Using the cup (see *The Cervical Cup,* page 76) maximizes the number of motile sperm that contact the cervical mucus and are allowed into the uterus. The cervical cup is beneficial when infertility results from low

THE CERVICAL CUP

After instruction by the nurse, the woman inserts the cervical cup and positions it over the cervix. She uses a syringe to introduce sperm into the cervical cup and an applicator to advance the ball up the cup's stem to prevent loss of sperm.

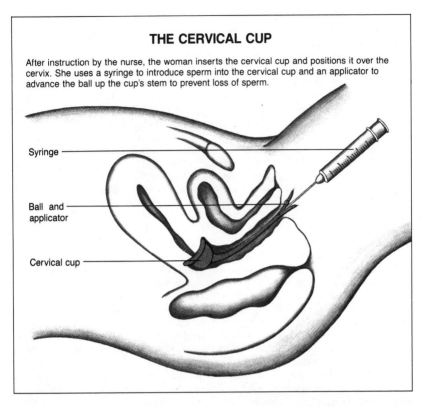

Syringe

Ball and applicator

Cervical cup

sperm count, motility, or volume. It's also effective in women who have poor postcoital tests with negative tests for antisperm antibodies.

The small plastic cervical cup, which comes in various sizes to allow for proper fit, is positioned directly over the cervix before insemination. The sperm, which was collected by masturbation, is placed in a syringe and then injected into the tube of the cervical cup. After insemination, the cup is left in place for 4 to 6 hours.

Using the cervical cup offers several advantages. It protects sperm from a potentially hostile environment; sperm can be collected in the privacy of the home; it allows insemination during sexual stimulation, timed by the couple according to the fertile period and unrestricted by the doctor's office hours; and the woman can resume activity immediately after insemination instead of lying with hips elevated for several minutes to an hour. In addition, the cup may be reused several times during a cycle, depending on the duration of the fertile period.

To promote effective use of the cervical cup, the couple is asked to see the doctor for a postcup test. The test indicates if the cup has been placed properly and if the sperm and cervical mucus are compatible. If findings are positive, the couple can reasonably expect to conceive within 6 to 12 months.

Intrauterine insemination (IUI). In this procedure, sperm are collected through masturbation, "washed" to remove the seminal plasma, then inseminated, using sterile technique, directly into the uterus during the fertile period (as evaluated by a basal body temperature chart, cervical mucus evaluation, home ovulation prediction test, or ultrasound).

IUI is helpful to couples with an abnormal sperm count, poor postcoital tests, male or female sperm antibodies, poor cervical mucus, or unexplained infertility.

Most recently, IUI has been used when a special egg-buffered solution to enhance sperm has been needed or for the couple with unexplained infertility who may not be financially or emotionally ready for IVF.

Since IUI is performed in the doctor's office and requires special equipment and trained personnel to prepare the sperm, it is expensive and time consuming. Preparation time is about 1 hour, and the woman must remain at the office for 20 to 30 minutes after insemination to allow cervical mucus to seal over the cervical os. Current fertility statistics with this method have not been encouraging.

Nursing intervention

• Help patients who are undergoing diagnosis or treatment of infertility understand how and why the various infertility tests and treatment techniques are done. Be able to clarify questions and concerns the couple might have about them, and provide appropriate support and encouragement. Be prepared to instruct them on how to conduct the test.

• Be prepared to assist with laparoscopy. Know the various uses of laparoscopy so you can assist with teaching and counseling the patient, as appropriate.

• With use of the cervical cup, your role includes fitting the cup; reviewing with the couple various methods for determining the woman's fertile period (for example, use of the home ovulation prediction kit); and instructing the couple in cup insertion, collecting the semen sample, doing the insemination, removing the cup, and caring for the cup to prepare it for reuse.

• Your role in IUI can include preparing the couple for the procedure, helping them plan an appropriate time in the woman's menstrual cycle for the

procedure, assisting the health care professional during the procedure, and offering the couple support and encouragement, as necessary.

CAROL SOLOMON DALGLISH, RN, MSN

SYNDROMES AND DISORDERS

Hypercholesterolemia and LDL receptors

Hypercholesterolemia, a high serum cholesterol level, may result from a high dietary intake of cholesterol and saturated fats, overproduction of cholesterol by the liver, or defective or reduced low-density lipoprotein (LDL) receptors. Cholesterol is insoluble in the serum and consequently circulates in lipoprotein particles as high-density lipoprotein (HDL) and LDL. Receptors for LDL, which are located on the cell surface, remove LDL from the bloodstream. When LDL receptors fail to remove these particles from blood, LDL levels rise. The result of elevated LDL levels is acceleration of atherosclerosis, in which cholesterol accumulates on arterial walls and forms plaques that inhibit blood flow.

The role of the LDL receptor was first appreciated when its absence was found to be responsible for familial hypercholesterolemia (FH). FH is an inborn error of metabolism transmitted as a dominant trait determined by a single gene. In the more common heterozygous form of FH, which affects about 1 in 500 people in most ethnic groups, one mutant gene is inherited. Among this population, the LDL level is twice its normal value, and heart attacks occur by age 35. In the homozygous form of FH, which affects about 1 in a million people, two genes are

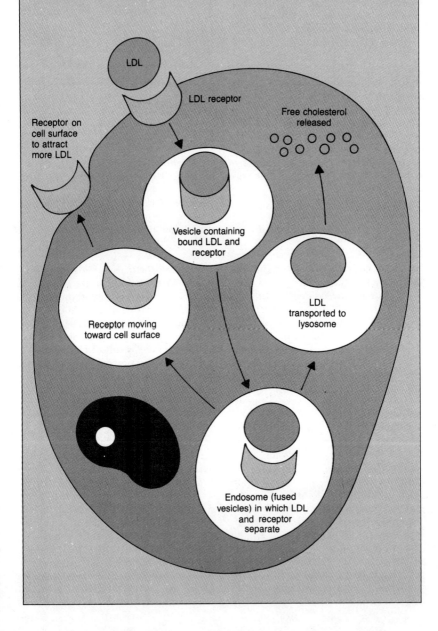

HOW L.D.L. RECEPTORS FUNCTION

Circulating low-density lipoprotein (LDL) enters a cell by binding to a special receptor. Within the cell, LDL separates from the receptor and is broken down into cholesterol for production of cell membrane, steroid hormones, and bile acids. The receptor is recycled to the cell surface to pick up more LDL.

LDL

LDL receptor

Free cholesterol released

Receptor on cell surface to attract more LDL

Vesicle containing bound LDL and receptor

LDL transported to lysosome

Receptor moving toward cell surface

Endosome (fused vesicles) in which LDL and receptor separate

mutant. Among this population, the LDL level is more than six times its normal value, and heart attacks may occur as early as age 2 and are inevitable by age 20.

Cause and pathophysiology
Cholesterol is a lipid that is essential to life. It is a necessary component of hormone synthesis and is part of the cell membrane structure. Cells receive cholesterol from LDL particles circulating in the blood. LDL receptors—specialized proteins found on the surface of animal cells—bind LDL particles and carry them to cells where they are broken down to yield cholesterol. (See *How LDL Receptors Function.*) The number of receptors on the cells' surfaces varies with their need for cholesterol. Consequently, as cholesterol accumulates in cells, cells stop synthesizing new receptors and take up LDL at a reduced rate. As a result, serum LDL levels rise.

Signs and symptoms
Patients with hypercholesterolemia may have xanthelasmas (soft yellow plaques on the eyelids), xanthomas (fatty yellow plaques or nodules over tendons), arcus lipoides corneae, or symptoms of coronary artery disease (chest pain, diaphoresis).

Treatment
Treatment for hypercholesterolemia involves the following:
• Reduced dietary intake of cholesterol and saturated fats to lower serum cholesterol levels. As a result, cells produce more LDL receptors and take up increased amounts of LDL.
• Administration of niacin or bile acid–binding resins such as cholestyramine to reduce cholesterol levels may be indicated if dietary measures are inadequate. Unfortunately, the liver may respond to the cholesterol "deficiency" by increasing cholesterol synthesis.
• Administration of mevinolin or compactin may reduce cholesterol synthesis. These investigational drugs act by blocking an enzyme necessary to cholesterol synthesis. Each shows much promise for future treatment of heterozygous FH, especially when used with dietary modification and administration of bile acid–binding resins. For patients with homozygous FH, liver transplantation to provide cells with active LDL receptors or plasmapheresis to clear the blood of LDL are the two investigational treatments at present.

Nursing intervention
Lifelong dietary modification and sometimes drug therapy are necessary to combat hypercholesterolemia.
• Educate patients about the need to have serum cholesterol levels checked regularly.
• Advise family screening of patients with known high cholesterol levels.
• Teach and counsel patients on the low-cholesterol, low–saturated fat diet.
• Teach patients about their medications, including common adverse effects (for example, flushing with niacin and constipation and bloating with bile acid–binding resins).
• Teach patients how to cope with adverse effects to improve compliance. For example, you might suggest a bulk laxative taken regularly to prevent the constipation commonly associated with bile acid–binding resins.
• Give patients long-term support and encouragement to make positive changes in their life-styles.

PATRICIA M. DEDRICK, RN, MS, NP

Prader-Labhart-Willi syndrome

Prader-Labhart-Willi syndrome is a developmental disorder that was first described in 1956. The prominent features of this disorder are congenital hypotonia, abnormal secondary sexual development, cognitive delays resulting in decreased sensitivity to pain, hyperphagia resulting in massive obesity when uncontrolled, occasional alterations in body temperature, and behavioral problems. This syndrome generally causes significant growth deficiencies: short stature, small hands and feet, and characteristic facies, including almond-shaped eyes, strabismus, triangular mouth, and narrow bifrontal diameter.

Prader-Labhart-Willi syndrome is an uncommon disorder, with incidence estimated at 1 in 24,000 to 30,000 live births.

Cause

Prader-Labhart-Willi syndrome is a congenital disorder of unknown etiology. Diagnostic tests and autopsy studies have failed to show an anatomic lesion; therefore, the defect is thought to be biochemical. This syndrome has been primarily linked to a spontaneous alteration in chromosomal material—a deletion on the arm of chromosome 15 at point q11 to q13—and has been generally classified as a hypothalamic disorder. It is not associated with maternal or paternal age, fetal exposure to drugs, or occupational exposure to known toxic chemicals.

Signs and symptoms

Since the pathophysiology of the syndrome is unknown, symptoms are best defined using a developmental framework.

Mothers of patients with this syndrome have reported a pregnancy marked by fetal inactivity. (Such inactivity is more apparent to mothers who previously had normal full-term pregnancies.) These mothers' birth histories also show a higher incidence of abnormal births and difficult deliveries necessitating special medical intervention.

Infants with Prader-Labhart-Willi syndrome characteristically show hypotonia, inability to breast-feed, and hypogonadism. Hypotonia causes weakness in suckling. Consequently, these infants require gavage feedings or special nipples to prevent severe growth retardation and failure to thrive. Feeding them requires extreme patience, since they may take an hour or longer to consume as little as an ounce of formula. Time-consuming, complicated feeding routines interfere with normal bonding; typically, parents suffer frustration and disappointment because of their inability to help these infants grow and thrive.

Hypogonadism is obvious in male infants, who have a small penis and/or undescended testes. In female infants, hypogonadism is more difficult to detect.

Despite their difficulties with feeding, these infants tend to be calm and happy. However, transition to early (ages 2 to 5) and later childhood is marked by profound confusion, disappointment, and turmoil for both parents and child. In most of these children, muscle tone improves by age 2 or 3, but appetite becomes voracious. Their parents, used to struggling to give their children adequate calories, may now inadvertently overfeed them as they suddenly begin to regularly clean their plates.

Motor milestones are significantly delayed. These children learn to sit at about age 1 and walk at about age 2 or 3. Their speech is commonly delayed, and they tend to have problems with articulation.

In middle childhood (ages 6 to 12), scoliosis and abnormal pubertal development are prominent. Behavioral problems may accelerate, and these children may show inappropriate eating and social behavior. They may forage for food, steal food, lie about eating, and raid the refrigerator at night. They may have tantrums and show subtler behavioral signs, such as marked perseveration (repetition of the same verbal or motor response to varied stimuli or continuation of the response after the stimuli are withdrawn) and poor impulse control. At school, they show learning problems as well as behavioral problems.

Adolescents may show severe behavioral deterioration marked by acceleration of tantrums, aggressive behavior, marked perseveration, and, rarely, hallucinations. These patients die as young adults due to obesity and its complications.

Diagnosis

The diagnosis of Prader-Labhart-Willi syndrome during infancy is crucial. The syndrome should be suspected in children who are born of pregnancies marked by intrauterine hypotonia and who show neonatal hypotonia, failure to thrive, weak ability to suckle, and hypogonadism. Chromosomal studies should be performed to help confirm the diagnosis, since most Prader-Labhart-Willi infants have a deletion on the proximal arm of chromosome 15.

Treatment

No specific medical treatment is available for Prader-Labhart-Willi syndrome. Management includes strict regulation of food intake and food-related behavior, limiting access to an appropriate caloric level. A carefully structured environment can help minimize poor behavior control. These children commonly need special residential placement in centers designed for such problems.

Nursing intervention

To prevent anxiety and confusion in the child with Prader-Labhart-Willi syndrome, promote a structured environment. Provide simple, clear, and firm guidelines for behavior, keeping in mind the wide spectrum of potential eating and behavioral disturbances. Not every child shows the desperate food-seeking behavior and significant cognitive dysfunction that characterize the syndrome.

Support and encourage the parents. Emphasize the importance of strict dietary controls. If necessary, encourage parents to place locks on the refrigerator door to prevent overeating. At the same time, try to understand and sympathize with their frustration over such restrictions. Be sure to explain that these extreme behavioral and eating problems result from a biochemical abnormality, not inappropriate parenting.

ROBERT WHARTON, MD

Preterm labor

Preterm birth, the major cause of infant death and disability, is the result of labor that occurs after 20 weeks' gestation and before 37 weeks' gestation. Contractions that occur during preterm labor are accompanied by cervical effacement and/or dilation.

Of every 100 births, 7 are preterm. Many of these infants must remain hospitalized for weeks after birth. Preterm infants are 40 times more likely than full-term infants to die in their first month. Those who survive are twice as likely as full-term infants to suffer lifelong handicaps, such as blindness, deafness, cerebral palsy, and learning disabilities.

Improvements in neonatal care have decreased the risks associated with preterm birth but have failed to reduce the number of preterm births. Fortunately, new approaches, such as programs of risk assessment, early identification of preterm labor, prompt medical treatment, and home uterine monitoring, are now showing great promise in reducing the number of preterm births.

Causes

Little is known about the specific causes of preterm labor. However, certain socioeconomic and medical factors place a woman at high risk for having preterm labor. *Socioeconomic factors* include poverty, stress, and cigarette smoking. Poor, nonwhite teenage females are more likely to deliver preterm infants. In addition, women who perform heavy physical or stressful work, who commute more than 30 minutes to work, and who smoke more than 10 cigarettes daily are also at higher risk for preterm birth.

Medical risk factors include a previous history of premature labor, spontaneous or induced abortions, cervical conization, pyelonephritis, uterine anomaly, diethylstilbestrol exposure, two or more stillbirths or neonatal deaths, and cyanotic heart disease or renal failure.

Pregnancy-related factors that place a woman at high risk for preterm labor include multiple gestation, abdominal surgery during pregnancy, hemoglobinopathies, placenta previa, inappropriate weight gain, uterine irritability, and cervical dilation or effacement. Other factors include oligohydramnios, hydramnios, and second-trimester bleeding.

Signs and symptoms

Many women who go into preterm labor experience a prodromal stage that lasts hours or even days before cervical dilation occurs. But if the woman's contractions aren't painful or if she has never experienced labor before, she may not realize that she's in labor. Therefore, all high-risk patients should know the warning signs of preterm labor, which include:

• uterine contractions that feel like a hardening or tightening of the abdomen

• pelvic pressure that feels like the baby is pushing down

• low, dull backache that continues even after rest

• abdominal cramping with or without diarrhea

• change in vaginal discharge. All pregnant women experience increased vaginal discharge. However, a sudden gush or leaking of clear fluid or a thick, blood-tinged mucous discharge is a warning sign of impending labor and should be reported to the doctor immediately.

A woman who suspects preterm labor should be advised to drink two or three glasses of water or juice, rest on her left side, and palpate her uterus for contractions. She should be instructed to call the doctor if the signs don't disappear after resting an hour or if the signs worsen.

Treatment to inhibit labor

Uterine contraction monitoring should be performed on all women who are admitted to the hospital for suspected preterm labor. The most conservative treatment for preterm labor is hydration and bed rest. Pharmacologic inhibition of labor involves significant maternal risks; therefore, a decision to arrest labor must be based on a careful assessment of maternal and fetal conditions. Labor should never be inhibited in the presence of fetal distress, isoimmunization, fetal growth retardation, or anomalies incompatible with life. Maternal factors that would prohibit arresting labor include chronic hypertension or heart disease, intrauterine infection, preeclampsia or eclampsia, diabetes mellitus, hypothyroidism, and, in some cases, ruptured membranes. Labor should never be inhibited in the case of abruptio placentae or placenta previa. Labor usually isn't interrupted past 34 weeks' gestation.

Drug therapy may be ordered when preterm labor has been diagnosed and when contraindications to an arrest of labor have been ruled out. Commonly used labor-arresting drugs include ritodrine, terbutaline, and magnesium sulfate. These drugs are effective only if the cervix is dilated less than 4 cm; therefore, early identification of preterm labor is extremely important. (Ritodrine or terbutaline shouldn't be given if the patient's pulse rate exceeds 140 beats/minute or if the patient is having trouble breathing.)

Home management

If labor has been successfully arrested, the patient may be managed at home on ritodrine or terbutaline and self-uterine palpation. Recently, an ambulatory monitor has been developed for home use. Patients using the Termguard Home Monitor are instructed to monitor uterine activity three to four times each day. Data is transmitted by telephone to a central station, where it is analyzed by specially trained staff. This new technology may detect labor early enough for effective drug therapy.

Nursing intervention

• Teach the woman at high risk for preterm labor to recognize its warning signs, and instruct her on what to do if it occurs. Such information is particularly important for the patient who has been admitted to the hospital for management of preterm labor.

• Teach the patient to palpate her uterus for contractions. Have her place her fingers lightly on her abdomen. It should feel soft. Next, have her sit up from a lying position, since a contraction will often result. Have her feel the hardness of her uterus. Explain to her that a contraction is a hardening or tightening of the uterus.

• If a patient is admitted to the hospital in preterm labor, immediately place her in the left lateral position to increase uterine blood flow. Take a history and evaluate her for signs of infection, as indicated by fetal tachycardia, and maternal fever and tachycardia, or for signs of urinary tract infection. Monitor uterine activity and fetal heart rate, and assess the patient's hydration level (for example, has she been voiding frequently or perspiring profusely?). After drug therapy begins, monitor vital signs, including breath sounds, every 15 minutes or until stable. Check reflexes if the patient has been receiving magnesium sulfate. Baseline laboratory studies, such as urinalysis, complete blood count, blood glucose levels, serum electrolyte studies, and EKG, may be ordered.

• If the patient is discharged on ritodrine or terbutaline therapy, instruct her to call her doctor if symptoms of labor recur. Stress the importance of continuing to take prescribed medi-cation. Explain that such side effects as agitation, palpitations, and dizziness are common with these drugs. Also stress the importance of decreased activity or bed rest.

• Assess the patient's psychosocial status. Is her family supportive and readily available? Has she experienced premature labor or fetal loss before? How has she dealt with such a crisis in the past? How is she handling the emotional stress caused by the threatened loss of her child? Should someone from the clergy be called in for pastoral counseling? Will she need homemaker service to help at home? With these factors in mind, offer the patient reassurance and support and suggest supportive counseling as appropriate.

SUSAN RUMSEY, RN, BSN, MPH

Postdate pregnancy

Postdate, postterm, or prolonged pregnancy occurs when gestation extends beyond 42 weeks. Postdatism occurs in 2% to 11% of pregnancies and represents one of the most common complications of pregnancy. Twenty percent to forty percent of infants born postterm suffer the effects of postmaturity syndrome, which can include asphyxia, cerebral edema, meconium aspiration, pneumothorax, pneumomediastinum, and polycythemia. These infants are three times more likely to die than term infants and are at greater risk of subsequent severe illness and delayed development.

Causes and pathophysiology

The cause of postdatism is unknown. Its effects are thought to be the result of an aging placenta, decreased amniotic fluid (oligohydramnios), inadequate placental and oxygen exchange between fetus and mother before or during labor, or a combination of these factors.

In low-risk pregnancy, the placenta

carries maternal oxygen and nutrients to the fetus and removes wastes. The placenta functions efficiently for 40 weeks, when it begins a gradual decline. Oxygen saturation of umbilical venous blood drops, and although the fetus can compensate partially by raising the hemoglobin concentration, fetal hypoxia eventually results unless delivery occurs.

As pregnancy progresses to term and beyond, the volume of amniotic fluid diminishes. The result is significantly increased vulnerability to compression of the umbilical cord, a major cause of fetal bradycardia and asphyxia.

Diagnosis

The diagnosis of postdatism is based on an accurate estimate of fetal gestational age. No dating method alone is completely reliable, but the date of the mother's last normal menstrual period is the single most important factor in determining gestational age. This date may be unreliable if the mother had no intervening menstrual period between pregnancies, if she confused postconceptional bleeding for a menstrual period, if she was using contraceptive drugs within 3 months of becoming pregnant, or if she forgot the date of her last menstrual period. Nägele's rule is used to calculate estimated date of confinement (EDC) by counting back 3 months from the first day of the last menstrual period and adding 7 days. Other dating methods that confirm EDC include:

• quickening. Fetal movement is usually felt for the first time by primigravidas at 18 to 20 weeks; by multigravidas at 16 to 18 weeks.
• uterine size. Determining uterine size by bimanual examination is most reliable for pregnancies of less than 12 weeks' gestation.
• fetal heart tones. Fetal heart tones may be heard at 12 to 16 weeks with a Doppler device and at 18 to 20 weeks with an unamplified stethoscope. This method is less reliable in obese patients.

• ultrasonography. Gestational age is assessed by measuring the biparietal diameter of the fetal skull or femur length. This method is more accurate if performed serially and before 30 weeks.

The status of the pregnancy is determined by three methods. Placental grading, an ultrasonic technique, is used to evaluate placental maturation. The biophysical profile is a battery of measurements that assesses fetal breathing movements, fetal movements, fetal tone, amniotic fluid volume, and response to fetal movement (nonstress test). The nonstress test (NST) and the oxytocin challenge test (OCT) are used alone or in combination with the biophysical profile. In the NST, fetal heart rate is monitored continuously for 20 minutes, during which time fetal movements are recorded. The test is considered reactive if at least two fetal movements are associated with heart rate accelerations in a 20-minute period. A reactive test implies fetal well-being.

OCT is usually performed when the result of an NST is considered nonreactive or equivocal, or in lieu of an NST. In an OCT, the fetal heart rate and uterine activity are monitored for 20 minutes. If no spontaneous contractions occur, oxytocin is administered I.V. and increased gradually until three uterine contractions occur in a 10-minute interval. In the absence of fetal decelerations, the OCT test is considered negative and fetal well-being is assumed.

Recently, some clinicians have advocated the use of nipple stimulation instead of exogenously administered oxytocin to induce contractions. This method is controversial because it may cause uncontrolled hyperstimulation of the uterus.

Signs and symptoms

After birth, the infant's gestational age may be calculated by using the Dubowitz or Ballard tests of infant development to evaluate physical and

DECELERATED FETAL HEART RATES AND UTERINE CONTRACTIONS

Unlike variable decelerations, early and late decelerations occur in a predictable pattern in relation to uterine contractions.

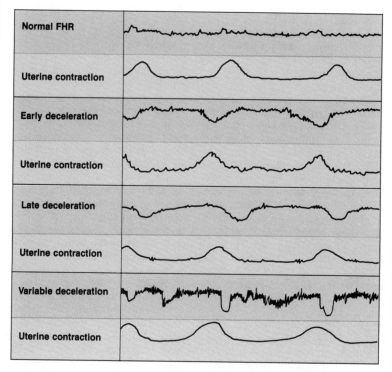

The three types of FHR decelerations—early, late, and variable—occur at different points in the contraction phase.

Early FHR decelerations occur at onset of uterine contraction and reach their lowest point at the peak of the contraction. FHR returns to the average baseline by the end of the contraction. FHR produces a smooth wave pattern that mirrors the uterine contraction. Early deceleration is usually benign and is most commonly caused by compression of the fetal head.

Late decelerations begin after onset of a contraction and reach their lowest point after the contraction has peaked. FHR recovery occurs after the contraction. Although the FHR tracing in late deceleration resembles the smooth wave of early deceleration, its implications are far more serious. Late decelerations usually result from uteroplacental insufficiency and

may lead to fetal hypoxia. When associated with increased variability or with tachycardia and decreased variability, late decelerations indicate fetal central nervous system depression and hypoxia.

Variable decelerations—sudden drops in FHR—may occur at any time during a contraction. Following the decline, baseline FHR recovery is rapid. Since the fall in FHR is unrelated to uterine contractions, wave patterns also vary. Variable decelerations are common, occurring in about 50% of all labors, and are usually associated with transitory umbilical cord compression. However, a severe drop (to less than 70 beats/minute for more than 60 seconds), numerous variable decelerations without recovery time, decreasing variability, and meconium staining may indicate fetal acidosis, hypoxia, and low Apgar scores.

neuromuscular maturation. Physical characteristics of postmature infants include:
- alert facies
- long, lean body
- abundant hair growth
- long fingernails that may be meconium-stained
- decreased subcutaneous fat
- cracked, peeling, parchmentlike skin
- mature genitals
- absence of vernix.

Treatment

Increased recognition of the morbidity and mortality associated with postdate pregnancy has prompted a more aggressive treatment approach. First, the pregnancy must be determined to be truly postdate. If it is, the cervix is examined for ripeness, or softening, and dilation. If the cervix is favorable, the next step is induction of labor. If not, NSTs, OCTs, amniotic fluid volume measurements, biophysical profile, placental grading, or any combination of these evaluative methods is used weekly or biweekly until the cervix confirms clinical conditions that favor induction of labor.

If any of these tests indicates fetal distress, either induction is cautiously attempted or cesarean delivery is planned. Induced labors are associated with increased incidence of fetal distress, higher rates of cesarean section, and prolonged labor in the absence of cervical ripening.

Nursing intervention

Meticulous surveillance is the key to nursing care for the postdate expectant mother and her baby.

Teach expectant mothers a gross screening method that each mother can perform daily when the pregnancy is postdate. The expectant mother can count fetal kicks. At least 10 kicks daily is adequate. Less than 10 kicks daily may indicate fetal hypoxia, in which case the woman should notify the doctor immediately. During labor and delivery, perform continuous electronic fetal monitoring. Interpret fetal heart rate tracings and report patterns of concern (late and variable decelerations, tachycardia, bradycardia, and decreased variability) to the doctor. Since the likelihood of cesarean section increases in postterm patients, you'll need to be prepared at all times for surgery.

Watch for meconium when membranes rupture and during labor. Notify the doctor if meconium is present. Because many postterm infants have passed meconium in utero, anticipate a pharyngeal aspiration of the neonate prior to delivery of the shoulders. Tracheal visualization and suctioning may be required if meconium is present in the amniotic fluid.

Many postterm infants are macrosomatic (weighing more than 8⅞ lb [4 kg]). These large infants are more likely to experience birth trauma, so be sure to assess such infants for fractured clavicles, brachial plexus, head injuries, facial nerve palsy, and bruising. Because of an increased risk of hypoglycemia, perform Dextrostix tests hourly until the infant is feeding and stable. Unless they are medically contraindicated, begin feedings as soon as possible (breast or bottle). Also observe the postterm infant for jitteriness, poor tone, and seizures—signs of hypoglycemia and hypocalcemia. Perform laboratory tests for blood glucose, hematocrit, and bilirubin levels as ordered.

Like premature infants, postmature infants are particularly vulnerable to cold stress. Thoroughly dry them after delivery and keep them warm during the first days after birth.

Monitor the infant carefully for signs of respiratory distress. Make sure that suction, oxygen hood, and bag and mask are available at the infant's bedside.

Postmature infants may be irritable and difficult to pacify. Supportive nursing care can help prevent possible problems in parent-infant bonding.

SUSAN RUMSEY, RN, BSN, MPH

Recognizing subtle seizures

Because different types of seizures require different drug therapies, accurate recognition of seizures is crucial to successful management. Using the wrong drugs can lead to patient injury if they fail to control the seizures or cause dangerous side effects.

According to the International Classification of Seizures, epileptic seizures can be divided into two categories: those that begin in one part of the cortex (partial seizures) and those that begin more diffusely (primary generalized seizures). Partial seizures, which most often result from a focal brain lesion (for example, a tumor, a stroke, an abscess, or trauma) in the part of the brain where the discharge arises, are further subdivided into those that impair awareness (complex partial seizures) and those that don't (simple partial seizures). Partial seizures may become generalized (secondary generalized seizures), especially if treatment is inadequate.

Signs and symptoms
Recognition of most generalized (grand mal) major motor seizures is fairly straightforward. But some generalized seizures, such as 3-second spike-wave absence or petit mal seizures, and some partial seizures can go undetected by the uninformed observer. Absence seizures are marked by a suddenly blank facial expression and cessation of all voluntary motor activity for several seconds or minutes. The resulting interruptions in speech and activity may be subtle and easy to overlook.

Partial seizures produce widely varying effects, but they do have some common manifestations. Since a seizure is a nonphysiologic discharge of groups of neurons, the manifestations depend on the anatomic connections and functions of that part of the cerebral cortex. Some patients hear noises, see flashes of light, or feel tingling sensations—symptoms that indicate a focus in the auditory, visual, or somatosensory cortex respectively. Muscle twitching beginning in the face, hand, or foot indicates a focus in the motor strip in the area corresponding to the body part affected.

A seizure can begin with markedly abnormal behavior (for example, arm jerking) or a sudden interruption of normal behavior (for example, the patient may stop speaking in mid-sentence). Electrodes placed deep inside the temporal lobe have indicated that even such complex behavior as compulsive water drinking may be accompanied by tiny seizure discharges without any other manifestation. Temporal lobe discharges may cause smelling or tasting hallucinations, laughter or fear, nausea or fullness, déjà vu or jamais vu (never experienced) sensations, or bizarre motor activity such as running or twirling of the arms.

Laboratory tests
The following tests can help to identify and manage seizures:
• Determining the serum levels of antiepileptic drugs is generally helpful whenever questions of toxicity or inadequate therapy arise; it may not be necessary for patients who are well controlled and who have no adverse drug effects. For such tests, blood samples must be drawn at trough levels (low point) for optimal interpretation. Therefore, blood samples must be taken just before the next scheduled dose.
• Serum prolactin levels are now known to rise, especially after a generalized or partial complex seizure. Therefore, determining prolactin levels can help to distinguish hysterical seizures involving generalized body movements from real generalized seizures. Elevated prolactin levels may confirm that a patient found unconscious, possibly after a fall, actually had a seizure.
• The electroencephalogram (EEG)

DIFFERENTIATING SEIZURE TYPES

DISORDER	AREAS INVOLVED (FOCUS)	CHANGE IN CONSCIOUSNESS
PARTIAL SEIZURES*		
Simple partial		
Focal motor	Motor strip on precentral gyrus in frontal lobe	Unilateral: No change in consciousness
Focal sensory	Postcentral gyrus in parietal or occipital lobe	No loss if unilateral
Complex partial		
Psychomotor	Temporal lobe	Impaired consciousness with confusion and amnesia; slow return to full consciousness
* Partial seizures may evolve to generalized tonic-clonic seizures.		
GENERALIZED SEIZURES		
Generalized tonic-clonic (grand mal)	Generalized	Loss of consciousness with postictal state
Absence (petit mal)	Generalized	Transient losses of consciousness; no postictal state; rapid return to full consciousness
Infantile spasms (salaam, head drop)	Generalized	Usually brief decrease in consciousness; no postictal state
Myoclonic	Generalized	Possible momentary loss of consciousness
Akinetic (drop attacks)	Generalized, with brain stem involvement	None; no postictal state

Focal motor

Psychomotor

E.E.G. FINDINGS	CLINICAL EFFECTS
Focal, slow waves or spikes	Convulsive movements and temporary disturbance in muscles controlled by that brain region; possible "marching" progression
Spikes and slow waves over epileptogenic focus	Subjective sensory experience; may be visual, auditory, olfactory, or somatosensory; possible "marching" progression
Temporal or frontotemporal spikes or slow waves or rhythmic theta discharges	Hallucinations, dyscognitive states (déjà vu), automatism, loss of awareness, running, laughing
Rapidly repeating spikes (over ten per second) in tonic phase; spikes interrupted by slow waves in clonic phase with postictal suppression	Major tonic muscular contraction followed by longer phase of clonic (jerking) contractions; possible loss of bowel and bladder control; possible tongue biting
Spikes and waves (three per second) bilateral and diffuse	Interference with conscious response to environment when uncontrolled; possible blinking and minor facial movements
Multiple spikes and slow waves of large amplitude (hypsarrhythmia)	Jackknife, flexor spasms of extremities and head; severe mental and developmental deficiencies usual
Multiple spikes or slow waves	Uncontrollable brief or repetitive jerking movements of extremities or entire body
Sudden flattening of EEG or low voltage fast activity or polyspike or multiple spike waves	Sudden postural tone loss; possible intellectual, perceptual, and motor impairments

Generalized clonic

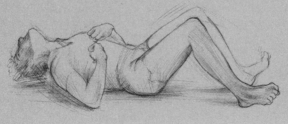

uses scalp electrodes to sample the electricity generated by the brain. Electrical seizure discharges seen on the EEG can reveal critical information regarding location, severity, and frequency of seizure discharges as well as other abnormalities. EEG with videotape monitoring provides a record of the patient's behavior during the EEG recording so that the patient's abnormal behavior during a seizure can be correlated with the EEG tracing.

• Depth electrodes, which are surgically implanted, are sometimes required to link certain seizures with focal electrical brain discharges. Patients with such seizures may be candidates for surgical therapy. Intraoperative recording from the surface or depths of the cortex may help to further localize the seizure focus at the time of surgery.

Nursing intervention

When you observe unusual behavior that suggests possible onset of a seizure, always make sure the patient's airway is patent, check vital signs, and carefully observe the patient throughout the incident. In a nonthreatening manner, encourage the patient to interact with you in conversation or to follow a simple command. When the seizure ends, check for orientation and ability to follow commands. A focal abnormality that's detected in the neurologic examination may persist for minutes to hours after a seizure (for example, Todd's postictal state). Therefore, look for subtle signs of asymmetry via arm drift and roll tests immediately after a seizure. Certain patients with partial seizures have periodic spells (for example, minor twitching of a hand or foot) that occur every 20 minutes or so. Accurate documentation of the abnormal behavior, its duration, and the intervals between seizures allows for evaluation of the therapy and the need for further intervention. Diminishing intensity and duration and a lengthening interval between seizures suggest that therapy is effective.

JOHN M. BERTONI, MD, PhD

Stevens-Johnson syndrome

Stevens-Johnson syndrome is a dermatologic condition characterized by target lesions with mucosal ulcerations and bullous skin lesions. These target lesions—erythema multiforme—generally precede skin sloughing. Bullae tend to be localized without extension to surrounding skin. Both types of lesions affect the skin as well as the internal mucous membranes. Because of the extensive skin loss, patients with Stevens-Johnson syndrome are best cared for at a burn treatment center. Stevens-Johnson syndrome was originally described in the 1800s as stomatitis with ophthalmia.

Causes

Drug reactions are considered the major cause of this disorder. Certain drugs, most commonly sulfa drugs, may act as antigens, evoking an allergic response that may be a type of delayed hypersensitivity reaction. In addition to sulfonamides (Septra, Bactrim), these drugs include phenylbutazone, the sulfonylureas (Orinase), phenytoin, and barbiturates.

Signs and symptoms

The primary manifestation is a dispersed, maculopapular rash. The rash is initially pruritic but becomes painful. Then bullous lesions develop, eventually open, and begin sloughing. The resulting ulcerations may involve the oral, rectal, genitourinary, conjunctival, respiratory, and GI tracts, and may lead to such complications as urinary sepsis, pneumonia, and GI bleeding. High fevers and marked facial and periorbital edema are also prevalent.

Diagnosis

Diagnosis is based on characteristic clinical manifestations and on tissue biopsy results. Patients with Stevens-

Johnson syndrome tend to have localized bullae and an infiltrate of inflammatory cells in the dermis.

Treatment

First, treatment with the offending drug
(if identified) must be discontinued; a
mild reaction may then require only
topical application of steroids.

In treatment of severe reactions, fluid
replacement is of primary importance
and depends on the extent of sloughing
and the patient's ability to take fluids
by mouth. Protein loss (as indicated by
hypoalbuminemia) through capillary
leakage is replaced by administering
colloids, blood transfusions, and nutritional supplements through intravenous hyperalimentation or enteral
feedings, or both.

Nutritional support usually begins
via tube feeding unless the severity of
tissue sloughing and the condition of
the GI tract contraindicate its use. Hyponatremia, resulting from skin
sloughing, can be managed by frequent
electrolyte measurements and salt replacement via I.V. fluids and by adding
salt to the water during daily hydrotherapy.

Steroid therapy may prevent progression of bullae, skin sloughing, and
mucosal erosions. But because such
therapy risks significant complications,
including G.I. bleeding and suppression of early signs of sepsis, it is tapered
off as soon as possible.

Septic shock is common in such patients, usually originating in the oral,
GI, respiratory, and genitourinary
tracts as well as in the wound surfaces.
Routine treatment of septic shock is
then initiated.

Treatment of patients with Stevens-
Johnson syndrome requires daily hydrotherapy. Once bullae begin to rupture, the involved skin is left in place
to act as a biological dressing or cover
for the wound surface. Loose tissue is
debrided daily and denuded areas are
covered with dressings of polysporin–
fine mesh gauze. Polysporin is applied
in small amounts to prevent systemic

absorption and toxicity. Polysporin can
also be applied to intact bullae, which
are then left open to the air. The use
of silver sulfadiazine is avoided to prevent hypersensitivity. Other useful
dressings are povidone-iodine foam,
0.5% silver nitrate soaks, homograft
applications, and Biobrane, a synthetic
skin substitute.

Nursing intervention

● Monitor the patient for hypothermia;
apply a radiant heat shield as needed.
● Ensure meticulous mouth care and
check for signs of oral thrush.
● Monitor for signs of sepsis: increased
heart rate, decreased blood pressure,
and hypothermia after high fever.
● Encourage a high-protein, high-calorie diet; supplement enteral feedings
with milk shakes.
● Secure feeding tube to face and nose
with Tegaderm or Op-Site to prevent
tape burns on edematous facial tissue.
● Perform daily hydrotherapy treatments.
● Rinse the eyes with saline solution,
or provide artificial tears to prevent
corneal abrasions.
● Check for occult blood, and monitor
the pH of tube feeding residuals every
2 to 4 hours for signs of GI ulceration.
● When applying a homograft, roll
grafts with sterile swabs soaked in normal saline solution to remove any
drainage underneath. This will help
prevent sepsis and promote healing.
● Provide emotional support to the patient and his family. Teach relaxation
techniques to use during painful procedures.
● Maintain adequate isolation. Protect
the patient from cross-contamination.

LAUREN A. GIANNAKOPOULOS, RN

Stress-related illnesses

An estimated 50% to 80% of all disease
is associated with stress. From tension
headaches to heart attacks, stress has

been identified as a causative factor in numerous diseases: peptic ulcer, ulcerative colitis, irritable bowel disease, hypertension, cardiac dysrhythmias, asthma, atopic dermatitis, urticaria, hay fever, arthritis, allergies, Raynaud's disease, enuresis, migraine headaches, cancer, impotence, general sexual dysfunctions, sleep-onset insomnia, alcoholism, and various neurotic and psychotic disorders.

Recently, attention has focused on female stress and the specifically female symptoms, such as amenorrhea, premenstrual tension/headache complex, postpartum depression, menopausal melancholia, vaginismus, problems in sexual arousal, anorgasmia, and infertility.

Given this long list of diseases and disorders associated with stress, the nurse is sure to deal with them sooner or later. Indeed, she may experience some of them herself.

Defining stress

Hans Selye, whose extensive physiologic research has provided a scientific basis for stress, defines it as a specific syndrome that consists of all the nonspecifically induced changes within a biological system. Simply stated, stress is the body's nonspecific response to any demand made upon it. Within the broad concept of stress, "distress," unpleasant or damaging, is differentiated from "eustress," good or pleasant. Stress, therefore, can result from anything happening around or within us. Consequently, it can't be avoided. Instead, it must be dealt with through coping mechanisms.

Fortunately, research has documented the generalized effects of stress on the body and the benefits of various interventions to manage stress and promote health. Such research indicates that an integrated and holistic approach to stress management is most effective. Nurses can help their patients adapt to stress through an integrated mind-body approach that involves counseling and teaching coping strategies; assisting with adaptation to illness through technical skills and physical care; and providing emotional support and helping the patient's family adjust to the impact of illness.

Physiology of stress

Stress stimulates the body's "fight or flight" system. It initiates the chemical,

---

STRESS RESPONSE: PHYSIOLOGIC PROCESSES

The short-term physiologic effects of stress enable the person to cope with its demands, but its long-term effects are detrimental.

BRAIN ACTIVITY	SHORT-TERM EFFECTS	LONG-TERM EFFECTS
Stimulation of motor nerves to activate muscle contraction	Prepares person for emergency	Muscle fatigue
Stimulation through autonomic nervous system of heart, lungs, intestines, blood vessels, endocrine system	Prepares the "fight or flight" system	Organ exhaustion/failure
Stimulation of hypothalamus activates secretion of hormones by pituitary gland, which stimulates the adrenal gland	Raises metabolic rate and energy production	Hormonal imbalances

STRESS REACTION:
THE GENERAL ADAPTATION SYNDROME

STAGE 1	STAGE 2	STAGE 3
Alarm reaction • enlargement of adrenal cortex • enlargement of lymphatic system • increase in hormone levels (corticosteroids and catecholamines)	**Resistance** • adrenal cortex shrinkage • lymph nodes closer to normal size • hormone levels sustained	**Exhaustion** • dysfunctioning of lymphatic system • increase in hormone levels • depletion of adaptive hormones

physical, and psychological changes that allow a person to cope with the demands placed upon him.

More specifically, all stressors, whether good or bad, place a demand on the body that results in stimulation of both the nervous and the endocrine systems. When the nervous system is activated, messages travel from the brain (1) through motor nerves that prepare the skeletal muscles for action; (2) to the autonomic nervous system, which raises blood pressure, heart rate, and blood glucose level and slows intestinal activity; and (3) to the adrenal medulla, causing release of epinephrine.

The hypothalamus receives messages from the brain that activate the endocrine system. Subsequently, the pituitary gland and adrenal cortex release hormones that help to raise the white blood cell count; change sodium and water balance; and stimulate the thyroid gland, which then raises the metabolic rate. The result is a body mobilized to take lifesaving action if necessary. If stress is brief, the body quickly returns to its usual state of functioning and rests. However, after prolonged stress, the body can't return to its normal functioning state; the result: wear and tear on the body's organ systems. When the body deviates too far from its normal functioning state, it becomes vulnerable to illness and death.

A more encompassing description is provided by the general adaptation syndrome, which explains the body's reaction to continuing stress. This syndrome has three distinct stages: (1) the alarm reaction, (2) the stage of resistance, and (3) the stage of exhaustion. The alarm reaction, as its name implies, is the generalized mobilization of the body's defenses. If stressors are damaging and overwhelming, death may occur during this stage. However, with prolonged exposure to stressors, the body can't maintain the physiologic processes in the alarm reaction stage. Then, a stage of resistance arises in which many of the processes reverse themselves. For instance, the adrenal cortex discharges granules of fatty secretion into the bloodstream during the alarm reaction and accumulates a reserve of them during the resistance stage. Continued exposure to the stressors eventually leads to failure of the adaptation gained during the resistance stage. The stage of exhaustion follows—a premature aging that results from prolonged wear and tear on the organ.

Kenneth Pelletier, who has studied stress-related illness and preventive techniques, finds that generalized, untreated stress places the person in a physiologic disequilibrium that may increase susceptibility to disease. During adaptation to prolonged stress, the constant challenge to an organ or organ system may cause it to lose some or all of its function. Combined with other factors, such as genetic predisposition, nutritional state, and age, stress may then lead to disease.

Effects of prolonged stress

In recent years, stress has been clearly linked to the development of various diseases:

• *Cardiovascular disease.* Partially attributable to other risk factors, such as smoking, elevated serum cholesterol levels, and sedentary life-style, the prevalence of coronary artery disease has continued to parallel society's increasing complexity. Stress is clearly a contributing factor in cardiovascular diseases. Essential hypertension, a major form of cardiovascular disease, has no discernible organic cause. Generally, hypertension may be regulated with tranquilizers or diuretics. However, destructive behavior patterns that probably contribute to the disease must also be corrected, or the patient may enter a cycle of escalating drug therapy to control rising blood pressure. Comprehensive programs are needed to detect essential hypertension early and to correct negative life-styles that contribute to this illness.

• *Cancer.* The link between psychological factors and cancer has been noted since ancient times but has been studied objectively only in recent years. Research suggests that cancer involves the breakdown of the body's immune system. This breakdown, according to many, can be precipitated by a stressor that triggers a cascade of physiologic changes that result in an internal environment of hormonal and immune system disequilibrium. While stress doesn't cause cancer directly, it may help establish conditions that permit cancer cells to grow unchecked.

Unfortunately, the proposed relationship between stress and cancer could cause patients to feel psychologically responsible for having cancer. Such feelings could interfere with their treatment and require appropriate counseling.

• *Arthritis.* Rheumatoid arthritis may be the result of an autoimmune response in which the body essentially turns against itself. Stress may be a factor in this immune system dysfunction. Also, among those patients for whom a complete history is possible, a correlation may be apparent between stress and arthritis attacks. Use of stress-reduction techniques may help reduce the severity of rheumatoid episodes or prevent them.

• *Migraine.* Migraine headaches seem clearly linked to emotional stressors. Studies have shown that migraine headaches are prevalent among people who can be described as perfectionists or people who are excessively competitive, rigid, and chronically resentful, and who tend to conceal their true feelings. When such persons learn to manage hostility and frustration more effectively, possibly through venting their feelings, they can sometimes avoid migraine headaches.

• *Peptic ulcers.* Peptic ulcers are the known outcome of prolonged stress that overcomes the defenses protecting the gastric lining from destruction by digestive enzymes. Prolonged stress stimulates the adrenals to increase secretion of anti-inflammatory hormones. Concurrently, the production of peptic enzymes increases, augmenting the challenge to the gastric lining. In addition, the stress response of nerves within the stomach may be a factor in ulcer formation.

Preventive measures

The relationship between stress and disease is reciprocal: stress has a role in causing disease, and disease may cause stress. Depending on the illness, the stress impact may range from slight to catastrophic. And, medical treatment for the disease may also cause stress.

According to recent research, stress-prevention measures promote health, enhance treatment and control of disease, and may reduce the incidence of illness. Various techniques and life-style approaches are suggested in the

FACTORS THAT INFLUENCE STRESS RESPONSE AND RESISTANCE

A stressor's impact on an individual is determined by the individual's perception of the stressor, his conditioning, and his repertoire of coping mechanisms. These factors determine the power of the stressor over the individual, the individual's resistance to stress, and general manifestations of the stress response. Nursing measures should focus on recognition of these factors and appropriate interventions.

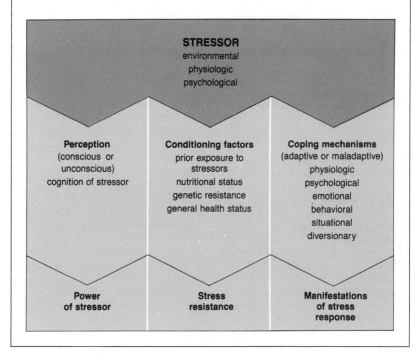

STRESSOR
environmental
physiologic
psychological

Perception
(conscious or unconscious)
cognition of stressor

Conditioning factors
prior exposure to stressors
nutritional status
genetic resistance
general health status

Coping mechanisms
(adaptive or maladaptive)
physiologic
psychological
emotional
behavioral
situational
diversionary

Power of stressor

Stress resistance

Manifestations of stress response

literature for managing stress and augmenting the person's coping ability.

Relaxation techniques, when practiced regularly, have been found effective in many settings. Four elements are common to all relaxation techniques: (1) a quiet environment; (2) a passive attitude; (3) a comfortable position; and (4) a neutral object to dwell upon. The success of relaxation techniques depends on the individual's willingness to practice the techniques regularly. During relaxation, the individual gains physiologic and psychological benefits as well as biochemical benefits—enhanced anabolic processes that promote cell growth and repair.

Relaxation techniques include progressive muscle relaxation, hypnosis, meditation, and biofeedback. For example, in progressive muscle relaxation, a person learns to control his skeletal muscles and thus lower the tone levels in the major muscle groups. The benefit lies in the fact that muscular relaxation opposes physiologic stress.

Meditation elicits the relaxation response and has the added benefit of gaining mastery over attention. In other words, the meditator develops the ability to interrupt, at will, his normal cognitive processes and directly perceive stimuli.

Relaxation techniques have a measurable effect in managing postoperative pain, test anxiety, chronic anger, tension headaches, and insomnia and are taught to patients with various diseases and disorders. Burish and Redd have done extensive work with people undergoing chemotherapy who develop conditioned side effects to their treatments. Their results suggest that behavioral relaxation techniques can relieve or minimize some of the side effects. In general, relaxation techniques do seem to offer some patients a way of managing conditioned side effects.

Techniques for stress management take in a broader area than the various relaxation strategies. While a specific technique—for example, biofeedback—may be beneficial to the person with Raynaud's disease, a broader approach combines life-style behaviors, diet, and relaxation to combat environmental stressors. For example, the Simontons and Norman Cousins have written popular books that advocate self-healing through the use of several interventions. Their premise is that the mind and body are inseparable in developing disease as well as in regaining health. Other authors advocate a broad approach to enhance one's ability to manage stress, including exercise, diet changes, relaxation techniques, learning assertiveness, recognizing stressors, anticipating stressors (such as the holidays) and preparing for them, and learning to use play and humor as part of one's life. For instance, cardiac rehabilitation programs include not only drug treatment but diet instruction, exercise programs, education on stressors and behavior changes, and support groups.

Although many questions about stress and its role in health and illness are still unanswered, the new holistic concept now receives increasing scientific support. A mind-body model of health and illness is consistent with the traditional focus of nursing practice—the whole patient.

BRENDA MARION NEVIDJON, RN, MSN

Treatment of spasms from upper motor neuron lesions

Many types of spasms occur in the presence of upper motor neuron lesions occurring in various disorders, including head and spinal injuries, multiple sclerosis, stroke, and brain tumors. Identifying these spasms correctly is crucial to an effective treatment plan. For example, when evaluating spasms in a spine-injured patient who has suffered significant cerebral trauma, the possibility of epileptic seizures must be considered.

Classifying spasms

Some patients show sustained, repetitive muscle contractions when holding a limb in a certain position; when the limb is repositioned, the contractions subside. Such contractions are a form of clonus and are due to exaggerated muscle tendon reflexes.

Another type of spasm is reflex withdrawal of the lower extremities, usually elicited by stimulation of the foot. This is due to an exaggerated Babinski's reflex and is usually accompanied by flexion, possibly sustained, of the hip, knee, and ankles. Such flexor spasms are often a sign of local irritation and may be the result of bedsores or urinary tract infections.

Other spasms resemble decerebrate rigidity, in which the elbows and knees are fixed in extension, usually for brief periods. Adductor spasms, which occur in the hip muscles, can prevent the patient's participation in physical therapy and make his bowel and bladder care extremely difficult.

Still other, more complex, movements can occur, such as writhing or repetitive motions that are similar to stimulation resulting from irritative foci in partially injured tissues.

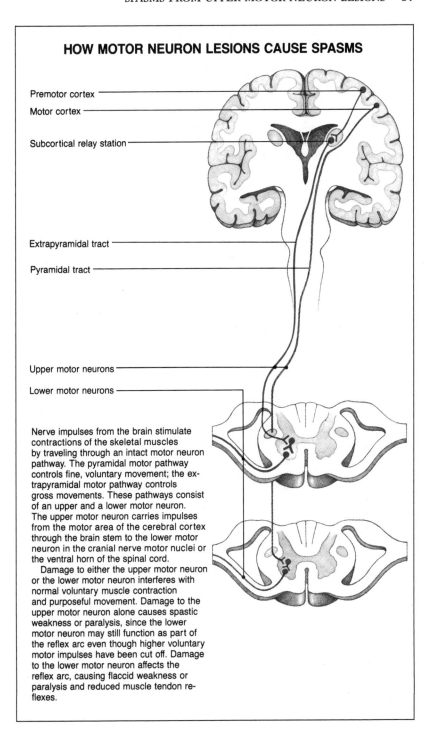

HOW MOTOR NEURON LESIONS CAUSE SPASMS

Premotor cortex

Motor cortex

Subcortical relay station

Extrapyramidal tract

Pyramidal tract

Upper motor neurons

Lower motor neurons

Nerve impulses from the brain stimulate contractions of the skeletal muscles by traveling through an intact motor neuron pathway. The pyramidal motor pathway controls fine, voluntary movement; the extrapyramidal motor pathway controls gross movements. These pathways consist of an upper and a lower motor neuron. The upper motor neuron carries impulses from the motor area of the cerebral cortex through the brain stem to the lower motor neuron in the cranial nerve motor nuclei or the ventral horn of the spinal cord.

Damage to either the upper motor neuron or the lower motor neuron interferes with normal voluntary muscle contraction and purposeful movement. Damage to the upper motor neuron alone causes spastic weakness or paralysis, since the lower motor neuron may still function as part of the reflex arc even though higher voluntary motor impulses have been cut off. Damage to the lower motor neuron affects the reflex arc, causing flaccid weakness or paralysis and reduced muscle tendon reflexes.

Treatment

After the spasm is identified, treatment can begin. Treatment can be classified as preventive, medical, or surgical.

• *Preventive therapy* consists of meticulous prevention of skin lesions and urinary tract infections to avoid spasticity and septic complications.

• *Medical therapy* consists of muscle relaxants, such as baclofen, diazepam, and dantrolene; anticonvulsants, such as phenytoin and carbamazepine; agents that induce muscle weakness; and antispasticity drugs.

• *Surgical therapy,* which may be directed at nearly any structure, from a muscle to the cerebral cortex, may be either ablative (removal or destruction of tissue) or stimulating. New approaches include the implantation of devices that relieve spasms by electrical stimulation. This approach offers distinct advantages over irreversible ablative procedures.

JOHN M. BERTONI, MD, PhD

White clot syndrome

White clot syndrome is a complication of heparin therapy that derives its name from the pale intravascular clots, consisting mostly of platelets, that are found during surgery or autopsy. This drug-induced immune response, which is associated with heparin-induced thrombocytopenia, occurs in about 10% of patients who receive heparin. White clot syndrome affects men and women of all ages.

Causes

White clot syndrome results in a thrombocytopenia that involves platelet aggregation. Apparently, heparin influences some change in the platelets that cause antibodies to recognize them as foreign (non-self); the antibodies then attack the body's own platelets, causing heparin resistance, intravascular clotting, and a dramatic decline in platelet counts. If severe, thrombocytopenia may result in hemorrhage.

Triggered by heparin, this syndrome is also heparin-dependent. When heparin is stopped, platelet counts rise and the syndrome resolves. If heparin is resumed, platelet counts plummet again.

Patients who receive heparin tend to develop white clot syndrome within 7 to 15 days after therapy begins. Patients with previous exposure to heparin may develop it sooner, within 2 to 3 days.

All forms and brands of heparin and all administration routes can induce this complication in susceptible patients. Moreover, this syndrome does not seem dose-related; it has developed after mini-prophylactic doses as well as after large doses used to manage patients after myocardial infarction (MI). And, it has occurred after use of heparin from both bovine lung and porcine intestinal mucosa. Bovine heparin has been linked with 28% incidence of white clot syndrome; porcine heparin, with 7%.

Signs and symptoms

During the period of susceptibility (after 7 to 15 days of heparin therapy), the patient with white clot syndrome may show clinical signs of an arterial or venous thrombus. Such a clot can form at any site and has occurred in the pulmonary, cardiac, cerebral, and peripheral vascular systems.

Thrombophlebitis may develop in the affected vessel, causing swelling, redness, tenderness, warmth, and induration. Pulmonary embolism may cause dyspnea, chest pain, tachycardia, productive cough with blood-tinged sputum, and low-grade fever. The effects of cerebral thromboembolism may range from such symptoms as intermittent weakness, numbness, visual deficits, ataxia, and speech difficulty with transient ischemic attacks to aphasia, hemiplegia, blindness, and loss of consciousness with some strokes. Embolism to the heart causes severe substernal chest pain, diaphoresis, dyspnea, and the dysrhythmias of an acute MI; embolism to a kidney may cause no symptoms or may occasionally cause flank pain and hematuria. Concurrently, the patient's platelet count drops to thrombocytopenic levels (between 5,000 and 54,000). The resulting coagulation defect may result in hematuria, melena, bleeding gums, and extensive bruising.

Diagnosis
Diagnosis is based on clinical signs and symptoms of emboli and low platelet counts related to heparin therapy. Heparin resistance—indicated by normal PT/PTT levels despite increasing doses of heparin—is also a clue.

Treatment
Until now, heparin therapy, once considered free of complications, has been used routinely to prevent pulmonary emboli after thrombosis of a peripheral vessel and after MI. However, recognition of white clot syndrome indicates that such treatment isn't completely without risk and mandates careful monitoring of platelet counts. Platelet counts below 5,000 or thromboembolism necessitates discontinuing heparin. Protamine, the heparin antidote, is ineffective against heparin's antigenic properties. Platelet transfusions may be given if acute bleeding develops; however, platelet counts return to normal spontaneously within several days after heparin is discontinued. To shorten the period of susceptibility to white clot syndrome, patients who require treatment with heparin should be switched to oral anticoagulant therapy as soon as possible.

Nursing intervention
• Routinely monitor platelet counts during heparin therapy to avert thrombocytopenia and major emboli.
• Emphasize to the hospitalized patient (and to the rare patient who receives heparin at home) the need for special precautions: the use of an electric razor to avoid shaving nicks and soft toothbrushes to avoid gingival

bleeding; inspection of urine and stool for blood; careful use of sharp objects; and the need to check for unusual bruising. The patient should immediately report any abnormal bleeding.
• Teach patients that chest pain, dyspnea, pain and swelling in an extremity, and any neurologic symptoms are signs of thromboemboli and should be reported immediately.
• Before giving heparin, ask patients if they have ever received heparin before or experienced a reaction to it. Advise sensitive patients to inform future health care providers of their reaction and to wear a Medic Alert bracelet.

JULIE TACKENBERG, RN, MA, CNRN

ADVANCES IN TREATMENT

Chemonucleolysis for herniated disk

Chemonucleolysis is the injection of an enzymatic chemical into the soft, gelatinous center of a herniated intervertebral disk to reduce its size and relieve pressure on the spinal nerve root.

This procedure was developed as an alternative to surgical decompression of the pinched spinal nerve. Chymopapain (Chymodiactin, Discase), a proteolytic enzyme derived from the papaya plant, is injected into the nucleus pulposus, where it causes the gelatinous chondromucoprotein to lose its water-binding capacity. As a result, the disk shrinks, reducing pressure on the nerve root and easing symptoms.

Though chemonucleolysis is not new, it remains controversial. Because clinical trials begun in 1964 produced conflicting results, chymopapain did not receive Food and Drug Administration approval until November 1982. However, the newest statistics seem to confirm the efficacy of chemonucleolysis for treating disk herniation.

Indications

Chemonucleolysis is indicated for treatment of herniated lumbar intervertebral disks in patients who would also be candidates for traditional surgical intervention. Usually, it's reserved for patients experiencing leg pain (sciatica) and back pain in whom conservative treatment (10 to 14 days of complete bed rest, weight reduction, physical therapy, oral analgesics, and muscle relaxants) has failed to relieve symptoms.

Chemonucleolysis isn't used to treat cervical disk herniation, and it's generally ineffective when disk fragments have ruptured through the posterior ligaments.

Contraindications

Chemonucleolysis is contraindicated in persons with the following conditions:
• allergy to papaya or related substances, such as meat tenderizers made from papaya or certain beers that use papaya as a clarifying agent
• previous treatment with chymopapain (previous exposure increases the risk of an allergic response)
• pregnancy (the effects of chymopapain on the fetus have not been determined)
• rapidly progressing neurologic deficit
• bowel or bladder dysfunction
• cauda equina syndrome
• severe spinal stenosis with moderate to severe weakness
• complete myelographic block
• history of severe allergic reaction to any substance or an elevated sedimentation rate. Both conditions increase the risk of anaphylaxis. Chymopapain must be used with extreme caution in such persons.

Method and procedure

Skin testing may be done before the procedure to rule out allergy to chymopapain. Most doctors order diphenhydramine (Benadryl) and cimetidine (Tagamet) for 24 hours before the procedure to reduce the risk of anaphylaxis; some also order a steroid drug to further suppress immune response. An I.V. line using a large-gauge needle is placed in case rapid fluid administration becomes necessary.

Chemonucleolysis is performed in the operating room under fluoroscopy and requires about 30 to 60 minutes to complete. General anesthesia is usually used, although the procedure can be performed under local anesthesia. (Recent studies have shown fewer incidents of anaphylaxis and inadvertent nerve root damage when the procedure is performed under local anesthesia.)

The patient is placed in a side-lying position and draped appropriately. Under fluoroscopic guidance, the surgeon places a 6", 16G to 18G needle into the center of the suspected disk(s). Some doctors insert a large-gauge needle through the skin and subcutaneous tissue, then thread a smaller 22G needle through the first needle to enter the disk. The two-needle technique supposedly reduces the risk of diskitis—infection of the intervertebral disk. Once the needle has been correctly positioned, a water-soluble dye may be injected into the nucleus pulposus to confirm herniation. After completion of diskography, 15 to 20 minutes are allowed for the dye to dissipate. Extreme caution must be taken to assure proper needle placement since chymopapain and radiopaque contrast media may be toxic if they contact the subarachnoid space. Although rare, acute transverse myelitis has been reported.

While the dye dissipates, the chymopapain can be prepared for injection. Because it quickly loses its enzymatic activity, chymopapain must be used within 30 minutes of reconstitution with sterile water. Once prepared, chymopapain is injected into the nucleus pulposus through the needle that was placed for diskography. Initially,

INTERVERTEBRAL DISK HERNIATION

Intervertebral disks act as cushions located between the bony vertebral bodies of the spinal vertebrae. Normally, each disk's soft center—the nucleus pulposus—is surrounded by a thick, fibrous tissue—the annulus fibrosus.

HERNIATED DISK

If the annulus is ruptured or torn, the nucleus pulposus bulges into the spinal canal and exerts pressure on the spinal nerve root. This produces pain and varying degrees of neurologic dysfunction.

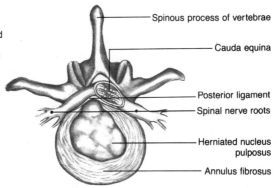

Spinous process of vertebrae

Cauda equina

Posterior ligament

Spinal nerve roots

Herniated nucleus pulposus

Annulus fibrosus

LUMBAR VERTEBRAE AND DISKS

The lumbar intervertebral disks—L3-4, L4-5, and L5-S1—are the most common herniation sites.

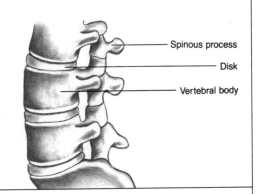

Spinous process

Disk

Vertebral body

PLACEMENT OF NEEDLE IN HERNIATED NUCLEUS PULPOSUS

Frequently, surgery (laminectomy or diskectomy) is necessary to decompress the spinal nerve and relieve symptoms. But by injecting an enzyme directly into the herniated nucleus pulposus, chemonucleolysis *chemically* decompresses the pinched nerve and thus offers an alternative to surgery.

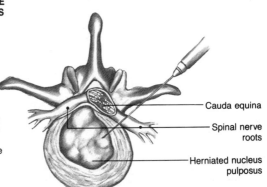

Cauda equina

Spinal nerve roots

Herniated nucleus pulposus

some surgeons will inject a small test dose—0.2 to 0.5 ml (500 to 1,000 units) and then observe the patient closely for signs of an allergic response, such as erythema or an unexpected drop in blood pressure. After 10 to 15 minutes, the surgeon can inject a full dose (1 to 2 ml, or 2,000 to 4,000 units) into each of the herniated disks. Some surgeons inject all abnormal disks; some treat only symptomatic herniations. After the injection is completed, the needle is withdrawn and a small dressing is applied to the puncture site.

For the first 2½ hours after chemonucleolysis, the patient must be observed closely (preferably, in the recovery room), since severe allergic reaction to chymopapain is most likely to occur during this time. If the patient remains free of signs and symptoms of drug allergy and vital signs are stable, he's returned to the general nursing unit. Some doctors order bed rest for 4 to 48 hours, depending on their own preference; some allow patients to resume activity as soon as they can tolerate it. Most patients can be discharged 48 to 72 hours after the procedure.

Effectiveness
Chemonucleolysis with chymopapain reduces the symptoms of herniated disk in 70% to 75% of those treated, as indicated by decreased leg pain, back pain, and disability. Chemonucleolysis is considered a failure if original symptoms persist or if disabling back or leg pain recurs 6 weeks after injection. About 50% of patients who had previous back surgery report improvement or relief of symptoms. In 1985, a long-term follow-up study of patients 9 to 12 years after treatment with chemonucleolysis reported that 75.2% of these patients continued to experience "marked improvement" of preprocedure symptoms.

Complications
By far the most serious risk of chemonucleolysis is anaphylaxis, which occurs in about 0.5% to 1% of those who receive chymopapain injection. (This incidence is about 10 times higher than that after administration of penicillin, a drug that's notorious for precipitating fatal anaphylaxis.) The first symptom of anaphylaxis is usually profound hypotension, but some clinicians report erythema before blood pressure falls. In 96% of the patients who develop anaphylaxis, its symptoms develop within 20 minutes after the chymopapain injection; in others, onset of symptoms may be delayed as long as 24 hours. Interestingly, anaphylactic reactions are more common in women and occur twice as often after use of a general anesthetic.

Less severe delayed allergic responses, such as skin rash, hives, and mild swelling of the mouth and eyes, may also occur. Severe muscle spasms at the injection site occur in about 20% of those undergoing chymopapain treatment; back pain and stiffness occur in about 50%. The latter discomfort usually resolves in 10 days to 3 months. Transient neurologic changes such as bowel or bladder disturbance or footdrop may also occur. Inflammation or infection of the arachnoid space (meningitis) or disk (diskitis) have been reported.

Paraplegia and subarachnoid or cerebral hemorrhage are rare.

Nursing intervention
Before chemonucleolysis, be sure to check for possible allergies to papaya products or iodine. Remember that patients with a seafood allergy may actually be allergic to iodine. Similarly, intolerance of meat tenderizers could indicate sensitivity to papaya. Also, prepare the patient to expect persistent pain and muscle spasms immediately after the procedure. Explain that pain and other symptoms will be gradually relieved as the enzyme slowly shrinks the disk.

After chemonucleolysis, remember to closely monitor the patient's vital signs, strength, sensation and movement of lower extremities, and ability to void. Watch for any delayed signs and symptoms of an allergic response, such as skin rash, pruritus, swelling of the eyes or lips, or changes in vital signs. Encourage normal activity, as ordered. Although many doctors restrict the patient to bed rest for a certain time, others encourage ambulation as soon as tolerated, since this may decrease the incidence and severity of muscle spasms. Many patients require I.M. narcotic analgesics during the first 24 to 48 hours after the injection. However, by the third day after the procedure, oral analgesics usually provide adequate pain control. Application of moist heat or ice to the injection site may also help reduce pain and spasm.

Instruct the patient about back care, and encourage him to avoid prolonged sitting, which can aggravate back pain. Usually, exercise is restricted for at least 3 weeks. The patient can return to work as soon as his doctor permits. Recuperation time at home varies with patient response to the procedure and the physical demands of his job; it may be complete in 2 weeks or may take as long as 3 months.

Investigational data

Though the controversy is far from resolved and the technique itself continues to be improved, chemonucleolysis may be an alternative to traditional laminectomy in selected patients.

Researchers are currently investigating use of a robot capable of placing needles, under computed tomography guidance, to within 1 to 2 mm of the desired location in the nucleus pulposus. Some areas of the nucleus pulposus may actually be better suited for contrast and enzyme injection, thus improving the quality of diskography and the effectiveness of chymopapain injection.

Clinical trials using the enzyme collagenase instead of chymopapain are also under way. It produces similar success rates (78%) and may produce fewer serious allergic reactions.

Advocates of chemonucleolysis suggest that it produces results similar to those of surgical treatment of herniated disk while reducing cost and length of hospital stay. Laminectomy requires an average 7- to 10-day hospitalization; chemonucleolysis normally requires only 1 to 3 days. However, because chemonucleolysis is performed in an operating room, under anesthesia; uses an expensive enzymatic drug (chymopapain costs about $500 to $1,000 per vial); and has a high incidence of severe postprocedure pain (which can prolong hospitalization), some authorities have questioned whether this procedure actually does save time and money. Researchers are currently gathering data to answer this important question.

KAREN E. BURGESS, RN, MSN

Closed vitrectomy in retrolental fibroplasia

Microsurgery is now being used to restore vision to neonates suffering from retrolental fibroplasia. More than 4,000 neonates annually develop this condition. Its consequences range from preretinal fibrosis to total retinal detachment and fibrosis, which cause impaired visual acuity or total blindness.

Causes

In the late 1950s, 300 cases of retrolental fibroplasia were reported annually. The recent dramatic rise in incidence has been attributed to the high arterial oxygen pressures used in neonatal intensive care units. Arterial oxygen pressures over 60 mm Hg cause the small peripheral vascular tree of the retina to contract. When oxygen levels return to normal, the arterial vessels respond with an overgrowth of fibrous tissue, causing traction on the retina and subsequent retinal damage.

Infants weighing less than 1,000 g are at greatest risk.

Although oxygen is considered the primary stimulus for neurovascularization in retrolental fibroplasia, this condition has been recorded in some neonates who had not received oxygen therapy or who received safe and closely monitored oxygen concentrations.

Treatment
The recently developed microsurgery technique is a closed vitrectomy procedure that is especially appropriate for the small eyes of neonates. The procedure involves removal of the lens, followed by careful dissection and suction removal of the fibrotic (scar) tissue. Fluid is then infused to maintain the intraocular pressure and to free the retina from the traction of the adhering scar tissue that initially caused the detachment. The now mobilized retina can settle to the back of the eye, where it will eventually reattach if the procedure has been successful. Usually, each eye is corrected separately, the second eye within weeks after the first.

Special considerations
Microsurgery for retrolental fibroplasia is most successful during the early stages of detachment, before the entire retina has been pulled to the center of the eye. Restoration of normal vision is not expected. This surgery is considered successful when any vision is salvaged.

JULIE TACKENBERG, RN, MA, CNRN

Diabetes treatment update

Standard treatment of diabetes mellitus attempts to control it through specific methods that control blood glucose levels. For Type I diabetes, treatment usu-ally involves insulin administration (single or multiple injections or insulin pump administration), a special diet and exercise program, blood glucose self-testing, urine ketone testing, and identification of and treatment for hyperglycemia and hypoglycemia.

For Type II diabetes, traditional treatment involves diet and exercise, possibly with insulin administration or an oral hypoglycemic agent, urine or blood glucose self-monitoring, and identification of and treatment for hyperglycemia and hypoglycemia.

New therapies
Current research is exploring the value of pancreas or islet cell transplantation, implantable probe and pump, autoimmune drug therapy, and the glycemic index to control diabetic diet.

Pancreas islet cell grafts. Such grafts are currently being performed in the hope that the grafted islet cells will control blood glucose metabolism and prevent or resolve microangiopathic complications. Such grafts require pure, undamaged pancreas islet cells for grafting; these are difficult to obtain. Another disadvantage is that isolated islet cells are more prone to rejection than islet cell grafts in an intact pancreas. The search continues for ways to obtain greater numbers of donor islet cells, human or animal, and to prevent rejection through drug therapy or implantation of new stem cells as the defense component of the immune system.

Pancreas transplantation. In the past 2 decades, 316 patients have received a pancreas transplant; approximately 18% of them have been found to secrete their own insulin. Pancreas transplantation is performed by segmental pancreatic transplantation, pancreaticoduodenal transplantation, and simultaneous pancreatic transplantation. Unfortunately, rejection of the transplant is common. As a result, patients are treated with immunosuppressive agents such as cyclosporine, antilymphocyte globulin, and prednisone—which may cause the following adverse effects to a greater or lesser degree: hepatotoxicity, nephrotoxicity, lymphoma, and increased susceptibility to infections.

Currently, patients selected for pancreas transplantation are those already receiving immunosuppressive agents because of a previous (nonpancreatic) transplant and those in whom diabetic complications are potentially more serious than the effects of chronic immunosuppression. At present, the success rate with this procedure isn't high enough to justify pancreas transplantation as a general treatment for diabetes. More research is also needed to improve immunosuppression therapy.

Implantable probe and pump. This has been designed to monitor blood glucose levels and automatically deliver the correct amount of insulin to maintain blood glucose levels within the normal range. However, several problems must be resolved before this device can be acceptable for long-term use in ambulatory diabetics. For example, the implantable probe tends to become clogged with protective body cells that prevent insulin secretion. Also, the pump doesn't reliably secrete the correct dose of insulin, thus causing hypoglycemia or hyperglycemia.

Cyclosporine therapy. This drug is being studied as a means of combating the destruction of islet beta cells by the immune system in the pathogenesis of Type I diabetes. Researchers have found evidence of circulating serum islet-cell antibodies associated with loss of beta-cell function. Accordingly, they suggest that the immunosuppressive action of cyclosporine may prevent these antibodies from attacking the islet cells.

Glycemic index (GI). (See *Glycemic Index*.) This method ranks blood glucose levels of fluctuation to various foods. It identifies low-fat, starchy foods that diabetics can use to increase carbohydrate intake without causing high postprandial blood glucose levels. Patients on a GI diet must accurately perform blood glu-

GLYCEMIC INDEX

The glycemic index (GI) helps diabetics select foods that provide carbohydrates without raising postprandial blood glucose levels. Foods that raise blood glucose levels slowly are the slowly absorbed starches identified in the GI by their low percentage ratings.

Least desirable foods for the diabetic raise blood glucose levels rapidly. These glucose-containing foods have the highest percentage ratings in the GI.

Special note: Because the GI doesn't evaluate other nutritional values, it should be used only with the American Diabetes Association's food exchange lists.

FOOD (1.75 OZ)	GLYCEMIC INDEX
Soybeans	15%
Fructose	20%
Kidney beans	29%
Lentils	29%
Black-eyed peas	33%
Whole milk	34%
Chick-peas	36%
Ice cream	36%
Yogurt	36%
Tomato soup	38%
Apple	39%
Orange	40%
Bran cereal	51%
Peas (frozen)	51%
Oatmeal	54%
Corn	59%
Banana	62%
Raisins	64%
Brown rice	66%
Shredded wheat	67%
Potato (new)	70%
White rice	72%
Cornflakes	80%
Instant mashed potatoes	80%
Honey	87%
Glucose (corn sugar)	100%

cose self-monitoring after every meal and snack. Consequently, many diabetic patients find compliance difficult.

CHRIS PLATT MOLDOVANYI, RN, MSN

Ether dissolution of gallstones

Cholelithiasis, the most common biliary tract disease, affects over 20 million Americans and accounts for the third most commonly performed surgical procedure—cholecystectomy. A new nonsurgical procedure—the use of methyl tertiary butyl ether (MTBE) to dissolve cholesterol gallstones—shows promise as an alternative to surgery.

Background

The concept of dissolving gallstones in situ dates back to the late 1700s when this was thought possible with oral administration of a combination of ether and turpentine. Since then numerous solvents have been administered orally or by direct infusion into the biliary system. But such agents as chenodiol and ursodeoxycholic acid usually require treatment for 1 to 3 years to complete dissolution of such stones. This, together with troublesome adverse effects, such as diarrhea and frequent recurrence of stones, has limited the use of these chemical solvents.

Monoctanoin (MO) is now the preferred agent for direct dissolution of the most common duct stones, which usually contain a mixture of cholesterol, bile salt, calcium, bile pigment, and other solids. (The less common pigment stones contain calcium bilirubinite, complex bilirubin polymers, and organic and inorganic solids.) Treatment with MO usually requires 3 to 21 days of therapy.

New treatment

MTBE is a potentially fast-acting, relatively complication-free procedure for patients with cholesterol gallstones. It may be especially useful for such patients who are high surgical risks because of other illness or debilitation. MTBE is liquid at body temperature, has a cholesterol-solubilizing capacity comparable to MO, and dissolves cholesterol stones five times faster, but it requires direct contact with the cholesterol stone. Therefore, this agent's therapeutic use is limited to a closed environment such as the gallbladder, which can contain MTBE and thus minimize systemic absorption.

Clinical studies report that MTBE can dissolve multiple human cholesterol stones implanted in dog gallbladders within hours of infusion and without serious adverse effects. Two case reports indicate that MTBE can rapidly dissolve cholesterol gallstones without causing acute toxicity. MTBE is more effective in dissolving gallbladder stones than common bile duct stones.

Procedures

Two methods for instilling MTBE are currently being studied: via transhepatic catheter and nasobiliary catheter.

• Transhepatic catheter instillation is used to dissolve gallbladder stones (see *Gallstone Dissolution*). Under sterile conditions, a catheter is fluoroscopically guided into the gallbladder, which is then observed for evidence of bleeding and is rechecked with cholecystography via catheter for placement. Maximal aspiration of the gallbladder is performed. To identify stones, 5 ml of contrast material is infused, then removed, and continuous infusion and aspiration of MTBE at 1-minute cycles begins. With each infusion, the volume of MTBE is gradually increased from 1 ml to a total volume of 5 ml. When the syringe is half-filled with bile, it's replaced with a fresh one containing MTBE. Cholecystograms are obtained at 2, 4, and 7 hours after treatment to check for stone dissolution.

• Nasobiliary catheter instillation is used to remove intrahepatic duct stones. After endoscopic placement of a nasobiliary catheter, infusion—either manual infusion or continuous syringe infusion—and aspiration of 0.5 ml MTBE via catheter occurs every 30 minutes. MTBE is reinfused in gradually increasing volumes to a maximum of 2.5 ml. After 4 hours of MTBE instillation (total volume of 7.5 ml), a second cholangiogram is performed to check for disappearance of the stone in the duct.

Complications

Toxicity with MTBE appears to be similar to that of diethyl ether. Ninety percent of the ether compound is excreted in breathing; a small residual of MTBE is metabolized to methanol. Intrahepatic infusion of substantial amounts can produce hemolysis or necrosis. MTBE can also cause duodenitis and is a powerful lipid solvent. Both MTBE and diethyl ether are explosive anesthetics at certain concentrations, but MTBE is less volatile (with a boiling point of 131.4° F. [55.2° C.] vs. 94.1° F. [34.5° C.] for diethyl ether).

Nursing intervention

Since MTBE therapy is still experimental and no protocol has yet been established for it, nursing care is extremely important. Follow the guidelines below:

• Obtain a baseline of liver enzymes in case the patient sustains liver damage.
• Frequently check the patient's mental status, since ether is an anesthetic and may cause somnolence.

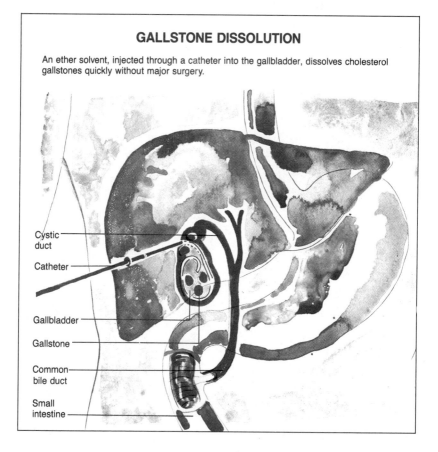

GALLSTONE DISSOLUTION

An ether solvent, injected through a catheter into the gallbladder, dissolves cholesterol gallstones quickly without major surgery.

Cystic duct

Catheter

Gallbladder

Gallstone

Common bile duct

Small intestine

• Frequently check the patient's breath for MTBE odor.

• Observe for signs of MTBE toxicity: change in mental status or vital signs, nausea, and vomiting. Check stool for blood and observe for signs of abdominal pain, since MTBE can cause duodenitis. Remember that necrosis or extravasation into the liver may also cause abdominal pain.

• To prevent explosion, prohibit smoking in the patient's room and make sure machinery is well maintained and grounded.

• Check that nasobiliary tube placement has been verified fluoroscopically before administering MTBE.

• Observe the patient for discomfort during MTBE instillation.

• Observe aspirated fluid for amount, color, consistency, and evidence of blood.

• Provide meticulous mouth care to reduce possible irritation from the nasobiliary tube.

• Observe the transhepatic catheter site for signs of infection, leakage, or drainage. Change the dressing daily.

• Offer the patient reassurance and emotional support. Teach him to identify the signs and symptoms of stone recurrence, which should be reported immediately. Emphasize the importance of follow-up care to detect stone recurrence.

TERRI B. ROSENBERG, RN, BSN
BARBARA S. HENZEL, RN, BSN, GIA

Interventional endoscopy

Flexible fiberoptic endoscopy has been a valuable diagnostic tool for the past 2 decades. With the development of sophisticated endoscopes and endoscopic accessories, endoscopy now has important therapeutic applications. For example, in the high-risk patient with biliary and GI disorders, endoscopy allows treatment without general anesthesia or surgical incision, thus ensuring faster and safer recovery. Moreover, because some endoscopic procedures can be performed on outpatients, therapeutic endoscopy is receiving wider acceptance as a safer, cost-effective alternative to surgery.

Endoscopic procedures

• *Endoscopic sphincterotomy* was introduced 12 years ago for treating retained common duct stones after cholecystectomy. This procedure has since been expanded to include treatment of high-risk patients with biliary dyskinesia and to produce drainage in obstructing bile duct tumors in which the endoscopic sphincterotomy precedes placement of a stent.

Sphincterotomy is accomplished by passing a cutting wire (papillotome) through the endoscope. Under fluoroscopic guidance, the wire is skillfully placed within the papilla of Vater and the cut is made. The papillotome is then attached to an electrical cautery unit and, with the patient properly grounded, the sphincter muscle tissue is cauterized. Often the stone drops out after cutting alone. If it doesn't, a wire basket can be passed through the endoscope and into the common bile duct. The assisting nurse opens and closes the basket around the stone upon the doctor's instruction. (See *Techniques for Removing Common Bile Duct Gallstones.*)

Stones can also be retrieved through the endoscope with a balloon. A deflated balloon is passed up the common bile duct beyond the stone. The nurse inflates the balloon, and the stone is forced down the duct as the inflated balloon is extracted. Extremely large stones that won't pass through the sphincterotomy have been handled with mechanical lithotripsy.

• *Endobiliary prosthesis,* or stenting, is used to treat both malignant and benign biliary strictures. Malignant strictures are common in patients with met-

TECHNIQUES FOR REMOVING COMMON BILE DUCT GALLSTONES

Several endoscopic techniques may be used to remove common bile duct gallstones. In the two techniques shown here, a fiberoptic endoscope is passed through the stomach and duodenum to the ampulla of Vater. In the first technique, a sphincterotomy is performed with a special cutting wire (papillotome), which has been introduced through the endoscope. An incision at this site allows the stone to pass into the duodenum. If sphincterotomy is unsuccessful, a second technique is used. This involves a Dormier basket, which is introduced through the endoscope to remove the stone. Another technique, used as a last resort, involves mechanically crushing the stone.

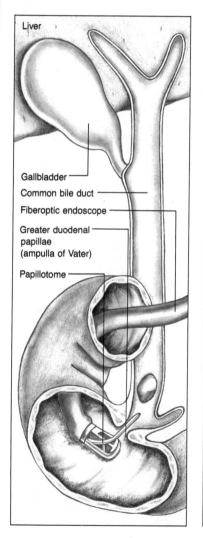

Liver
Gallbladder
Common bile duct
Fiberoptic endoscope
Greater duodenal papillae (ampulla of Vater)
Papillotome

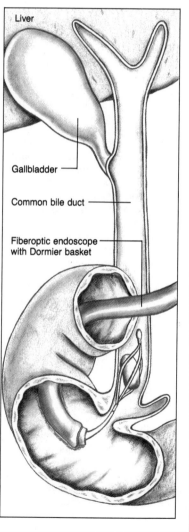

Liver
Gallbladder
Common bile duct
Fiberoptic endoscope with Dormier basket

astatic liver disease and cancer of the pancreas. Complete obstruction of bile flow can lead to sepsis and death. Endoscopic intervention to relieve the obstruction offers palliative treatment for the high-risk surgical candidate with an obstructed biliary tree who would otherwise receive a relatively blind attempt at percutaneous drainage or no treatment at all.

Benign bile duct strictures are less common. They result from injury during surgery, periductal fibrosis secondary to chronic pancreatitis, cholangitis due to choledocholithiasis, primary sclerosing cholangitis, and congenital defects. Surgical correction in such patients has been largely abandoned because of the high incidence of restenosis. In these strictures, stenting relieves jaundice and prevents recurrent cholangitis.

The procedure is performed by inserting an endoscope into the common bile duct. Usually, a sphincterotomy is performed to ease the passage of the stent through the ampulla of Vater. The distal end of the stent must be above the obstruction, and the proximal end must be visualized in the duodenum. Continuity of the duct is then established and bile can flow freely.

After sphincterotomy for stone removal, a nasobiliary catheter may be used temporarily to decompress the biliary tree or to ensure an accurate cholangiogram. Generally, large-diameter catheters (#10 and #12 French) are preferred. The distal portion of the catheter is in the common bile duct; the proximal portion is pulled out through the patient's nose and attached to straight drainage. Bile can then flow freely through the catheter tip.

• *Esophageal sclerotherapy*, also known as injection sclerotherapy, is commonly used to stop bleeding from esophageal varices, which can develop in patients with liver disease. Of the nonneoplastic diseases of the GI tract, variceal rupture causes the most life-threatening form of hemorrhage because of the massive volume of blood lost. Esophageal sclerotherapy is now preferred over treatment with the Blakemore tube, Pitressin drip, or portacaval shunt. The Blakemore tube, once used to control such bleeding with pressure, is now seldom used since the amount of pressure it requires can cause esophageal necrosis. Pitressin drip can be used to treat bleeding varices by vasoconstriction, but its effect is temporary. Surgical intervention with portacaval shunts has a high mortality because of the patient's poor condition. A safer procedure, injection sclerotherapy can be used therapeutically to control emergency esophageal hemorrhage and prophylactically to control rebleeding.

To perform this procedure, the doctor passes the endoscope into the esophagus to visualize the varix. A sheathed needle is passed through an open channel in the endoscope. The needle is unsheathed mechanically and placed either alongside the varix or directly into it. A sclerosing agent, usually morrhuate sodium or sodium tetradecyl sulfate (Sotradecol), is then injected in a volume of 0.5 to 3 ml. The sclerosing agent damages the venous intimal endothelium, causing inflammation and thrombus formation. The blood clot occludes a varix, and deep tissue necrosis occurs, followed by fibrosis, which prevents recurrent hemorrhage. This procedure may need to be repeated every 2 to 6 weeks until all varices have been occluded. Patients who are not actively bleeding may be treated prophylactically on an outpatient basis.

Nursing intervention

Following these procedures, frequently monitor vital signs and complaints of nausea, vomiting, and abdominal pain. With nasobiliary stenting, the catheter is attached to straight drainage and will require special care. Secure the catheter to the nose as for a nasogastric tube. Irrigate to ensure patency according to doctor's orders, usually with 10 ml of normal saline solution every 12 hours. Normally, the nasobiliary catheter is removed within 24 to 72 hours by gently pulling the catheter through the nose.

Complications

Complications after sphincterotomy include bleeding, pancreatitis, and perforation. Monitor the patient's vital signs every 15 minutes for the first hour, every 30 minutes for the next hour, then every 4 hours for 24 hours. Promptly report any complaints of severe abdominal pain and any sign of abdominal rigidity to the doctor.

After sclerotherapy, substernal chest pain is common, and hematemesis and fever may occur. If the patient isn't in an intensive care unit, he should be monitored closely and reassured that his discomfort will subside soon. Major complications of sclerotherapy may include pleural effusions, pulmonary embolism, bacteremia, and excessive blood loss, but they're rare. Long-term complications are still unknown but may include esophageal ulceration and stricture formation. Repeated injections cause progressive inflammation, ulceration, and subsequent fibrosis that may progress to stricture formation.

CAROL LORENZO, RN

Radial keratotomy

Radial keratotomy (RK) was first conceived in Japan 30 years ago and was further developed in the Soviet Union. It is now available to help persons suffering with myopia or moderate astigmatism. Myopia, or nearsightedness, results from a common but abnormal elongation of the eyeball or, occasionally, from too much power in the eye's lens system. Consequently, light rays from distant objects focus in front of the retina instead of on it. Astigmatism is an uneven curvature of the cornea or lens that causes horizontal and vertical rays to focus at different points in the eye. By changing the shape of the cornea, RK can improve the eye's optical power, often correcting vision as poor as 20/1600 to 20/20.

Candidates for RK must be over age 18 and without ocular pathology. The degree of stability of the patient's myopia or the severity of astigmatism are also important considerations.

Procedure

RK is a 3- to 8-minute procedure performed on an outpatient basis under a local and topical anesthestic. A standby general anesthestic is available, depending on the patient's degree of anxiety. A series of 8 to 16 precise incisions are made through 90% of the cornea's thickness. The resulting scars change the corneal shape and therefore its optical power. The globe of the eye is left intact to avoid permanent damage. Each eye is treated separately, the second within 1 week after the first. The outcome depends on the surgeon's skill.

Posttreatment care

Patients are discharged approximately 1 hour after the procedure. After 5 hours, the patient can remove the eye patch and resume normal activities. The patient's vision is evaluated to determine the need for corrective lenses.

Adverse effects and complications

The patient may experience mild discomfort in the affected eye, such as a dull ache that may last up to 24 hours, photophobia, and scratchy irritation. His vision may initially be blurry. Antimicrobial eye drops and pain medication are prescribed to prevent infection and ease discomfort.

The most frequently reported complications include undercorrection or overcorrection of the myopia. If the wound is irrigated too vigorously during surgery, epithelial cysts or abraded incisions may occur. Scleral cuts can cause red blood cell debris in the wound. Asymmetrical incisions can lead to astigmatism.

DIANE COCHET, RN, BSN

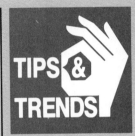

Seasonal affective disorder

Patients who suffer from recurrent winter depressions may have seasonal affective disorder (SAD). Researchers have attributed this disorder to an abnormality of neurotransmitters such as serotonin and melatonin.

SAD is triggered by changes in climate, geographic latitude, and intensity of environmental light. It produces a cluster of depressive symptoms that commonly includes a depressed mood, excessive sleeping, overeating, and craving of carbohydrates. These symptoms have traditionally been treated with antidepressants and psychotherapy, but they are now known to respond dramatically to new and still experimental treatment—phototherapy. Patients are encouraged to walk outside in the fresh air and sunshine for at least 30 minutes a day. They receive supplemental light therapy by daily exposure to a bright artificial light, such as Vita-Lite, which closely mimics sunlight. The beneficial effects of phototherapy are usually evident within 4 days.

SIDS update

Sudden infant death syndrome (SIDS) is the leading cause of death among infants aged 1 month to 1 year, with deaths occurring at a rate of 2 in every 1,000 live births. In the United States, 7,000 infants die of SIDS annually. Although SIDS has been described since ancient times, its causes are still obscure.

Formerly, SIDS was believed to be caused by accidental suffocation of infants during sleep or as a result of abuse. Diagnosis continues to be based on exclusion, but researchers believe that SIDS probably has more than one cause. They have uncovered the following information:

• Peak incidence occurs between the 2nd and 4th months of life; incidence declines rapidly between 4 and 12 months. Sixty-one percent of SIDS victims have been boys.

• Infants die suddenly in their sleep, without warning, sound, or struggle.

• Incidence of SIDS is slightly higher in preterm infants, native Alaskan infants, disadvantaged black infants, infants of mothers under age 20, and infants of multiple births. Incidence is 10 times higher in SIDS siblings; slightly higher in infants whose mothers smoke; and up to 10 times higher in infants whose mothers are narcotic addicts.

• Some SIDS-diagnosed infants show postmortem changes that indicate chronic hypoxia, hypoxemia, and large airway obstruction.

• *Clostridium botulinum* toxin has been linked to a few SIDS deaths.

• Infants commonly succumb to SIDS in the fall and winter. Many have a history of respiratory infection, suggesting viral infection as an etiology.

• Studies show conflicting data about abnormal hepatic or pancreatic processes in SIDS infants.

• The link between apneic episodes and SIDS is unclear. But about 60% of infants with near-miss respiratory events have second episodes of apnea; some succumb to SIDS.

When an infant dies of SIDS, assure parents that they were in no way responsible for the death. Answer questions about autopsy, and explain it as a benefit in achieving peace of mind as well as furthering knowledge of SIDS. Encourage parents to seek counseling about the risk of SIDS to siblings and their possible evaluation with cardiopneumogram and apnea monitoring. Parents can seek help from health care providers, clergy, and the National Sudden Infant Death Syndrome Foundation (1-800-221-SIDS).

For parents of healthy infants who worry about SIDS, explain that apnea/cardiac monitoring is generally recommended only for siblings of SIDS victims because of its high cost and often disruptive effects on family dynamics.

The Penn State heart

The Penn State heart is a recent development in the search for ways to prevent death from cardiac disease. This temporary air-powered artificial heart is the outcome of 13 years of research at the Pennsylvania State University's Colleges of Medicine and Engineering.

The Penn State heart has two primary purposes. First, to provide temporary total mechanical support for postoperative open-heart surgery patients who can't be separated from the heart-lung machine because of pre-existing heart disease and for whom left ventricular mechanical support is not an option. Second, to sustain patients with end-stage heart disease while they await a suitable heart organ donation.

The fully constructed heart is similar in weight to a natural heart and is designed to fit inside the chest of a man weighing at least 155 lb.

Mechanics

The Penn State heart features two artificial ventricles, the two major pumping chambers of the natural heart. Made of hard plastic, each covers a soft plastic sac that stretches to allow the artificial heart to beat. The smooth, seamless inner sacs allow blood to flow through them without collecting on their surfaces, thus reducing the risk of thrombus formation. As the sacs fill with blood from the body, air pres-

FILLING PHASE

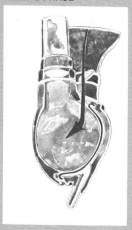

PUMPING PHASE

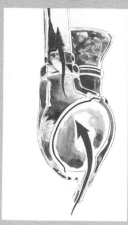

sure, injected through tubes into the space between the soft sac and the hard case, pumps blood in and out of the heart.

Unlike other artificial hearts that must be manually adjusted to adapt to the blood flow demands

of various activities, the Penn State heart automatically adjusts to increased blood flow demand.

Artificial heart candidates

The potential candidate for the Penn State heart must be age 55 or younger with good vital organ function (excluding the heart), no evidence of infection or lung damage, and no insulin-dependent diabetes. He must also have a healthy mental state and strong family support. He must have failed to benefit from all conventional treatments, such as cardiac drugs, intraaortic balloon pump, and mechanical ventricular support.

Before surgery, the patient must sign a four-page consent form that details the potential risks: blood clot formation, air embolus, equipment/artificial heart failure, and infection.

Postimplantation care

Postoperatively, the patient requires intensive nursing care until an organ donor is found. Nursing responsibilities are as follows:
• Counsel the patient and his family preoperatively and postoperatively.
• Closely monitor the patient's clinical status.
• Develop expertise in the operation of the artificial heart and other life-support equipment.
• Provide the daily supportive nursing care required by all surgical patients.

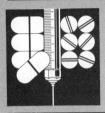

Drugs

Calcium: Real hope for osteoporosis?

The latest in a seemingly endless series of "miracle" drugs is one of the most abundant minerals in nature—calcium. The National Institutes of Health (NIH) has called calcium, along with estrogen, the "mainstays of prevention and management of osteoporosis." Others go even further, suggesting that calcium may also lower blood pressure and help prevent cancer of the colon.

The result of these claims? A dramatic rise in the sales of calcium supplements (with total sales expected to top $200 million in 1987) and growing evidence that women, the primary victims of osteoporosis, are changing their dietary habits to include more high-calcium foods.

And it's no wonder. For osteoporosis afflicts up to 20 million Americans, most of them women over age 45, predisposing them to potentially dangerous fractures—particularly of the vertebrae, femur, and hip. In fact, about 20% of women with such hip fractures develop a fatal complication such as infection or pulmonary embolism, and another 20% become permanently crippled, making osteoporosis a leading cause of disability and death in older women. In this group, osteoporosis strikes more frequently than heart attacks, strokes, diabetes, rheumatoid arthritis, or breast cancer.

How does osteoporosis develop? We don't know for sure, but we do know that it's a slowly progressive process that may take decades to develop fully. During childhood and adolescence, the rate of bone formation far outstrips the rate of bone resorption, so the bones become larger and denser. But after bone mass reaches its peak density, at about age 35, resorption begins to overtake formation, and the bones become lighter and weaker.

In women, bone resorption increases markedly after menopause, mainly because of a sharp reduction in estrogen secretion. Men also lose bone density with age, but this isn't nearly as severe a problem for them, since they have considerably more bone density than women to begin with and don't experience the sudden drop in estrogen levels associated with menopause.

Osteoporosis particularly affects the porous trabeculae of the lower thoracic and lumbar vertebrae and the epiphyses of the femur, tibia, and the other long bones of the arms and legs. It can develop insidiously, with gradually increasing bone deformity, kyphosis (the

DIETARY SOURCES OF CALCIUM

FOOD	CALCIUM CONTENT (mg)
Bread, white (1 slice)	21
Broccoli, cooked (½ cup)	88
Cheese, cheddar (1 oz)	213
Cheese, cottage (1 cup)	138
Collard greens, cooked (½ cup)	152
Cream pie (1 slice)	62
Hot chocolate (1 cup)	298
Ice cream, vanilla (½ cup)	88
Milk, nonfat (1 cup)	296
Milk, whole (1 cup)	288
Oysters, raw (6)	81
Peanuts, roasted (⅔ cup)	69
Salmon, canned, with bones (3 oz)	222
Sardines, canned, with bones (3 oz)	258
Spinach, cooked (½ cup)	73
Yogurt, low-fat, plain (1 cup)	415

CALCIUM, ESTROGEN, AND OSTEOPOROSIS

Osteoporosis is a metabolic bone disorder in which there is a gradual loss of bone matrix. Primary osteoporosis usually becomes apparent after menopause due to a decrease in circulating estrogen resulting from atrophy of the ovaries. Decreased estrogen circulation adversely affects bones by increasing their sensitivity to parathyroid hormone (PTH). PTH stimulates reabsorption of calcium and phosphorus from bone by activating bone-removing osteoclast cells and transiently depressing bone-renewing osteoblast cells. This reabsorption raises circulating calcium levels. Through a negative feedback mechanism on the parathyroid glands, increased blood calcium level causes decreased PTH secretion. Decreased PTH causes reduced absorption of dietary calcium and phosphorus in the intestines as well as increased excretion of calcium in the renal tubules. As calcium is continually washed from the body, osteoporosis may manifest itself in fractures.

Besides menopause, other risk factors for osteoporosis include white race, lean build, short stature, smoking, alcoholism, high-fiber diet, high intake of phosphorylated beverages, sedentary lifestyle or prolonged bed rest, and long-term therapy with steroids, diuretics, thyroid hormone, or tetracycline.

Prevention of osteoporosis is far more effective than any attempt to cure it. Menopausal and postmenopausal women should increase calcium intake to 1.5 grams a day. Therapy with estrogen replacement, calcium, and vitamin D (to enhance absorption and facilitate the action of calcium) may help prevent or treat osteoporosis.

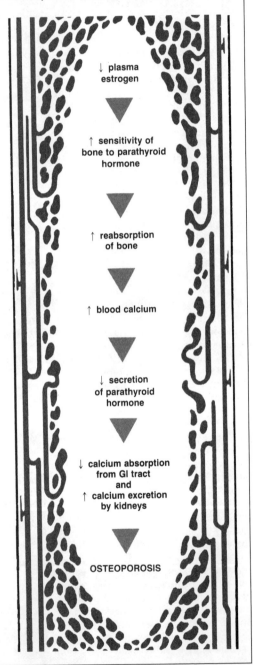

↓ plasma estrogen

↑ sensitivity of bone to parathyroid hormone

↑ reabsorption of bone

↑ blood calcium

↓ secretion of parathyroid hormone

↓ calcium absorption from GI tract
and
↑ calcium excretion by kidneys

OSTEOPOROSIS

classic "dowager's hump"), and an aged appearance. Or it can produce sudden fractures; vertebral collapse from a series of small fractures can cause a profound loss of height—up to 2 inches in just a few weeks. Hip fractures, caused by loss of bone density in the ball-and-socket joint of the femur and pelvis, are also common. Once osteoporosis sets in, the simplest body movement, such as bending over to pick up a book, can cause a fracture.

But how can calcium help prevent osteoporosis? Calcium is the most abundant mineral in the body, with almost all of it contained in bone. The rest of the body's calcium circulates in the bloodstream and is necessary for such important functions as the transmission of nerve impulses, muscle contraction and relaxation, regulation of cardiac rhythm, and the chemical activity in all body cells. If the circulating calcium level falls too drastically, bone resorption increases to restore it. This resorption causes bones to lose calcium and phosphate salts and thus become porous, brittle, and abnormally susceptible to fracture. Replacing the bones' depleted calcium stores strengthens their structure and inhibits resorption. However, calcium replacement and other therapies for osteoporosis (estrogen, fluoride, and vitamin D therapy, with moderate amounts of weight-bearing exercise) can only slow, not stop, the progression of bone degeneration. Thus, one key to successful prevention of osteoporosis is early initiation of a high-calcium diet.

How much calcium is needed to achieve these effects? The NIH has recommended that women increase calcium intake to 1,000 mg/day before menopause and 1,500 mg/day after menopause if they don't take estrogen. (On average, Americans get only 450 to 550 mg/day from food sources.)

What can you do to help your patients maintain an adequate calcium intake? Start by pointing out good food sources of calcium (see *Dietary Sources of Calcium*, page 115). Unfortunately, some of the best sources of dietary calcium—dairy products—are also high in calories and saturated fats, making them unattractive to weight-conscious adults. Fortunately, you can advise a patient who's counting calories that low-fat dairy products contain as much, if not more, calcium as whole-milk products. At the same time, advise your patient to limit her intake of alcohol, which interferes with calcium metabolism, and caffeine and sodium, which increase calcium excretion in the urine. If she's taking any medication that increases calcium excretion, such as prednisone or other corticosteroids, advise her to increase calcium intake to compensate. Also tell her that stress and prolonged inactivity may reduce her body's ability to utilize calcium; advise her to exercise regularly, as her condition permits, and to take time out to relax each day.

You may also advise the patient to take a calcium supplement. If you do, remember to teach her how to differentiate the amount of elemental calcium from the total amount of calcium compound in these preparations to help her get the most protection for her money. For example, the popular supplements Os-Cal, Caltrate, and the antacid Tums contain calcium in the form of calcium carbonate—which is only 40% elemental calcium. This means a 1.25-gram tablet contains only 500 mg of elemental calcium. Other calcium compounds contain even less elemental calcium: calcium glubionate, 6.5%; calcium gluconate, 9%; calcium lactate, 13%; and dibasic calcium phosphate, 23%.

While teaching your patient to increase calcium intake, remember to warn her of the dangers of too much calcium. Excessive calcium can disrupt levels of other nutritionally important minerals, including iron, zinc, and manganese. It can also cause hypercalciuria, which can lead to formation of painful renal calculi and other problems.

LARRY NEIL GEVER, RPh, PharmD

Adult vaccination—new recommendations

Recently, the Centers for Disease Control and the American College of Physicians both published guidelines for routine immunization of adults living in the United States. These guidelines

VACCINE	INDICATIONS/DOSAGE
Hepatitis B—chemically inactivated hepatitis B surface antigen particles	For all high-risk persons—susceptible male homosexuals, intravenous drug abusers, household and sexual contacts of hepatitis B carriers, dialysis patients, persons receiving clotting factors VIII or XI, mortuary workers, medical or laboratory workers frequently exposed to blood or blood products, and residents and staff of institutions for the mentally retarded: three doses (each 1 ml I.M. in the deltoid muscle), with the second dose given after 1 month, the third after 6 months; double doses for immunocompromised patients
Influenza—inactivated whole virus or subunits grown in chick embryo cells	For all high-risk persons—patients with diabetes or other metabolic diseases, severe anemia, or chronic pulmonary, cardiovascular, or renal disease; immunosuppressed patients; patients in chronic care facilities; all persons over age 65; and doctors and other personnel who have contact with high-risk persons: one dose (0.5 ml I.M.) annually
Measles—attenuated live virus grown in chick fibroblasts*	• A single dose (0.5 ml S.C.) of live measles vaccine for every person born after 1956 who didn't receive live measles vaccine after age 1 and who doesn't have absolute proof of immunity (a documented history of measles infection or laboratory evidence of immunity) • A single dose of live vaccine for all persons vaccinated between 1963 and 1967 with inactivated measles vaccine, to prevent severe atypical measles
Pneumococcal—polysaccharides from 23 types of *Streptococcus pneumoniae*	For all high-risk persons—patients with chronic cardiac or pulmonary disease, alcoholism, cirrhosis, diabetes, Hodgkin's disease, nephrotic syndrome, renal failure, cerebrospinal fluid leaks, immunosuppression, and other conditions that predispose to pneumococcal infection, particularly asplenism and sickle-cell anemia; and all persons over age 65: one dose (0.5 ml S.C. or I.M.)
Rubella—attenuated live virus grown in numan diploid cells (RA 27/3 strain)*	One dose (0.5 ml S.C.) for all unimmunized women of childbearing age and all pediatric or obstetric care workers who don't have laboratory evidence of immunity
Tetanus-diphtheria (Adult Td)—adsorbed tetanus and diphtheria toxoids	• A primary series of immunizations (two doses of 0.5 ml I.M., given 1 to 2 months apart; then one dose 6 months later) for all unimmunized persons • One Td booster injection every 10 years for everyone

*May be given as combined measles-rubella or measles-mumps-rubella vaccine.

recommend six vaccinations for routine use. Of these six vaccines, three—influenza, pneumococcal, and hepatitis B—are especially underused and should be given more frequently.

The chart below summarizes the indications, dosage, possible adverse reactions, contraindications, and other considerations for these six routine vaccinations.

ADVERSE EFFECTS	SPECIAL CONSIDERATIONS
Local pain	• Hepatitis B vaccination doesn't predispose recipients to acquired immunodeficiency syndrome (AIDS); in fact, HTLV-III virus, the causative agent of AIDS, is inactivated during the preparation of hepatitis B vaccine. • Infants born to mothers who test positive for hepatitis B surface antigen (HBsAg) should receive both the vaccine and hepatitis B immune globulin (HBIG). • Pregnancy isn't a contraindication; the vaccine poses no risk to the fetus, and hepatitis B infection in a pregnant woman can cause problems for the mother and fetus.
Fever, chills, myalgia, malaise	• Adverse reactions are rare from today's influenza vaccines. • Influenza and pneumococcal vaccinations can be given concomitantly at different sites with no loss of safety or effectiveness. • Influenza vaccination is contraindicated in patients who are allergic to eggs. • Whole virus vaccine is contraindicated in patients under age 13.
Low-grade fever	• Persons born in or before 1956 are likely immune to measles. • About 1 in 10 patients develop mild symptoms of attenuated measles (fever, malaise, anorexia, characteristic rash) within 5 to 10 days after vaccination. • Live measles vaccination is contraindicated in pregnancy, allergy to eggs, hypersensitivity to neomycin, and immuno-compromised status.
Local pain and erythema	• Pneumococcal vaccine is effective in 60% to 75% of patients with normal immune function, but severely immuno-compromised patients apparently aren't protected. • Vaccination is contraindicated in previously immunized patients, even those who received an older vaccine that contained fewer pneumococcal types; adverse reactions are much more severe following a second vaccination. • Pneumococcal and influenza vaccinations may be given concomitantly at different sites with no loss of safety or effectiveness.
Low-grade fever, rash, lymphadenopathy, sore throat, arthralgia, and arthritis	• About 40% of patients develop joint pain, usually in the small distal joints, after vaccination; frank arthritis is rare. • Arthralgias generally begin 3 days to 3 weeks after vaccination, persist for up to 11 days, and rarely recur. • Incidence of arthralgias and arthritis increases with age. • Rubella vaccination is contraindicated in pregnant women, patients with hypersensitivity to neomycin, and immunocompromised patients.
Local pain and swelling	• Arthus reaction—severe local pain and swelling—can result from too-frequent Td booster injections. • Pertussis vaccine, combined with diphtheria and tetanus for children under age 7, isn't recommended for adults. • Adult Td is contraindicated in any patient who has experienced hypersensitivity reaction to a previous dose.

Update—adverse drug reactions and interactions

As a nurse, you know that keeping up with all potentially adverse drug reactions and interactions is increasingly difficult. This chart can help. It presents recently documented adverse reactions and interactions for some commonly prescribed drugs, with nursing considerations for preventing and managing such effects.

DRUG REACTIONS

DRUG	POSSIBLE ADVERSE REACTION	NURSING CONSIDERATIONS
captopril (Capoten)	Cholestatic jaundice: itching, fever, chills, jaundiced skin	Monitor the patient's serum bilirubin levels; notify the doctor of any significant rise.
doxycycline (Vibramycin)	Dysphagia/esophagitis	To minimize adverse effects: • Have the patient remain standing for at least 90 seconds after taking the drug. • Give doxycycline with at least 100 ml of liquid. Give the drug in liquid form, whenever possible.
metoclopramide (Reglan)	Extrapyramidal symptoms ranging from mild restlessness to severe dystonia	Monitor the patient for mild adverse effects, such as insomnia or restlessness, which could herald a more severe future reaction.
metronidazole (Flagyl)	Peripheral neuropathy when used to treat patients with Crohn's disease	Monitor patients with Crohn's disease for early manifestations of peripheral neuropathy, such as paresthesias and loss of sensation; notify the doctor if they occur.
minocycline (Minocin)	Tooth staining in adolescents and young adults	Advise the patient to watch for early signs of discoloration and to immediately notify the doctor if it begins. (Unfortunately, discoloration will persist and may require cosmetic dental treatment, such as bleaching.)
penicillin G procaine	Psychosis and seizures	Screen patients for a history of psychiatric disturbance or drug or alcohol abuse; if it exists, ask the doctor to consider an alternative antibiotic.
psyllium-containing bulk laxatives (Hydrocil)	Esophageal obstruction	Help the doctor remove the gelatinous obstruction with forceps, and vigorously irrigate the throat. To prevent this reaction, make sure the patient drinks plenty of water when taking a dry bulk laxative.
sustained-release theophylline (Theo-Dur)	Diffuse macropapular skin rash	Remember to obtain a complete allergy history before administering the drug to identify any allergy to each of the drug's constituents—particularly beeswax and cornstarch.

DRUG REACTIONS *(continued)*		
DRUG	**POSSIBLE ADVERSE REACTION**	**NURSING CONSIDERATIONS**
tocainide (Tonocard)	Agranulocytosis	Monitor the patient's hematologic studies for evidence of decreasing granulocyte count; notify the doctor of any significant downward trend.
valproate sodium (Depakene syrup)	Enuresis	Reduce the total dosage and/or change scheduled administration times to give smallest dose early at night and largest dose first thing in the morning. Reassure the child and his parents that bed-wetting should stop after the dosage is adjusted.

DRUG INTERACTIONS		
DRUGS	**POSSIBLE ADVERSE INTERACTION**	**NURSING CONSIDERATIONS**
phenytoin and rifampin	Decreased seizure prevention from phenytoin (rifampin speeds up the metabolic breakdown of phenytoin, possibly blunting its effect)	Monitor the patient's neurologic status; he may need increased doses of phenytoin to keep him seizure-free. Be sure to take standard seizure precautions.
phenytoin and sucralfate	Decreased seizure prevention from phenytoin (sucralfate decreases gastrointestinal absorption of phenytoin, possibly blunting its effect)	Monitor the patient's neurologic status; he may need adjustment of phenytoin and/or sucralfate dosages to keep him seizure-free. Also, be sure to take standard seizure precautions.
warfarin and erythromycin	Increased bleeding	Monitor the patient's prothrombin time. If it's prolonged, notify the doctor; he may decrease warfarin dosage to minimize bleeding risk.
warfarin and ibuprofen	Increased bleeding	Urge the patient taking warfarin to take ibuprofen sparingly, if at all, to minimize bleeding risk.

Ribavirin—new treatment for RSV infection

Respiratory syncytial virus (RSV) infection poses a significant threat to infants and young children, affecting an estimated 800,000 each year, 100,000 of whom require hospitalization. The single most important cause of bronchopneumonia, tracheobronchitis, and pneumonia in infants and young children, RSV infection is a major cause of fatal respiratory tract disease in the first year of life, with the mortality rate for hospitalized infants approaching 5%. It's particularly dangerous in premature infants or those with an underlying cardiopulmonary disease.

Until now, no drug has proven

effective in treating RSV infection; standard treatment has consisted of supporting respiratory function, maintaining fluid balance, and relieving symptoms. But a new drug—ribavirin (Virazole)—promises effective treatment of the infection, not just its symptoms. Ribavirin, a synthetic analog of guanosine, inhibits RNA—and hence protein—synthesis. The drug, indicated for treatment of certain hospitalized infants and young children with severe lower respiratory tract infections from RSV, is delivered directly to the lungs in an aerosol mist form by a specially designed small-particle aerosol generator (pictured below), with the patient in a hood or tent.

Ribavirin therapy consists of 12 to 18 hours of aerosol delivery per day, for 3 to 7 days. It's most effective when started within the first 3 days of RSV infection and when combined with a total treatment program that includes standard supportive measures to maintain respiration and fluid balance. Ribavirin shouldn't be administered with other aerosolized medications (the small-particle aerosol generator is de-signed specifically for ribavirin) and shouldn't be given to patients requiring assisted ventilation (ribavirin can precipitate in respiratory equipment, interfering with ventilation). Serious adverse reactions—among them apnea and hypotension—have occurred in severely ill infants with life-threatening underlying disorders, many of whom required ventilatory assistance, but the role of ribavirin in these reactions is unclear. Minor adverse effects, such as rash and conjunctivitis, have also been documented.

Besides treatment of infants and young children with RSV infection, ribavirin may have other important clinical applications. In world-wide studies, this broad-spectrum antiviral has proven effective against influenza A and B, parainfluenza, measles, chicken pox, herpes simplex, herpes zoster, hepatitis A, and hemorrhagic fever. Use of ribavirin for these applications in the U.S. is pending FDA approval, however. Currently, ribavirin is widely used by victims of acquired immunodeficiency syndrome (AIDS), who obtain the drug in Mexico. Clinical trials to

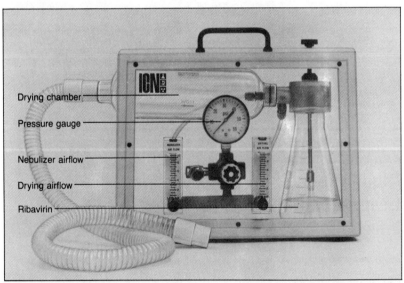

Drying chamber

Pressure gauge

Nebulizer airflow

Drying airflow

Ribavirin

The SPAG-2 small-particle aerosol generator (shown above) is used to deliver an aerosol mist of ribavirin directly to the lungs.

ribavirin
(Virazole)

MECHANISM OF ACTION
Inhibits viral activity by an unknown mechanism. Thought to inhibit RNA and DNA synthesis by depleting intracellular nucleotide pools.

INDICATION & DOSAGE
Treatment of hospitalized infants and young children infected by respiratory syncytial virus (RSV)—
Infants and young children: Solution in concentration of 20 mg/ml delivered via a small-particle aerosol generator (SPAG-2). Treatment is carried out for 12 to 18 hours per day for at least 3, and no more than 7, days.

ADVERSE REACTIONS
• Blood: anemia, reticulocytosis
• CV: *cardiac arrest,* hypotension
• Other: *worsening of respiratory status, bacterial pneumonia, pneumothorax, apnea, ventilator dependence*

INTERACTIONS
None known

NURSING CONSIDERATIONS
• Contraindicated in women or girls who are or may become pregnant during exposure to drug.

• Ribavirin aerosol is indicated only for lower respiratory tract infection due to RSV. Although treatment may be started while awaiting diagnostic test results, existence of RSV infection must eventually be documented.
• Most infants and children with RSV infection don't require treatment because disease is often mild and self-limited. Those with underlying conditions such as prematurity or cardiopulmonary disease will benefit best from treatment with ribavirin aerosol since they get the disease in its most severe form.
• This treatment must be accompanied by, and does not replace, supportive respiratory and fluid management.
• Ribavirin aerosol *must* be administered by the Viratek SPAG-2 small-particle aerosol generator. Don't use any other aerosol generating device.
• The water used to solubilize the drug must not have any antimicrobial agent added. Use sterile USP water for injection, *not* bacteriostatic water.
• Discard solutions placed in the SPAG-2 unit at least every 24 hours before adding newly reconstituted solution.
• Store reconstituted solutions at room temperature for 24 hours.

test this drug's effectiveness in treating AIDS are now under way.

LARRY NEIL GEVER, RPh, PharmD

Somatrem—new biosynthetic growth hormone

Until 1985, children with growth hormone deficiency were routinely treated with human pituitary-derived growth hormone (pit-hGH) to help them achieve normal adult height. This therapy proved effective, but was associated with certain problems. The most serious surfaced in the 1980s, when researchers first linked administration of pit-hGH to at least three cases of Jakob-Creutzfeldt disease, a rare, invariably fatal viral infection that causes spongiform cerebellar degeneration. After this report, use of pit-hGH was curtailed and finally discontinued entirely by September 1985.

But the estimated 10,000 to 15,000 growth hormone-deficient children in the United States need not be deprived of effective treatment. For a new biosynthetic growth hormone—somatrem (Protropin)—gained FDA approval in October 1985 and is now available for use.

Somatrem is a polypeptide hormone

RECOMBINANT D.N.A. PRODUCTION TECHNIQUES

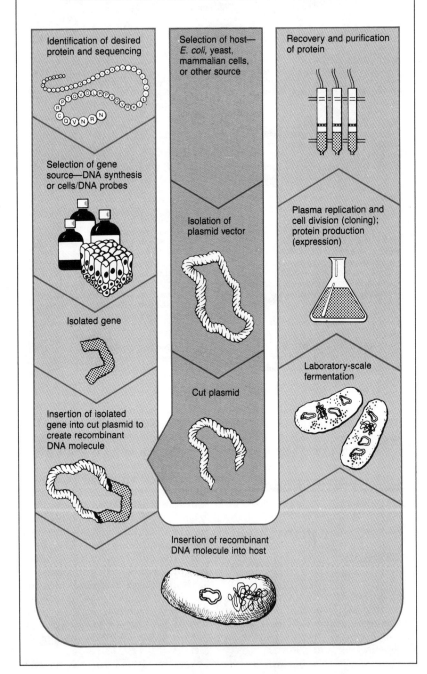

Identification of desired protein and sequencing

Selection of host—*E. coli*, yeast, mammalian cells, or other source

Recovery and purification of protein

Selection of gene source—DNA synthesis or cells/DNA probes

Isolation of plasmid vector

Plasma replication and cell division (cloning); protein production (expression)

Isolated gene

Cut plasmid

Laboratory-scale fermentation

Insertion of isolated gene into cut plasmid to create recombinant DNA molecule

Insertion of recombinant DNA molecule into host

somatrem
(Protropin)

MECHANISM OF ACTION
Purified growth hormone of recombinant DNA origin which stimulates linear, skeletal muscle, and organ growth.

INDICATION & DOSAGE
Long-term treatment of children who have growth failure due to a lack of adequate endogenous growth hormone secretion— *Children* (pre-puberty): 0.1 mg/kg I.M. given 3 times weekly.

ADVERSE REACTIONS
• Endocrine: *hypothyroidism, hyperglycemia*
• Other: *antibodies to growth hormone*

INTERACTIONS
Glucocorticoids: may inhibit growth-promoting action of somatrem. Glucocorticoid dose may need to be adjusted.

NURSING CONSIDERATIONS
• Contraindicated in patients with closed epiphyses; in patients who have an active underlying intracranial lesion; in patients with known sensitivity to benzyl alcohol.
• Use cautiously in patients whose growth hormone deficiency results from an intracranial lesion. Patient should be examined frequently for progression or recurrence of the underlying disease process.
• Observe patient for signs of glucose intolerance and hyperglycemia.
• Monitor periodic thyroid function tests for hypothyroidism. If hypothyroidism occurs, doctor will treat with a thyroid hormone.
• This drug replaces pituitary-derived human growth hormone, which was removed from the market in 1985 because of an association with the development of a rare but fatal virus infection (Jakob-Creutzfeldt disease). Reassure your patient and his family that somatrem is *pure* and that it is *safe*.
• To prepare the solution, inject the bacteriostatic water for injection (which is supplied) into the vial containing the drug. Then swirl the vial with a gentle rotary motion until the contents are completely dissolved. *Don't shake* the vial.
• After reconstitution, vial solution should be clear. Don't inject into the patient if the solution is cloudy or contains particulate matter.
• Store reconstituted vial in refrigerator. Must use within 7 days.
• Be sure to observe product's expiration date.

synthesized through the use of recombinant DNA techniques. In this process, the gene responsible for human growth hormone production is isolated and introduced into a vector, the bacterium *Escherichia coli,* for cloning in a bacterial culture. Because somatrem is a synthetic hormone produced under strict laboratory controls, it's much "cleaner" than growth hormone derived from human pituitary glands, which is often subject to viral contamination, as happened in the transmission of Jakob-Creutzfeldt disease. Synthetic growth hormone can be produced in abundance, whereas production of pit-hGH relied on the availability of healthy human pituitary glands.

Somatrem, the second recombinant DNA-produced drug to gain FDA approval for human use (the first was human insulin [Humulin]), has performed well in clinical trials, tripling the average growth rate of children with growth hormone deficiency during the first year of therapy and more than doubling growth rates during the second and third years. Approximately 30% of patients treated with somatrem in these trials developed persistent antibodies to growth hormone; however, this response hasn't been associated with toxicity, and only one patient demonstrated interference with the growth response to somatrem.

Caution required
Several considerations apply to somatrem therapy, however. Since somatrem may induce a state of insulin resistance, you should observe any

patient receiving somatrem for signs of glucose intolerance. Because the concurrent use of a glucocorticoid, such as dexamethasone, hydrocortisone, or prednisolone, may inhibit the growth-stimulating effects of somatrem, patients with coexisting growth hormone and adrenocorticotropic hormone deficiencies need precise adjustment of glucocorticoid replacement doses to ensure optimal growth rate. And because hypothyroidism can develop from somatrem therapy, interfering with growth rate, patients taking somatrem need periodic thyroid function tests and treatment with thyroid replacement hormone when necessary.

The sooner somatrem therapy begins, the more likely the child is to achieve normal adult height. Somatrem is effective only until linear bone growth ceases and the epiphyses close, usually at the end of puberty. It's contraindicated for use after this period, and is also contraindicated when evidence exists of underlying progressive intracranial lesions.

LARRY NEIL GEVER, RPh, PharmD

Aldose reductase inhibitors for diabetes complications

Late complications of diabetes mellitus primarily affect the eyes, kidneys, nervous system, and large blood vessels. With the exception of large blood vessel complications (coronary artery, cerebrovascular, and peripheral vascular disease), the development of these complications seems related to the metabolic abnormalities associated with hyperglycemia, since they generally develop in tissues in which glucose transport doesn't depend on insulin. Although the exact mechanism by which hyperglycemia causes damage in individual tissues remains un-

known, growing evidence suggests that the enzyme aldose reductase plays an important role. Based on this evidence, regulation of aldose reductase through the use of potent inhibitors of this enzyme appears to provide a promising new method of treating these insulin-independent complications.

Ocular complications

Chief among these complications, in terms of seriousness and number of patients affected, are those involving the eyes, specifically diabetic retinopathy and cataracts. (Blindness is 25 times more common in diabetic persons than in nondiabetic persons.)

But how does hyperglycemia cause these ocular complications? Briefly, it begins when, in response to a hyperglycemic state, aldose reductase converts excess glucose to sugar alcohol, or sorbitol. Because lens membranes are fairly impervious to sorbitol, sorbitol builds up, eventually creating a hypertonic condition that draws water into the lens fibers to maintain osmotic equilibrium. This osmotic swelling sets off a chain reaction that causes ruptured blood vessels and other damage and ultimately results in retinopathy and/or cataracts.

New drug offers hope

Once the role of aldose reductase in the development of these complications became clear, researchers set out to develop a drug that would block or inhibit its action. After years of research and development, a potent new aldose reductase inhibitor, sorbinil, was approved for use in clinical trials on humans. Early results of these trials are promising, suggesting that sorbinil can, in fact, delay and possibly prevent the osmotic changes that cause ocular damage and loss of sight. Although the drug doesn't appear to reverse existing damage, it does seem to offer real hope for prevention and early treatment of diabetic retinopathy, cataracts, and other ocular complications.

LARRY NEIL GEVER, RPh, PharmD

Drug therapy in the elderly

Nowadays, you're probably caring for more and more people over age 65. Chances are, you're also seeing more serious drug reactions and interactions than with younger patients.

Why are the elderly so susceptible to adverse reactions? And why are these reactions so much more serious than in younger patients? For answers, you must consider several factors.

To begin with, the aging process produces physiologic changes that can significantly alter drug actions and effects, possibly causing an adverse reaction. If such a reaction occurs, many of the same physiologic changes that contributed to the reaction also limit the patient's ability to cope with it. As a result, an adverse reaction may have more serious consequences for an elderly patient than it would for someone younger.

Further complicating the picture is the fact that many elderly patients develop chronic illnesses requiring drug therapy. Most of these patients take several different prescription medications daily; they may regularly use over-the-counter drugs as well. Each time a patient adds a new drug to his daily regimen, he increases his risk of experiencing adverse drug reactions and interactions.

How aging influences drug action

The aging process changes anatomy and physiology in ways that alter many body functions. Though age-related changes aren't always apparent, they can significantly alter the absorption, distribution, metabolism, and excretion of drugs.

Absorption. Some studies suggest that aging reduces the absorption rate for several reasons. First, decreased hydrochloric acid secretion may reduce the acidity of stomach contents. As a result, oral drugs that require an acid medium for absorption are either absorbed more slowly or not at all. These drugs include iron, salicylates, oral anticoagulants, nitrofurantoin (Furadantin), probenecid (Benemid), digoxin, and tetracycline (Achromycin, Tetracyn).

Second, intestinal villi become shorter and broader with age, decreasing the intestine's surface area. Finally, reduced GI motility and blood flow may also decrease absorption.

Distribution. Drug distribution changes for several reasons. First, plasma protein levels (particularly albumin levels) decrease, reducing the number of protein-binding sites. As a result, the amount of free drug increases, and the drug remains active in the patient's system longer.

In addition, an elderly patient's active and passive transport systems function less efficiently. This impedes drug transfer across tissue membranes.

Changes in body mass also affect drug distribution. With aging, water volume and lean tissue diminish. Since water-soluble drugs normally distribute to body fluid and lean tissue, the reduced availability of either increases the concentration of these drugs in their free (active) forms. Conversely, because the proportion of fatty tissue increases with age, the aging body tends to retain lipid-soluble drugs, which prolongs their action.

Metabolism. Decreased hepatic blood flow, smaller liver size, and reduced production of enzymes that break down most drugs slow drug metabolism in the elderly. As a result, drugs remain active in their systems longer. These metabolic changes can be further aggravated by certain medical conditions, such as congestive heart failure.

Excretion. The kidneys are the primary excretion site for most drugs (or their metabolites), including such commonly ordered drugs as digoxin, most antibiotics, and many antidiabetic agents. But because renal blood flow

RECOMMENDED DRUG DOSAGES FOR ELDERLY PATIENTS

DRUG NAME (generic)	DOSAGE
albuterol	Initial dose: 2 mg t.i.d. or q.i.d. If bronchodilation is inadequate, dosage may be increased gradually to 8 mg t.i.d. or q.i.d.
alprazolam	Initial dose: 0.25 mg b.i.d. or t.i.d. This dosage may be gradually increased if needed and tolerated.
amitriptyline	10 mg t.i.d. with 20 mg at bedtime may be satisfactory in elderly patients who do not tolerate higher dosages.
amitriptyline/ perphenazine	Initial dose: Triavil 4-10 t.i.d. or q.i.d.; adjusted as required.
chlorpropamide	Initial dose: 100 to 125 mg daily.
clorazepate	Initial dose: 7.5 to 15 mg, adjusted as required by patient's response. Lower doses may be indicated.
diazepam	Initial dose: 2 to 2.5 mg q.d. or b.i.d., increasing gradually as needed and tolerated.
diflunisal	Initial dose: Half of usual adult dose in persons over age 80.
digoxin	Usual dose: 0.125 mg P.O. q.d. Frail or very small elderly and those with diminished kidney function may require only 0.0625 mg P.O. q.d., or 0.125 mg P.O. every other day.
flurazepam	Initial dose: 15 mg at bedtime.
haloperidol	Optimal response is usually obtained at lower dosage, 0.5 mg to 2 mg b.i.d. or t.i.d.
levothyroxine sodium	Initial dose: As little as 25 mcg (0.025 mg) per day, increased by 25 mcg at 3- to 4-week intervals, depending on patient response.
lorazepam	Initial dose: 1 to 2 mg per day, in divided doses, adjusted as needed and tolerated.
NSAIDs	Initial dose: Half of usual adult dose in persons over age 80.
oxazepam	Initial dose: 10 mg t.i.d. If necessary, increase cautiously to 15 mg, t.i.d. or q.i.d.
oxyphenbutazone	Initial dose: Half of usual adult dose, increased as needed and tolerated. Therapy should not exceed 1 week.
prazepam	Initial dose: 10 to 15 mg daily in divided doses.
temazepam	Initial dose: 15 mg at bedtime.
thioridazine	Initial dose: 25 mg t.i.d.
thyroid hormone	Reduce replacement by 25% in persons over age 60.
tolazamide	Initial dose: 100 mg once daily.
triazolam	Initial dose: 0.125 mg at bedtime. Dosage range: 0.125 to 0.25 mg at bedtime.

SENILITY OR DRUG REACTIONS?

Many drugs can cause symptoms often attributed to senility, such as confusion and forgetfulness. Review the chart below and be alert for drugs (or drug combinations) that may cause such symptoms. If you suspect that your patient's problem is drug-related, alert the doctor so he can adjust drug therapy.

SYMPTOMS	POSSIBLE CAUSES
Confusion	Methyldopa, digoxin, and cimetidine
Depression	Reserpine
Anorexia	Digoxin
Weakness	Certain diuretics, such as furosemide and hydrochlorothiazide, which can deplete potassium
Lethargy and drowsiness	Various antianxiety agents, analgesics, antihistamines, and sleep medications, including chlorpromazine and pentobarbital
Ataxia	Phenytoin, very high doses of flurazepam (and other sedatives), or hypnotics
Forgetfulness	Barbiturates and methyldopa
Constipation	Medications with anticholinergic properties, such as belladonna-containing drugs, narcotics, tricyclic antidepressants, and iron preparations
Diarrhea	Antacid preparations containing magnesium; quinidine

diminishes during the aging process, the elderly patient's kidneys filter and excrete these drugs more slowly. And because fewer of his renal tubules continue to function, glomerular filtration, tubular reabsorption, and active tubular secretion progress more slowly. The combined effect of these age-related changes is a longer half-life for most drugs, a factor that can cause drug toxicity in the elderly patient.

Other influences

As a patient ages, tissue sensitivity changes, heightening the effects of some drugs. As a result, more of these drugs remain active in the patient's system. This is especially true of barbiturates, which are especially potent for elderly patients.

Decreased hormonal secretion may inhibit drug action at receptor sites. Replacement therapy may be necessary to counteract the decline. However, replacement therapy can increase the sensitivity of receptor sites.

Finally, keep in mind that aging can affect a patient's compliance as well as his physiologic response to drug therapy. Cerebral arteriosclerosis, for example, can cause many behavioral disorders, including memory loss, confusion, and lethargy. These problems, in turn, can lead to poor compliance, accidental overdose, or use of the wrong drug. But don't make the mistake of assuming that a patient exhibiting behavioral disorders associated with old age is senile. He may be experiencing adverse reactions from one or more of his drugs. For guidelines on distinguishing between senility and adverse drug reactions, see above.

LARRY NEIL GEVER, RPh, PharmD

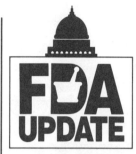

FDA UPDATE

Fluoride rinse precautions

Although regular use of an over-the-counter fluoride rinse can help prevent dental caries, excessive consumption can lead to mottling of the teeth. This is a problem particularly for young children, who tend to swallow rather than spit out rinses and mouthwashes. Because of this possible adverse effect, the FDA recommends that children under age 12 use fluoride rinses only with adult supervision, and that children under age 6 not use them without a dentist's or doctor's approval.

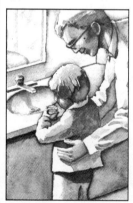

Burns from Hibitane Tincture

Patients prepped with Hibitane Tincture before electrocautery can suffer serious thermal burns if the preparation isn't allowed to dry properly. An antimicrobial preparation containing 0.5% chlorhexidine gluconate in 70% isopropyl alcohol, Hibitane Tincture is used to cleanse operative sites before surgery or skin puncture. Although manufacture of the product has been discontinued, some hospitals are still using residual supplies.

To avoid burns, follow these precautions while prepping patients with Hibitane Tincture:
• Make sure the skin is *completely* dry.
• Remove excess liquid with a sterile towel; don't allow Hibitane Tincture to pool around the patient.

Failure to follow these directions may cause the alcohol in the preparation to ignite during electrocautery, burning the patient's skin.

Safety of hepatitis B vaccine confirmed

Fears that the hepatitis B (HB) vaccine could somehow cause acquired immunodeficiency syndrome (AIDS) are unfounded, according to the FDA. Recent studies have confirmed that HTLV-III, the human retrovirus identified as the etiologic agent for AIDS, isn't transmitted by HB vaccine. These concerns arose from the fact that HB vaccine is produced from the pooled plasma of persons with asymptomatic chronic hepatitis B infections—some of whom could be in high-risk groups for AIDS. But careful inactivation procedures used in the manufacturing process, along with strict testing of each lot for sterility, antigenicity, and immunogenicity (including inoculation

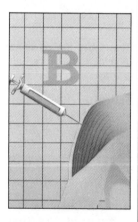

into mice, guinea pigs, and human-derived cell cultures), ensures safety of the HB vaccine. Researchers found that after these inactivation procedures, the vaccine contained no detectable HTLV-III virus.

DES Task Force recommendations

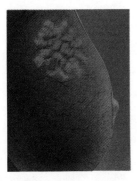

Research on the long-term effects of diethylstilbestrol (DES) prescribed during pregnancy continues. The U.S. Department of Health and Human Services (HHS) 1985 DES Task Force has reviewed recent studies showing a possible increased risk of breast cancer in women who were given DES while pregnant (DES mothers) and a possible excessive rate of precancerous cervical and vaginal abnormalities in women who were exposed to DES *in utero* (DES daughters). Based on this research, the Task Force has recommended that doctors continue attempts to locate and notify women for whom they prescribed DES during pregnancy, and that the HHS continue to support and encourage research on the possible adverse effects of DES. (Although the Task Force didn't review recent studies on DES-exposed males [DES sons] in depth, it stated that previous recommendations—careful medical history and thorough physical examination—still seemed appropriate.) In addition, the Task Force recommends the continued dissemination of DES research information to all doctors and DES mothers and their offspring, and continued surveillance of DES mothers, daughters, and sons.

Minoxidil for baldness

As you may know, topical reformulations of oral minoxidil (Loniten) have gained widespread use for the treatment of male pattern baldness. This use follows the discovery that hypertrichosis occurs as a side effect in 80% of patients who take minoxidil for hypertension, its approved application.

But because the safety and effectiveness of applying this drug topically for treating baldness hasn't yet been clinically established, the FDA has asked doctors and pharmacists to refrain from recompounding the oral tablets for topical use. And until much more is known about the side effects and long-term safety of these preparations, the FDA urges individuals not to use them.

Reye's syndrome and salicylates

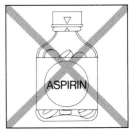

Mounting evidence continues to link the use of aspirin and other salicylates to treat influenza or chicken pox to the development of Reye's syndrome (RS) in children and adolescents. But, on a brighter note, recent evidence also points to a greater public awareness of this link. In a telephone survey recently conducted by the FDA, only 12% of the 1,155 parents surveyed said they would give their children aspirin for the flu or chicken pox. This compares quite favorably to a 1981 Centers for Disease Control survey, in which 69% of parents were likely to give aspirin to children with these conditions. The FDA attributes this increased public awareness of the RS-salicylate link to its own public education campaign, as well as to the efforts of drug manufacturers, pharmacists, doctors, and nurses.

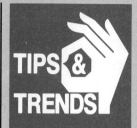

REDUCES RISK

Aspirin for MI prophylaxis

According to recent U.S. and foreign studies, an aspirin a day can help prevent heart attacks. The studies, involving more than 12,000 patients with myocardial infarction (MI) or unstable angina, concluded that the use of aspirin can greatly reduce the risk of new or recurring MI in such patients. Based on these studies, the FDA has issued new guidelines on aspirin prophylaxis for MI. Recommended dosage is 300 to 325 mg per day of any conventional aspirin product (higher doses can cause gastrointestinal bleeding and possibly other GI disturbances). However, because of buffered aspirin's high sodium content (over 500 mg per tablet), this form is contraindicated in patients with sodium-retaining disorders such as congestive heart failure or renal failure.

ANTIHYPERTENSIVE AGENTS

Calcium channel blockers: A new application

Quick quiz: What are the characteristics of the ideal antihypertensive drug? First, it should be monotherapeutic—not requiring the assistance of other drugs for effectiveness. Second, it should cause minimal side effects. Third, it should be effective in a single daily dose to help ensure patient compliance with drug therapy. And finally, it should be affordable; after all, antihypertensive therapy is a lifelong proposition that can be quite expensive.

Wishful thinking? Maybe not; some doctors think the ideal antihypertensive drug is available now—and has been since the early 1980s. The drug? It's actually a class of drugs—calcium channel blockers. Originally developed to treat certain cardiac dysrhythmias and angina pectoris, calcium channel blockers are now being touted as effective agents in the treatment of essential, or primary, hypertension as well.

But despite widespread clinical evidence of its effectiveness in this application, calcium channel blockers have not yet received FDA approval for use in the treatment of hypertension. However, many doctors are currently prescribing them for their hypertensive patients regardless of the official FDA position, and are quite pleased with the results.

Based on clinical results to date, calcium channel blockers seem a particularly good choice for patients who sometimes experience problems with currently approved modes of therapy, particularly beta-adrenergic blockers and diuretics. These patients include insulin-dependent diabetics with hypertension, hypertensive patients with a history of bronchospasm, and, perhaps most importantly, patients with low-renin hypertension—a category that includes the elderly and blacks.

CALCIUM BINDS ACTIN AND MYOSIN

Calcium is stored in a muscle fiber's sarcoplasmic reticulum. When muscle cells depolarize, they release calcium. Calcium permits binding between two protein filaments called actin and myosin, causing the fiber's sarcomeres to shorten and the fiber to contract.

The illustration at right is a conceptual representation of the cross-bridges that form when actin and myosin bind together.

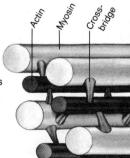

Nitroglycerin spray for acute angina

Angina sufferers now have an alternative to sublingual nitroglycerin tablets for relief of their pain. A new drug formulation, nitroglycerin lingual aerosol (Nitrolingual Spray), has been introduced in the United States after almost two decades of successful use in Europe. The new drug, indicated for the management of acute angina pectoris due to coronary artery disease, is a metered-dose aerosol containing nitroglycerin in propellant. The spray canister contains 200 metered 0.4-mg doses of nitroglycerin, the same

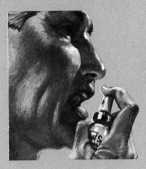

dose as in most sublingual tablets. The spray seems to have several key advantages over tablets, however. Unlike tablets, which need a short time to

dissolve, the aerosol spray is rapidly absorbed through the oral mucosa, providing almost instant pain relief. The canister may be easier to handle than tablets during an acute angina attack, particularly for sight-impaired, arthritic, or otherwise disabled patients. The canister also protects the nitroglycerin from contact with heat and light, prolonging its potency for up to 3 years. In contrast, tablets begin to deteriorate immediately upon contact with air, and usually retain potency for no longer than 3 to 6 months.

Amitriptyline for pathologic crying and laughing

Some victims of multiple sclerosis, stroke, brain trauma, or other disorders causing damage to the subcortical forebrain structures that mediate emotional expression experience a bizarre and troubling symptom: unpredictable paroxysms of laughing and crying. These emotional outbursts are totally involuntary and unpredictable, bearing no relationship to the patient's underlying mood. For the victim, this can be an annoying and embarrassing problem that can interfere with social interaction and adjustment.

Until now, little could be done for such a patient.

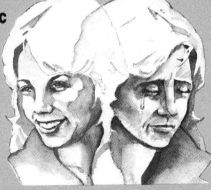

But a recent study reports some success in controlling these symptoms using low doses of the antidepressant drug amitriptyline. Of the 12 patients who completed the study, 8 showed significant improvement within 48 hours. Because doses of amitriptyline given during the

study were lower than those usually required to affect mood, and because the patients scored no differently on depression-rating scales during the test than they did before it, researchers believe that some mechanism of amitriptyline other than antidepressant must be responsible for this effect.

Buspirone—an alternative antianxiety drug

Despite the long-standing popularity of diazepam (Valium) and other benzodiazepine antianxiety agents, problems with addiction, adverse effects, and dangerous interactions with alcohol and other drugs have caused a gradual decline in their use over the last decade. Now, a unique new antianxiety agent—buspirone (Buspar)—may prove to be an attractive alternative to the benzodiazepines.

According to recent studies, buspirone is at least as effective as diazepam in reducing anxiety. But because it belongs to a new class of drugs, the azaspirodecanediones, that is structurally dissimilar to the benzodiazepines, its mechanism of action is entirely different. Whereas benzodiazepines reduce anxiety by inhibiting the central nervous system—producing sedation, euphoria, and other effects of CNS depression—azaspirodecanediones seem to act more selectively, reducing anxiety without overall CNS depression. This gives buspirone a wider safety margin in patients who consume alcohol or other depressants while on antianxiety drug therapy, those who need large doses of antianxiety agents and thus risk dependence or addiction, and those who cannot tolerate the sedative effects of diazepam.

Neuroleptic malignant syndrome

Neuroleptic drugs—antipsychotic agents and "heavy" tranquilizers—are among the most commonly prescribed drugs today. They're widely used to treat psychotic disorders and Tourette's syndrome, as antiemetics, and for dissociative anesthesia. Neuroleptics have many well-known side effects, such as extrapyramidal symptoms. But they also can cause an often-fatal reaction that's frequently overlooked: neuroleptic malignant syndrome (NMS). Most common in young men—although it can strike all ages and both sexes—NMS produces hyperthermia, muscle rigidity and akinesia, altered consciousness, and autonomic symptoms such as pallor, diaphoresis, tachycardia, cardiac dysrhythmias, and blood pressure instability. Mortality is as high as 30%, typically from cardiopulmonary and/or renal complications. Onset of NMS is rapid, usually over a period of 24 to 72 hours. Deaths generally occur between 3 and 30 days after symptoms first appear.

You can guard against NMS in patients receiving neuroleptic drugs by carefully monitoring vital signs and neurologic status. If you detect any of NMS's characteristic signs, immediately discontinue the drug, call the doctor, and begin necessary supportive measures. The drugs dantrolene, pancuronium, amantadine, and bromocriptine have all shown promise in treatment of NMS.

Alpha-2-interferon for the common cold

Often claimed but never realized, effective treatment and prevention of the common cold may finally be at hand. Results of two major clinical studies have shown that alpha-2-interferon nasal spray effectively combats rhinovirus, the most prevalent cold virus. Because colds spread largely through contact—usually hand-to-hand—between family members, the two studies employed entire families as their subjects. Randomized, double-blind, and placebo-controlled, the studies used large doses (5 million units) of alpha-2-interferon nasal spray. Whenever one family member developed cold symptoms, the other family members used either the interferon spray or an identical-looking placebo spray once a day over a 7-day course of treatment.

The results? Researchers found that family members who used alpha-2-interferon spray developed about 40% fewer colds than those who used the placebo. The interferon proved especially effective against rhinovirus, producing an approximate 87% reduction in rhinovirus-related colds.

Two problems with earlier interferon sprays—high incidence of nasal bleeding and high cost—seem solved. In the recent studies, only 12% to 14% of patients experienced minor nasal bleeding. And recently developed recombinant DNA production methods have reduced the price of interferon dramatically; with increased demand, it should drop even further. One alpha-2-interferon spray—Intron—is currently awaiting FDA approval. Similar products will surely follow.

Beta blockers for stage fright

Stage fright (or, more accurately, *performance anxiety*) doesn't affect only performers: it strikes many people in many different situations far removed from the footlights. Virtually everyone feels a little nervous when speaking in public. Students may suffer symptoms of performance anxiety before an important test, athletes before a big game or competition, and job seekers before an interview. Some people seem able to not only cope with this anxiety, but to actually perform better under pressure. But for many others, performance anxiety can cause problems at work and in social situations.

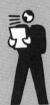

Some doctors are now prescribing beta blockers such as propranolol (Inderal), commonly used to treat angina and hypertension, for their patients suffering from performance anxiety. They've found that beta blockers inhibit sympathetic peripheral activity at the beta-adrenergic receptors, decreasing and, in some cases, eliminating the autonomic symptoms of performance anxiety—diaphoresis, tachycardia, tremor, and palpitations.

Beta blockers may be especially useful for musicians such as pianists and violinists, for whom trembling hands and sweaty palms could spell disaster. However, their most widespread benefit is probably in treating the many people who fear public speaking.

Unlike heart patients, who must take a prescribed beta blocker every day, persons suffering from performance anxiety need take only a single dose of the drug a few hours before the event or performance and so are unlikely to experience adverse reactions.

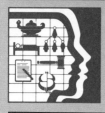

Law, ethics, and professional practice

COMPUTERS
IN NURSING
PRACTICE

"Chances are,
as a nurse, you're
using computers
now in some aspect
of your practice.
You can bet
you'll be using them
more and more
in the future."

SHARON C. NILSEN, RN, BSN

By now, most hospitals and health care agencies have installed computer systems to keep track of everything from billing to patient care information. Chances are, as a nurse, you're using computers now in some aspect of your practice. You can bet you'll be using them more and more in the future. Here's some of what you can expect.

What computers can do

Today's computers can perform a remarkable number of functions: store, categorize, and quickly retrieve patient information; standardize patient assessments; help prepare patient care plans; calculate equivalent drug doses and monitor medication schedules; organize and file educational materials; and provide instant communication with several departments, among many other possible applications. A nurse-manager can use a computer to monitor costs of patient care, classify patient acuity, and make staffing decisions. A staff nurse could possibly check a patient's laboratory test results, document his care, order drugs from the pharmacy, call up a doctor's orders, check when the operating room is ready for a patient, or alert the dietary department about a patient's dietary restrictions—all within minutes and without leaving the nurses' station.

Basically, computers streamline paperwork, giving nurses more time to do what they do best: provide patient care. They also save money—an important consideration in today's cost-constrained health care environment. Because of these attributes, computers are changing the way we work.

Some practical applications

You've probably already experienced the great usefulness of computers in medical record keeping, where they can save you a lot of time and reduce the chances of error and misinterpretation of orders and information. But besides record keeping, computers also offer nurses other important advantages in such areas as patient care planning, patient teaching, nursing management, and quality assurance.

Patient care planning

Computerized patient care planning can save you time and help you provide better patient care. A computer system can store standard care plans that you can use as the foundation for planning individual care. Such care plans might contain the minimal care requirements of patients in certain groups and list various options, from which you can choose the most appropriate. You can develop an individualized care plan by modifying one of these standard plans or by building the plan from the patient's nursing diagnosis.

With a computer-generated patient care plan, you and the patient's doctor can see at a glance the patient's status, present and future orders, and the care already provided. If the doctor requests a comprehensive review of all patient orders throughout the length of stay, you don't have to search through a chart or Kardex; with the computer, you can produce this information in minutes. Unlike the manual Kardex, which is discarded after a patient's discharge, the computer-generated care plan becomes part of the patient's permanent record. This not only provides valuable data for patient care conferences, but also serves as an excellent reference for reassessing the patient's needs upon any subsequent readmission.

Patient teaching

Using computer-assisted instruction as a tool for self-directed learning, you can help patients understand more about their physical condition, surgery, medications, and medical treatments than ever before. The patient can learn at his own pace and in a relaxed environment, thereby increasing understanding and, ultimately, compliance.

This application can also reduce the amount of teaching time you need to spend with a patient and his family, freeing you for other duties.

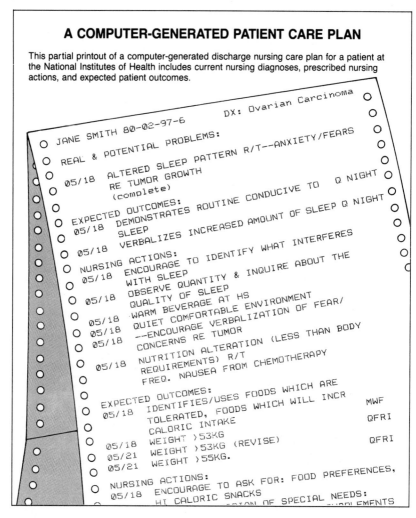

A COMPUTER-GENERATED PATIENT CARE PLAN

This partial printout of a computer-generated discharge nursing care plan for a patient at the National Institutes of Health includes current nursing diagnoses, prescribed nursing actions, and expected patient outcomes.

```
                                        DX: Ovarian Carcinoma   O
                                                                O
  O  JANE SMITH 80-02-97-6                                      O
  O  REAL & POTENTIAL PROBLEMS:                                 O
  O   05/18  ALTERED SLEEP PATTERN R/T--ANXIETY/FEARS           O
  O          RE TUMOR GROWTH                                    O
  O          (complete)                                         O
  O   EXPECTED OUTCOMES:  ROUTINE CONDUCIVE TO   Q NIGHT         O
  O     05/18  DEMONSTRATES                                     O
  O          SLEEP                                              O
  O     05/18  VERBALIZES INCREASED AMOUNT OF SLEEP Q NIGHT      O
  O   NURSING ACTIONS:                                          O
  O     05/18  ENCOURAGE TO IDENTIFY WHAT INTERFERES            O
  O          WITH SLEEP                                         O
  O     05/18  OBSERVE QUANTITY & INQUIRE ABOUT THE
  O          QUALITY OF SLEEP
  O     05/18  WARM BEVERAGE AT HS
  O     05/18  QUIET COMFORTABLE ENVIRONMENT
  O     05/18  --ENCOURAGE VERBALIZATION OF FEAR/
  O          CONCERNS RE TUMOR
  O     05/18  NUTRITION ALTERATION (LESS THAN BODY
  O          REQUIREMENTS) R/T
  O          FREQ. NAUSEA FROM CHEMOTHERAPY
  O   EXPECTED OUTCOMES:
  O     05/18  IDENTIFIES/USES FOODS WHICH ARE
  O          TOLERATED, FOODS WHICH WILL INCR       MWF
  O          CALORIC INTAKE                          QFRI
  O     05/18  WEIGHT >53KG
  O     05/18  WEIGHT >53KG (REVISE)                 QFRI
  O     05/21  WEIGHT >55KG.
  O   NURSING ACTIONS:
  O     05/18  ENCOURAGE TO ASK FOR: FOOD PREFERENCES,
  O          HI CALORIC SNACKS
                        ...ION OF SPECIAL ...PPLEMENTS    NEEDS:
```

Nursing management

As you know, in today's financially constrained Diagnosis-Related Group (DRG) environment, nursing departments are expected to provide more skilled nursing care with fewer resources. To make sure nursing gets an adequate share of the health care dollar, nursing administrators need to convince hospital administrators of nursing's financial worth to the hospital organization by clearly showing them that the nursing department is an income-producing area of the hospi-

tal's operations.

To claim the actual cost of nursing services—beyond the traditional "room and board" charge—nurses need precise indexes of individual patient care requirements, care delivered, and resulting effects on patient status. Computer-generated patient care plans provide this information. The care plan details the patient care required and the nursing care given. The information provided by the care plan helps answer the question "What do nurses really do?"

By systematically analyzing these plans in relation to specific DRGs, nurse-managers can determine patterns of nursing interventions and patient outcomes, and analyze how they relate to factors such as length of hospital stay, incidence of complications, and the need for patient teaching in preparation for discharge. The result is objective and readily available data that shows patterns of activity and provides an accurate index for costing out nursing care for specific patients.

A by-product of computer-generated patient care plans, computerized patient classification and scheduling systems give nurse-managers a tool for defining staffing requirements based on patient acuity and nursing task information. Such a system can:

• match patient needs with available nursing resources

• identify temporary and permanent staffing needs

• project future staffing needs for the nursing budget

• track nursing utilization and resource management

• provide more information to help cost out nursing services.

Quality assurance

Computers also contribute much to quality assurance in patient care. Previously, since the Kardex, the nursing care plan, and the nurses' notes were separately located, getting a clear picture of all patient care requirements was often difficult. Because of this, inconsistencies or omissions in care were not so noticeable or so easy to identify. But with a computer-generated patient care plan, a quick glance at the screen or a printout tells you what care measures have been completed and what you have left to do. This promotes accountability among the nursing staff. For example, if a nursing service wanted to audit care provided to patients with a particular nursing diagnosis that cut across medical diagnoses, it could use a computer to quickly sort through stored patient abstracts and list

DEVELOPING AND USING COMPUTERIZED CARE PLANS

The computer-generated care plan is an effective tool for planning, providing, and documenting patient care. This flowchart represents available components for developing and using such a care plan. Its core components include the patient's medical problems, assessment data, and the resulting nursing diagnoses. The care plan also documents difficult-to-measure nursing actions, such as patient teaching and psychological support; easily measured tasks, such as suctioning and turning; and ongoing nursing assessment and outcomes.

Interrelated components
Certain interrelated components provide immediate assistance in devising the care plan. The tickler file reminds the nurse of omissions and tasks to be done. The help system (a standardized computer function) provides more information, for example, about a nursing diagnosis, and decision support checks the nurse's choices, guiding her in proper care.

Other possible components—such as the nursing diagnosis code, management review, and standards of care—allow quick retrieval of information to help evaluate nursing care and ensure its quality.

Related components may also help project staffing requirements. For example, patient acuity values, which classify patients by the severity of their illness, are used for census information and short- and long-term staffing projections. In addition, coded time factors and frequency components help document nursing care for cost justification of nursing services.

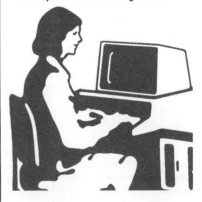

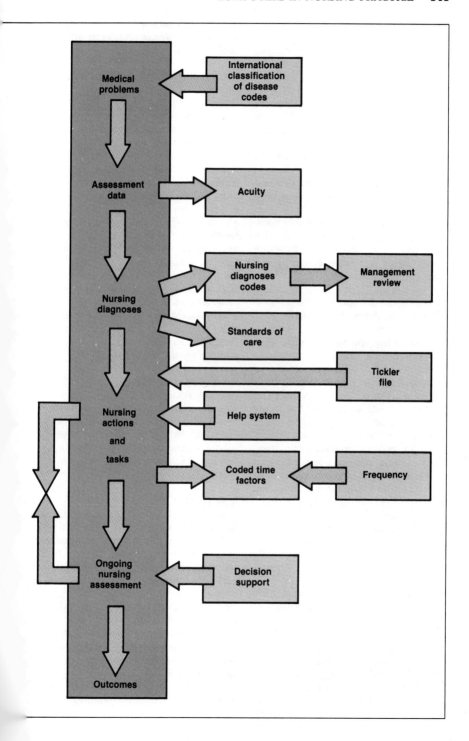

those that fall within a defined category.

By using a computer to store patient care standards—including both nursing process standards and expected patient outcomes—for easy reference, you can compare the care that was documented with the care that was planned, and compare the actual status of the patient with the projected outcome of the planned care measures.

The computer's rapid data processing capabilities can also help you keep track of equipment and supplies. And the communication function of a computerized information system can eliminate errors caused by illegible handwriting, repeated copying, and poor communications.

Security and legal concerns with computerized records

Clearly, computerized health data systems have the potential to make confidential medical information available to many sources, both authorized and unauthorized. To protect confidentiality, most systems have programmed-in signature controls to limit the information available to each nurse or other user of the system. Your personal identification number or password identifies you to the computer and gives you access to the types of information you're authorized to view. For example, you may be able to call up a patient's chart, but not your unit's annual budget. Gaining unauthorized access to confidential files and sharing passwords or identification numbers are typically grounds for dismissal in most hospitals.

Because paper copies of records are eliminated, computerized record keeping is much more efficient. But no computer system is foolproof; all are subject to breakdowns and data loss. So besides planning for computer system downtime, all nursing departments should develop procedures for safely storing critical data to prevent irretrievable loss in case of power surges or outages. A backup system is essential to ensure completeness and continuity of all records.

Computers mean new jobs for nurses

Computers aren't only changing the way nurses work. They're also creating new jobs for nurses. These new jobs, all of which require computer literacy, include:

• *nurse liaison*—a staff nurse who works with computer technicians and other nurses to smooth the installation of computers on a unit

• *nurse systems analyst*—a nurse who works closely with system users to define problems with and opportunities for system application

• *nurse programmer*—a nurse responsible for developing practical computer programs for use on the unit

• *nurse educator*—a nurse who teaches other nurses about the applications of computers in health care

• *nurse researcher*—a nurse who investigates the possibilities for enriching nursing practice through computerization and refined data bases

• *nurse consultant*—a nurse with extensive knowledge about computer applications in health care who assists others in the preparation, development, and implementation of computer systems.

The future

Computer use in nursing and other areas of health care has come a long way in recent years. But the future holds even more startling developments. For instance, imagine computerized robots that assist with patient care and transportation, instant translators for non-English-speaking patients, and other improvements, such as nurse consulting and patient teaching through a linkup between the hospital computer system and a personal computer in the patient's home.

You'll benefit greatly from these and other future innovations—and so will your patients.

MANAGEMENT ISSUES

Health care is nurses' business

The sweeping changes in health care delivery have added a new dimension to nursing. We now must see the nursing profession as an integral and critical part of the health care business.

To do this, we must recognize that nursing provides valuable, independently marketable services. Nursing supports hospital profitability primarily by providing direct patient care, but nurses also provide public relations, risk management, coordination of ancillary services, product evaluation, and cost-effective management.

Decentralization of authority and accountability in health care has placed greater responsibility for managing these various functions at every level of nursing practice. We will increasingly be called upon to make financial decisions using such techniques as network flow planning, budgeting, managing staff, and improving productivity. Mastering these

FACTORS AFFECTING NURSING

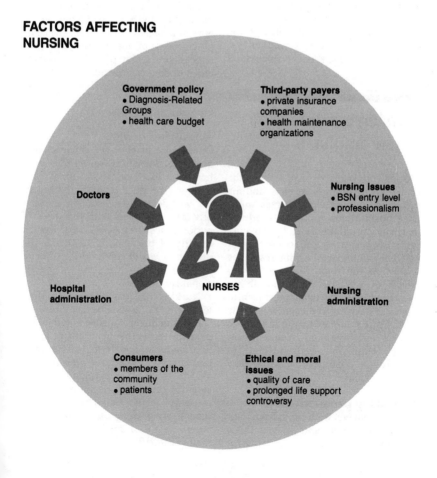

Government policy
• Diagnosis-Related Groups
• health care budget

Third-party payers
• private insurance companies
• health maintenance organizations

Doctors

Nursing issues
• BSN entry level
• professionalism

Hospital administration

NURSES

Nursing administration

Consumers
• members of the community
• patients

Ethical and moral issues
• quality of care
• prolonged life support controversy

techniques, we can place nursing in a favorable position to bargain for greater economic return for the services we provide—for our fair share of the health care dollar. To do so, we need to learn the language of the health care business so we can express our viewpoints and convince those who wield administrative power of our true economic worth to health care organizations. Most importantly, we need to take responsibility for determining nursing's economic future. We can't leave this vital task to others, hoping the outcome will be favorable. It won't be unless we make it so.

In this section, you'll find some business principles you need in managing health care today. These concepts are easy to learn and, once learned, easy to apply to your nursing practice. If you take the time to learn them, you'll be ready to help nursing claim its rightful place in the health care revolution.

JOANNE PATZEK DaCUNHA, RN, BS

Nursing productivity: A new emphasis

Through our primary responsibility for coordinating hospital services and for providing patient care, nurses influence hospital productivity—and, by extension, profitability. In light of current cost constraints, nurses have a special obligation to use hospital resources wisely. At the same time, as patient advocates, we have the responsibility to protect patients from the harmful effects of ill-conceived economies. The challenge for nurses in the late 1980s will be to deliver quality patient care in less time and with limited resources—in other words, to become more productive.

Measuring productivity
Nurse-managers, with input from their staffs, must create and select reliable systems for measuring nursing productivity and for determining the true cost of health care delivery. Productivity measures the efficiency with which labor, materials, and equipment are converted to goods and services; simply stated, it's the ratio between input and output. In nursing, productivity is usually measured in terms of man-hours (input) and services rendered (output). Input is easily quantified by staff time sheets. But measuring output is more difficult.

Lately, hospitals are measuring nursing output by the number of points derived from a patient classification system (PCS), which measures patient acuity, or the amount and complexity of care needed by hospital patients. (See also "Financial concepts in nursing," pages 154 to 156, for a more detailed discussion of PCS.) The PCS data allow nurse-managers to transform the complex process of nursing care into a financial scale that provides an easily understood measurement of productivity. This puts nurses in a better position to define patient care in objective terms for hospital administrators.

Measuring quality
Output also involves the efficiency and quality of nursing care, as measured by the number of "work units" processed or produced and by the degree of "zero defect" reached. The number of work units deals with the speed of performance; zero defect considers the quality of performance. Measuring quality in health care is quite difficult because health care involves professional services.

Nursing care involves more than technical and manual tasks; it also involves judgment, intellect, and interpersonal skills that are difficult to define and measure in terms of both speed and quality. Quality of nursing care also takes in other intangible dimensions of care, such as the needs and responses of individual patients, even though these dimensions make measurement of the quality of performance doubly difficult.

To measure the quality of care, standards of nursing practice must be defined for the entire nursing staff. Once these standards are in place, quantitative measurement of quality is possible through tools such as audits.

Increasing productivity

The two obvious ways to increase productivity—increasing staff and spending more money for better equipment and supplies—are severely limited in most institutions today. Consequently, nurse-managers must find ways to increase productivity while using available resources. First, they must make their staffs conscious of the need for maximum productivity and encourage them to seek new ways to improve nursing efficiency—for example, through specialization, use of all-professional staffs, practical improvements in nursing techniques, positive interactions with other health care agencies, standardization of work procedures, and improvements in staff management.

How does nursing specialization promote greater productivity? The more specialized a nurse becomes, the better she can deal with a specific group of patients. Because she knows exactly what to expect in these patients, she can intervene faster and more efficiently. Nurses who float to various departments or generalists obviously can't function as smoothly and therefore can't be as productive.

Another factor that influences productivity is the educational level of the nursing staff. The complexity of nursing practice mandates a need for an all-professional staff for greatest efficiency and flexibility. Staffing with registered nurses, whose education has prepared them for self-direction, produces higher-quality patient care with fewer personnel. An all-professional staff requires less supervision and can achieve greater output.

The nurse-manager should encourage her staff members to draw on all of their knowledge and expertise to increase productivity through practical improvements in daily nursing tasks. Staff nurses can devise creative, time-saving innovations for nurses' notes, better ways to write care plans, simpler methods for patient teaching, faster discharge planning strategies, and smoother interfacing with home health care agencies. Working together, staff members can coordinate and eliminate duplication of effort for such projects as patient care rounds, development and distribution of staff and patient educational materials, and evaluation of new equipment and supplies. We can also achieve greater productivity through standardization of certain work procedures. For example, although patients with the same diagnosis require individualized nursing care plans, staff nurses can enhance productivity by building diagnosis-specific care plans on the framework of a standard care plan, using pre-printed standard care plan forms. This strategy is particularly useful when caring for patients with diagnoses associated with short hospital stays.

Applying human resources management techniques can also increase staff productivity. Formal recognition of individual accomplishments and regularly scheduled staff evaluations provide regular assessment of staff productivity and allow the opportunity to discuss ways of improving efficiency and quality of care. The resulting improvements in morale and motivation can move the entire staff toward higher standards of productivity.

JUNE M. BUCKLE, RN, MSN

Marketing nursing services

Most hospitals and other health care agencies now have marketing departments to promote their health care services to the public. An important and highly visible part of these services, nursing is now recognized as key to any hospital's marketing potential. Nurses must become aware of their marketing role to claim their equitable share of the health care dollar. To do so, nurses must learn how to market nursing services.

Clearly, today's nurses must be sellers as well as providers of health care services. But selling successfully requires careful planning to make a product desirable and accessible to the buyers—in the case of health care, to patients and their families, to doctors, to preferred provider organizations, to insurance companies, and to health maintenance organizations. Planning a successful marketing program takes into account the four Ps: product, price, place, and promotion. To become effective marketers, nurses must provide access to a quality product at a reasonable price and promote related services.

How to develop a marketing plan

As a first step, nursing administrators can set up a task force to develop a marketing plan. Staff nurses can participate in this task force or offer information and suggestions. Developing a marketing plan involves several steps:
• identifying the target population the hospital wishes to reach with its services
• determining what services this population needs and what they are willing to pay for quality service
• identifying the competition and how their services compare
• identifying services that need improvement and planning how to make these improvements within a reasonable time.

Defining the quality hospital

An essential early step in any hospital marketing plan is a market survey to identify what health care consumers want in a hospital. Why does a consumer choose one hospital over an-

other? In market surveys, consumers consistently identify the following factors in order of importance:
• prompt, efficient service
• competent, caring, personable nurses
• concerned, compassionate doctors
• efficient, detail-oriented support staff
• clean, modern facilities
• good food.

Because doctors decide to which hospital they'll send their patients, doctors too are health care consumers. So, successful hospital marketing also involves making the hospital more attractive to doctors. Factors that influence a doctor's choice of hospital include:
• high-quality, well-staffed nursing department
• up-to-date, well-maintained equipment and facilities
• efficient, readily available emergency services
• central, easily accessible location for both patients and doctor
• a hospital administration responsive to doctors' needs
• staff doctors in a wide range of medical specialties
• competitive hospital rates.

Of course, nurses can't exert much influence on the quality of hospital equipment and facilities, hospital rates, or most other factors on these lists. They can only influence the quality of nursing care—but this factor is one of the most important in determining both patients' and doctors' choice of hospitals.

Clearly, to compete successfully, a hospital must attract and retain top-quality nursing staff. Thus, the comprehensive marketing plan must address nursing recruitment and retention. This begins with another survey, which asks present staff nurses what they like and dislike about the hospital. In addition, exit interviews with members of the staff who resign can provide much useful information about areas that need improvement. Head nurses can define hospital expectations and demands and describe the overall atmosphere on the nursing units in nursing departments. Successful nursing departments now apply a marketing perspective to recruitment techniques. They select staff nurses with good technical and communications skills as well as an awareness of their responsibility for containing costs and for contributing to favorable public relations.

Defining nursing products

Nursing is primarily responsible for patient care, but it also enhances a hospital's marketability by offering other services as well. Quality patient care includes not only accurate and timely clinical judgment and intervention, but also accountability for cost of services and patient satisfaction. A patient admitted to a hospital expects medical and nursing care that helps him recover quickly. Because he has the most direct contact with nurses, nursing interaction contributes to or detracts from his overall satisfaction with his hospital stay and influences his subsequent health care choices.

Other nursing product lines include continuing nursing education programs, patient education programs, consumer wellness programs, nurse-directed clinics in ambulatory care, home health care, and various specialized nursing care programs (such as perinatal nursing care, critical nursing care, emergency and trauma nursing care, and operating room nursing care). Each product line should have a separate marketing plan and a separate pricing structure. For example, the nursing department could develop a marketing plan for a cardiac rehabilitation patient education program, for which the patient would be billed separately. As another example, the nursing department could develop a marketing plan for packaging and selling nursing protocols and procedures for special areas such as burn care. Nurses who know such services are available and who are sensitive to their patients' needs can stimulate the use of these services—and contribute to the hospital's profitability—by promoting them to patients, their families, and doctors.

What price nursing care?

All nurses share a concern for quality patient care. But new costing procedures require that this concern take into account whether the patient is getting the best care possible for his money. This is necessary because costing systems can now identify the cost of nursing care for individual patients. In the past, most hospitals included the cost of nursing care in the patient's general room charge. A nurse-manager knew her department budget, but not the actual cost of nursing care for a specific patient or even what portion of the room charge reflected that nursing care. Today, through the use of patient acuity classification systems (PCSs), a nursing department can accurately identify the cost of nursing services for each individual patient. Consequently, many hospitals are using PCS data to set prices for different levels of nursing care.

Staff nurses on quality assurance committees help monitor PCS data to ensure that it accurately reflects the value of nursing services in terms of time and nursing judgment. Every staff nurse can contribute to reliable evaluation of nursing services through accurate, reliable reporting and documentation. As more hospitals begin to charge separately for nursing care, accurate documentation and PCS audits by staff nurses will determine appropriate prices for nursing care. In such institutions, nursing can then be positively identified as a cost-effective source of revenue.

Planning for place: Access to care

An effective marketing plan must involve concern of place—access to services. For inpatient care, place refers to the availability of hospital beds when needed. A nurse-manager needs to plan staffing levels to meet seasonal and other variable demands. For example, the demand for psychiatric services is greater in the winter than in summer; this variable demand must be planned for. Place also refers to continuity of care, for example, for patients who need different nursing services during a single hospitalization. For instance, an elderly patient admitted from the emergency department with a hip fracture is likely to need nursing care on the surgical unit, in the operating room, in the intensive care unit, and possibly at home after discharge. Delivering quality nursing care means coordinating the entire duration of the hospital stay and discharge planning for maximum benefit at the least cost to the patient.

Promotion is the key

How can the nursing department promote its services successfully? One basic step is in-house programs to increase staff nurses' awareness of marketing and public relations principles. These programs should help nurses to know more about the public they serve and to understand and remember that they represent the hospital and the nursing profession in every professional interaction.

Effective promotional methods also include advertising both to recruit nurses and to increase the community's recognition of the quality of nursing services. Such advertising can appear in various media—newspapers, magazines, radio, newsletters, posters, brochures, and various patient education materials. New services can receive free publicity through news releases and special promotional events. Speaking to the community on health care issues offers nurses another opportunity to promote their services.

Promotion within the hospital can be just as important to the marketing of nursing services as outside advertising. Educational programs for nurses in other departments and for other health care professionals can expand the use of special nursing services.

Is marketing a nurse's job?

Many nurses are uncomfortable with marketing nursing services. Some feel that it's inappropriate or even unethical. These nurses aren't used to thinking of patient satisfaction as a measurement of quality care. But it's an important consideration. A patient doesn't usually have the skills or background to evaluate a nurse's clinical judgment and technique—qualities that are reliably measured only by her professional peers and superiors. A patient can judge nursing care only by his personal experience. He measures nursing quality according to perceived credibility and concern for his welfare. A nurse shows concern for the patient's welfare through courtesy, promptness, responsiveness, and compassion. She acquires credibility by dressing professionally, appearing confident, speaking and acting with assurance, and clearly explaining procedures and policies. A patient is more likely to refer other patients and to return to a hospital where he received good nursing care. Broadening marketing awareness to include the patient's point of view also enhances the quality of the nurse-patient relationship and helps improve the overall quality of care.

The implications for nursing are clear. Since the health care consumer is becoming more aware of health care options and more selective in his choices, we need to work harder at selling ourselves to the public. We need to polish our image so that we always look and sound like the professionals we are. Above all, we must take every opportunity to let the public know just how much nurses do—what services we provide and how they can get those services more cheaply from us than from other health care providers.

Our message is simple and direct: No other group of health care professionals does more for people who are ill than nurses do. Let's get this message out!

JACQUELINE DIENEMANN, RN, PhD

Human resources management: Motivating staff

Effective staff management begins with recruiting and hiring the best-qualified nurses, matches their talents and strengths to fit the available work assignments, sets reasonable goals for staff performance, and provides support that helps the staff accomplish those goals. To a nurse-manager, helping the staff achieve stated performance goals is all-important. How to do it? By stimulating their desire to meet the goals and by clearly defining the steps necessary to do so. This is motivation, the key to achieving any goal.

Measuring motivation

Expectancy theory indicates that the strength of desire for something, modified by the probability of achieving it with a certain action (expectancy),

REMEMBER TO USE THE GRAPEVINE

The effective nurse-manager understands the importance of formal and informal channels of communication within her department and uses them both to best advantage. Formal channels—departmental meetings, memos—often prove slow and ineffective at spreading information throughout an organization. The informal channels—the "grapevine"—are subject to distortion but are often the best way to quickly disseminate important information. So, keep in touch with the grapevine and don't hesitate to use it yourself. To help you decide when the grapevine can be more effective, familiarize yourself with its common characteristics and learn to use it effectively. Remember that:

• People talk most about recent news.
• People talk most about things that affect their work.
• People talk most about people they know.
• People working near each other are more likely to be on the same grapevine.
• People in direct contact on the organizational chain tend to be on the same grapevine.
• People who distort news may be revealing their underlying fears and attitudes.

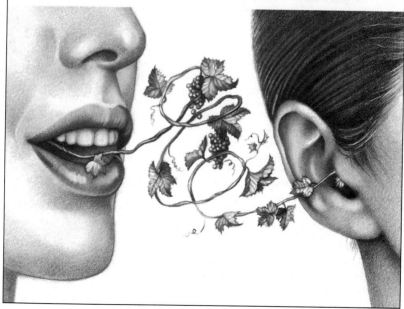

equals motivation, or the strength of drive toward a goal. In other words, if a person really wants something and believes she can obtain it through certain actions, her motivation will be strong to perform the needed actions. But if either desire or expectancy is high while the other is low, motivation will be only moderate. And if both desire and expectancy are low, motivation will also be low.

Understanding and applying this theory can help you motivate your staff. For example, if you would like a staff member to do staff-development teaching, you should clearly communicate your expectations and what she can expect from you in return for meeting them. If you offer something she desires, such as compensatory time or formal recognition, she'll be more likely to do a good job on the staff-development session.

Recognizing staff accomplishments
Encourage high-quality work and co-operation from your staff by providing specific and timely feedback on positive ideas and behavior and by acknowledging the value of these ideas and behavior to yourself and to the organization. By recognizing a staff member's good work, you reinforce management values, making the staff member more likely to repeat that behavior. You can offer such recognition in many ways: by noting an idea or praising behavior at a staff meeting; by praising a special achievement in a memo to your superiors, with a copy sent to the staff member; and by posting such a memo on the staff bulletin board. Recognizing and praising a staff member's achievements shows your awareness of positive behavior, reinforces it, and presents it to other staff members as a desirable performance model.

Recognize a staff member's achievements or progress at several stages: when she shows the first signs of improved performance, when she meets minimum performance standards, when she exceeds standard requirements, and when she provides a useful idea. To offer recognition appropriately at any of these stages, your feedback must be immediate and directly related to the behavior. To be most effective, you must have an awareness of your staff member's motivation—for example, was her behavior motivated by a concern for the patient, by the desire for personal professional growth, or by regard for your and the hospital's administrative goals? Mentioning and commending the motivation behind her behavior will make your recognition more personal and therefore more effective. By commending personal qualities, you reinforce those qualities and earn goodwill and support from your entire staff.

Formal recognition may be possible on a unit, divisional, or departmental level. For example, establishing a "Nurse of the Week" award or a similar type of formal recognition allows each staff member the chance to earn recognition for her efforts. Recognizing accomplishments helps a staff member feel important and valued, helps her realize that her efforts have an impact in the organization and are valued by others, and helps motivate her to continue contributing.

Using reinforcement techniques
Reinforcement techniques can stimulate motivation, encourage desirable behavior, and discourage undesirable behavior. *Positive reinforcement* is generally the most effective. It provides a favorable consequence that encourages repetition of desirable behavior. Positive reinforcement is a powerful motivational tool. When applied, it strengthens positive behavior; when withheld, it weakens it. For example, formal recognition of high-quality work encourages your staff to continue such performance, because people generally like recognition for their efforts. Absence of such recognition weakens motivation and may lead to apathy.

Negative reinforcement occurs when positive behavior is followed by removal of a negative consequence. (This isn't punishment, which usually adds some unfavorable consequence.) Behavior responsible for the removal of an unpleasant consequence is likely to be repeated under similar circumstances. For example, by not complaining when a staff member comes into work on time for a change, you've used negative reinforcement to encourage punctuality.

Negative reinforcement changes un-

UNDERSTANDING THE MOTIVATIONAL CYCLE

Staff motivation difficulties can plague even the most experienced and competent nurse-manager. After all, each staff member behaves differently in any given situation. But despite such disparity, all motivation for behavior follows a general pattern—the motivational cycle. As shown below, this cycle begins with a perceived need, moves through the steps necessary to meet this need, and after meeting it identifies another need. Understanding this pattern can help the nurse-manager identify effective strategies for influencing staff behavior. For instance, if a nurse-manager wants her staff to be certified in advanced cardiac life support (ACLS), she can identify and stimulate staff members' needs for greater confidence in caring for cardiac patients. She can motivate them by withholding merit raises until they demonstrate proficiency in cardiac care, and she can give them time off to attend ACLS classes, which can help them achieve their goal.

Nurse's perceived need

Motivating force or tension (internal or external)

Activity toward a goal

ACHIEVEMENT OF GOAL

RECOGNIZING
COPING BEHAVIORS

When reviewing a staff member's problem behavior, consider that such behavior may be a coping mechanism in response to stress. This chart can help you to recognize some common coping mechanisms and to understand their psychological causes.

COMPENSATORY MECHANISM	PSYCHOLOGICAL PROCESS	EXAMPLE
Compensation	Abnormal devotion to a particular pursuit to make up for a real or imagined inadequacy	A nurse who never advances beyond a staff position invests her energy into working as president of the Twenty-Five Year Club.
Conversion	Emotional conflicts expressed in muscular, sensory, or somatic symptoms of disability, illness, or pain	A disabling headache keeps a staff member off the job the day after a troubling or unresolved conflict.
Displacement	Redirecting pent-up emotions to swing toward persons, ideas, or objects other than the primary source of the emotion	A nurse brusquely rejects a simple request from a peer after receiving a rebuff from a colleague or a reprimand from her manager.
Fantasy	Daydreaming or other forms of imagining to escape from reality and find imagined satisfactions	An overworked nurse who considers her head nurse's demands unreasonable daydreams about "telling off" the head nurse in a staff meeting to enthusiastic applause by her peers.
Negativism	Active or passive resistance, operating unconsciously	A nurse, after failing to get out of an inconvenient staff-development assignment, picks apart every suggestion made in the staff meeting.
Projection	Avoiding awareness of one's own undesirable traits or unacceptable feelings by attributing them to others	An unsuccessful person wishes to block the rise of other staff members and continually feels that others are out to "get" her.
Rationalization	Justifying and explaining away inconsistent or undesirable behavior, beliefs, statements, or motivations	A nurse frequently comes in late because "everybody does it."
Repression	Completely excluding from consciousness all impulses, experiences, and feelings that are psychologically disturbing because they arouse guilt or anxiety	A nurse "forgets" to tell her manager the circumstances of an embarrassing incident.
Resignation, apathy, and boredom	Breaking psychological contact with the environment; withholding all emotional or personal involvement	An employee who receives no reward, praise, or encouragement loses interest in doing a good job.

desirable behavior more slowly than positive reinforcement. So, depending on the behavior you wish to change, select your reinforcement strategy carefully. A serious behavior problem (for example, consistent mismanagement of medications) requires a stronger, more urgent approach; a minor inefficiency, such as writing overlong sign-off reports, can allow slower correction.

Other reinforcement techniques include shaping, punishment, and extinction. *Shaping* is particularly useful for teaching complex tasks or behaviors by reinforcing desired behaviors only when improvement is noted. For instance, if a staff member consistently has problems completing all her assigned tasks before the end of her shift, you would reinforce behaviors that help her do so, such as combining patient teaching with routine nursing procedures, asking for help when necessary, organizing equipment and supplies, making better use of time, or collecting report information earlier.

Punishment occurs when a behavior elicits unfavorable consequences. Punishment does tend to discourage undesirable behavior, but it doesn't encourage desirable behavior. Using punishment tends to make desired behavior unpredictable and inconsistent. A staff member who is punished may be confused as to which aspects of her behavior are undesirable; this confusion may prevent her from recognizing and changing the undesirable behavior and may even discourage some desirable behavior.

Extinction tends to occur when a staff member's behavior produces no significant consequences—either favorable or unfavorable. Behavior that isn't reinforced tends to disappear, to be replaced by behaviors that are reinforced.

Reinforcement may be continuous or partial. Continuous reinforcement accompanies each desired behavior. Although it encourages quick learning of desired behaviors, continuous reinforcement is difficult to maintain in a work situation and tends to lose effectiveness over time. Partial reinforcement reinforces only the most important desired behaviors. With partial reinforcement, learning is slower but tends to be retained longer.

Motivation through evaluation

When handled correctly, staff evaluation is another effective method of reinforcing desired behavior and stimulating motivation. An evaluation that promotes improvement considers positive aspects of behavior; it's not an occasion for unrelieved criticism. When evaluating a member of your staff, begin by specifying merits, whenever possible. This indicates that you have listened and observed carefully enough to consider all aspects of behavior and performance and suggests that your evaluation will be objective and fair. This makes it easier for the staff member to accept your evaluation. You may start by saying something like "I particularly like..." or "This helps because..." or "I'm worried about this because..." Invite reactions and suggestions for improved performance, and request feedback on your evaluation.

When evaluating a job performance that doesn't include negative concerns, specify the merits and suggest ways to extend them to other areas. For example, you could say "You did a specific teaching plan as part of your nursing care plan for this patient. Could you do this for your other patients as well?" To get the most motivational benefit from a formal evaluation, focus on desirable behavior, set goals for the future, plan strategies for achieving them, and discuss problem-solving techniques.

When the nurses on your staff understand the importance of a management goal, want to achieve it, and know everything they must do to achieve it, you've set the stage for high-level motivation—an important achievement for any manager.

ANN MARRINER, RN, PhD

Financial concepts in nursing

Nurses are now expected to provide quality patient care and to exercise fiscal responsibility while doing so. Quality patient care now includes cost-effective care.

Responsibility for costs demands the application of financial skills and knowledge that aren't taught in most nursing schools. Such skills include judicious use of human and financial resources, planning and monitoring budgets, and aggressive negotiation for the resources necessary to develop and maintain a quality nursing practice.

In the current climate of cost containment, improved business practices have resulted in decentralization of the budgeting process, bringing it closer to the area where resources are consumed and revenues generated. To keep an equitable share of the health care dollar, nurses need budgeting skills and an understanding of the fiscal policies and mechanisms in their organization. They need this information to validate their contribution to the institution's profitability.

Because of their intimate knowledge of day-to-day activity on the nursing unit, staff nurses provide the most reliable information about the actual costs of delivering patient care. Their observations and suggestions can help ensure cost-effective use of supplies, pharmaceuticals, and procedures, while still maintaining high-quality patient care standards.

Identifying resources

In a health care institution, resources for nursing care depend on income from patient services and other revenue-producing areas of the institution. Income from patient services comes from several sources:

• *Medicare*—payment is now prospective, meaning a fixed rate or reimbursement depending on classification, as determined on discharge.

• *Private insurance*—payment is retrospective, based on charges for the hospital stay. Payment by the policy is usually partial; it is either a fixed percentage of the bill or is based on a fee schedule for different services. The patient pays the remainder not covered by the policy.

• *Preferred provider payment*—payment is retrospective, using a lower group rate negotiated with the hospital by the insurer in return for exclusive use of the hospital by the insured. The patient may or may not be a co-payer, depending on the policy. Many health maintenance organizations have preferred provider agreements with hospitals.

• *Self-pay*—the patient pays for services received.

Generally, a hospital's income is dependent on its case mix—the number of patients in each payment plan. Today, all hospitals are trying to stabilize income through increased use of financial planning and cost accounting. Planning includes seeking a profitable case mix; marketing profitable services while eliminating unprofitable ones; and diversifying the organization by adding new products (such as a medical supply business or a doctors' office building) or by expanding to new geographic areas through mergers, by opening new facilities, or both.

Cost accounting identifies the cost of each service and relates it to the price charged for it, forecasts inventory and staffing costs by volume of services, and then monitors actual expenses. The resulting figures are used to evaluate the use of resources and to improve forecasting of future costs. Implementing such methods requires computerization to create a data base of information for use in generating quick feedback, planning, and cost accounting.

Costing nursing care

One benefit of cost containment for nursing is the growing practice of costing nursing services separately from other overhead expenses charged in a patient's daily room rate. This allows nursing administrators to defend their budgets more aggressively and helps demonstrate the true economic value of a strong nursing department to hospital administrators. Most hospitals cost nursing services through a patient acuity classification system (PCS), such as Medicus or GRASP. Under a PCS, nurses on each unit perform an audit either daily or during each shift to classify each patient into one of four or more acuity categories. The audit then goes to a central office, where the data are used for making staffing decisions and, in some hospitals, for billing patients. In an integrated management information system, the nursing department can also use PCS data for preparing its annual budget and for tracking nursing costs for each Diagnosis-Related Group (DRG) category. This information helps nursing administrators negotiate a fair percentage of each DRG payment for nursing services.

Choosing a PCS

Obviously, accurate PCS data is essential to ensure accurate identification of costs and enable realistic financial planning. Thus, when helping their hospital choose a PCS, nurses must validate its rating criteria by considering the following questions:

• Were actual time and motion studies done?

• Will any studies be done at their hospital to check for significant differences due to the physical layout of floors, patient population, staffing, or other factors?

• Will nurses be consulted as to whether criteria make sense?

• How many hospitals now use this PCS?

• How do those hospitals compare to this hospital?

• Will the vendor assist in implementing the PCS?

• How much does it cost to purchase and maintain it?

• How much time does an audit take?

• How quickly will a unit get feedback for staffing?

• What computing equipment is needed to use the PCS and computer program?

• Who is responsible for providing the necessary training?

• Who will be responsible for entering data?

The answers to these questions will help determine whether the system is valid and feasible. The training, commitment, and periodic monitoring of nurses performing audits will determine if the system is reliable. Unless staff nurses believe the audit is honest and reliable and are thoroughly trained in rating patients, any PCS will produce misleading information. To maintain the integrity of the PCS, nurses need feedback on the quality of their audits and how the audits affect their work. Without such feedback, staff nurses will view the audits as meaningless, time-wasting rituals.

Understanding budgets

The recent trend toward decentralized budgeting makes many nurse-managers or head nurses responsible for developing a budget, defending variances, and controlling costs. Most hospitals use a fixed budget on a yearly cycle called the fiscal year. The budget makes financial projections for 1 year, using current objectives and statistics based on past costs to predict future costs and revenues. These projections are used as a standard for accounting during the entire fiscal year. A few hospitals use variable or flexible budgets, in which projections are also made for 1 year but are reevaluated and possibly changed during the fiscal year as income or cost changes occur.

Whether using a fixed or flexible budget, the nurse-manager or head nurse usually develops two budgets— one for capital expenses and one for operating expenses. A capital budget includes costs for building maintenance and repair, building construction, and equipment purchases above a stated amount or with payments extending over 1 year.

An operating budget includes both revenues and expenses, which ideally balance or show a profit. In nursing department budgets, revenues are monitored by patient census and acuity data from the PCS. Operating expenses include payroll and supplies. Most hospitals use a specific chart of accounts to track all operating expenses for reporting to the accounting department. Such a chart usually breaks down supplies and payroll into specific line items; for instance, under payroll, it may list RN base pay, vacation days, sick days, travel expenses, health insurance, inservice hours, and other items. The nurse-manager or the head nurse has a budget for each item. She receives a monthly report identifying the expenses incurred for each line item compared to the amount budgeted for the month. This report may also summarize revenues, expenses, and any variances (over or under) for the fiscal year to date. The nurse-manager or head nurse may consult with her operating revenues report, unit staff nurses, and the hospital accountant to explain the variances in the report to her superior. Some hospitals reward nurses in units that consistently have lower-than-projected operating expenses with bonuses or by allowing the nursing unit to spend a percentage of the savings on capital improvements for the unit.

Budgets and the nursing process

Nurses can master the budgeting process easily—if they remember that it encompasses the familiar elements of the nursing process: assessment, planning, implementation, and evaluation. In budgeting terms, *assessment* means evaluation of the hospital's sources of income, community needs, competition from other health care providers, standards of care to satisfy payers and patients, and working conditions to satisfy nurses. *Planning* involves preparation of the nursing budget as a part of the hospital's master budget. The nursing budget should reflect nursing department priorities and objectives for the next year, taking into consideration the impact on costs of desired changes, such as flextime or primary nursing. *Implementation* refers to the costs and revenues associated with patient care, including fixed expenses, which stay the same regardless of patient acuity and census (for example, the minimum number of nurses needed to staff a hospital unit regardless of patient census), and variable expenses, which change with patient census and acuity. *Evaluation* is based on data derived from quality assurance and utilization reviews and on cost data from records of patient charges and payments. Together, all these reports and data are known as the Nursing Information System (NIS).

A successful budgeting process realistically predicts the resources needed to achieve the nursing unit's stated goals. Staff nurses need continuous feedback so they can know whether their attempts to deliver quality, cost-effective care are successful.

JACQUELINE DIENEMANN, RN, PhD

Public relations: A critical nursing responsibility

Increasing competition for patient admissions is forcing hospitals to become more concerned about patients' perceptions of the quality of their hospital care. Because of this trend, successful hospitals have incorporated marketing strategies into their plans for delivering health services. One important facet of marketing—public relations (PR)—directly involves staff nurses on a daily basis.

As the most visible hospital staff members—the ones patients see the most—nurses usually influence a patient's memorable impressions of the hospital. Like it or not, nurses are in a pivotal position to promote hospital PR because of our close contact with patients, doctors, and other health care professionals; the impressions we make can even influence hospital visitors (who constitute 70% of all people entering a hospital and who are all potential customers). We're not yet used to thinking of ourselves this way, but we *are* largely responsible for the public's view of our hospitals.

Hospital PR: Giving the customer what he wants

Supporting your hospital's PR means giving your patient—the customer—what he wants, a concept known formally as demand management. Because they directly control the quality of nursing services (the product) provided to the patient (the health care customer), nurse-managers are responsible for demand management at the unit level—the level that shapes the patient's hospital experience, since this is where he spends most of this time while hospitalized.

Whether the patient perceives this experience as negative or positive depends largely on your interpersonal skills. When asked their impressions about a hospital experience, many people remember an emotional dimension of their care rather than the technical expertise of the staff. They mention someone who noticed their personal concerns and "really seemed to care." Clearly, what counts the most in the patient's mind is the human element— what used to be called bedside manner. This was a lot easier when patients stayed in the hospital longer and nurses' schedules allowed more time to get to know their patients.

As health care becomes more mechanized and impersonal, maintaining the "human" side of health care while providing the best treatment medical

PRINCIPLES OF GOOD CUSTOMER RELATIONS

To ensure good public relations, nurses must deal with health care consumers the same way any industry deals with its customers. The following principles of customer relations apply to any business setting.

- A customer is the most important person in any business.

- A customer is part of our business, not an outsider.

- A customer is not dependent on us. We are dependent on him.

- A customer can never interrupt our work, for he is the reason for our work.

- A customer brings us his wants; it's our job to fill those wants.

- A customer does us a favor when he calls; we do not do him a favor by serving him.

- A customer deserves the most attentive and courteous treatment we can give him.

- A customer is not someone with whom to argue or match wits.

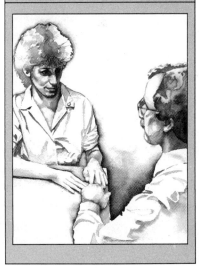

technology can offer becomes an even greater challenge. And your traditional role as patient advocate takes on even greater importance. Now, because you have so little time for it, you have to make positive interaction with your patients a conscious priority and pursue it in a purposeful way.

Find out what the patient wants

Obviously, before you can give the patient what he wants, you must first find out what it is. Does he want information, action, or understanding involvement? Watch the patient's expression and attitude, and listen carefully for the question behind the question. A

DEALING WITH AN ANGRY PATIENT

Because of the many pressures people feel today, nurses often have to deal with patients who, while trying to overcome severe illness, are distressed by overwhelming personal problems. This double burden of anxiety can strain coping mechanisms to the breaking point—triggering irritability, anger, and perhaps even violent behavior. As the primary care giver, you're the person who's most likely to feel the patient's anger. How you deal with it can calm the patient and help him cope, or it can give him another incident to feel angry about. To make sure your interaction with an angry patient is helpful and appropriate, follow these guidelines:

• Remain calm and speak softly.

• Address the patient by name.

• Closely observe his body language and monitor your own for signs of hostility; keep your stance relaxed and as neutral as possible.

• Listen carefully to his complaints; give him your undivided attention and maintain eye contact.

• Review his complaints and restate what he's said to try and identify his real concern.

• Demonstrate your concern for his welfare by explaining your intended actions.

• Never promise something you can't deliver.

• Explain your limitations in resolving a problem, and call for help if the situation is beyond your authority or control.

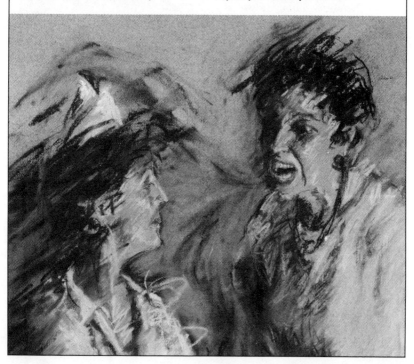

straightforward question deserves a prompt and direct answer, unless it's inappropriate in some way. Generally, you should tell the patient what he wants to know; if you don't know the answer, tell him you'll find out, and don't forget to follow through in a reasonable time. Similarly, you can communicate caring by honoring reasonable requests for action—perhaps another blanket, some juice, or an allowable change in diet—as promptly as possible.

Responding to a request for concerned understanding is commonly more difficult, mainly because the patient often masks his real question. If he asks you several times with increasing agitation what time his surgery is scheduled for, you can assume he's not asking about time; he's worried about undergoing surgery. At this point you should take the time to listen to the patient's fears and concerns. You might say "You seem worried about your surgery. Do you want to talk about it?" The patient who tells you "My doctor says I'm doing well, but it seems to me I'm getting worse every day" clearly wants reassurance and support. How can you best serve his needs? Not with an off-hand cheery remark like "You seem to be doing fine. Don't worry, you'll be out of here soon." Such a remark—while it may truly reflect the patient's clinical status—trivializes the patient's concerns. It ends the conversation without letting the patient explore his feelings. Such a response doesn't communicate caring. A better response would be something like "You seem worried. Why do you think you're not getting better? Would you like to talk about it?" This response gives the patient permission and the opportunity to explore his fears and concerns.

Remember, more than anything, an anxious patient usually wants someone to listen to his concerns. Listening is the first phase of a good nurse-patient relationship. During this first phase, you refrain from making suggestions or presenting options for his consid-

eration. This is often difficult because nurses are action-oriented and instinctively want to do something to solve problems immediately. But your personal interaction with a hospitalized patient is now likely to be brief, often not allowing the relationship to progress to the phase of understanding or resolution. Even so, if you truly listen when a patient wants to talk, he will remember your caring attitude and leave the hospital with a positive impression of his stay.

If you truly listen, you'll treat each patient like a valued customer—the best way to support your hospital's PR.
ROBERTA M. CONTI, RN, MS, FAAN, CNAA
JENNIFER BURKS, RN, MSN

CAREER CONSIDERATIONS

Advanced nursing practice update

When it comes to nursing practice, each state has different rules and regulations. The following chart, a state-by-state survey, lets you compare your state's regulations for advanced nursing practice to those of other states. *Advanced nursing practice* designates specialty areas of nursing practice, usually guided by state or national certification following an educational or training period, frequently (but not necessarily) at a master's degree level. Advanced nursing practice may include nurse practitioners in a variety of specialties, nurse anesthetists, nurse-midwives, and nurse clinicians or clinical nurse specialists. In most states, both medical and nursing boards must approve licensing of advanced nursing practitioners.

STATE-BY-STATE DEFINITIONS OF ADVANCED NURSING PRACTICE

The following state-by-state review shows the current definitions and requirements of advanced nursing practice.

ALABAMA

Nurse anesthetist: the performance of or the assistance in any act involving the determination, preparation, administration, or monitoring of any drug used to render an individual insensible to pain for surgical and other therapeutic or diagnostic procedures. The nurse anesthetist functions under the direction of a duly licensed doctor or dentist.

Nurse practitioner: the provision of primary health care services in institutional, occupational, and public and private community settings consistent with the definitions of practice published by national nurse practitioner specialty organizations approved by the board of nursing. Such nurse practitioner practice includes but is not limited to the following functions: to evaluate current health status and risk factors of individuals based on physical, psychosocial, and environmental assessment; to counsel, teach, and assist individuals to assume responsibility for self-care in prevention of illness, health maintenance, and health restoration; to collaborate and consult with other health care providers in the provision of patient care, including evaluation and management of disease states at the direction of a licensed doctor; and to plan, implement, and evaluate therapeutic regimens to promote positive patient outcomes.

ALASKA

Advanced nurse practitioner: a registered nurse authorized to practice in the state who, because of specialized education and experience, is certified to perform acts of medical diagnosis and the prescription of medical, therapeutic, or corrective measures under regulations adopted by the board of nursing.

Nurse anesthetist: a registered nurse authorized to practice in the state who, because of specialized education and experience, is certified to select and administer anesthetic agents and give anesthesia care under regulations adopted by the board.

ARIZONA

Nurse practitioner: a registered nurse who has been certified by the board of nursing and who, by virtue of added knowledge and skill gained through an organized program of study and clinical experience, has extended the limits of practice into specialty areas authorized by these rules and regulations. The nurse practitioner shall function with an organized system for the delivery of health care with members of the health team and in collaboration with and under the direction of a licensed physician in this state.

Nurse-midwife: a registered nurse licensed in Arizona who has extended the limits of practice in the area of management of care of mothers and babies throughout the maternity cycle.

Pediatric nurse associate: a registered nurse licensed in Arizona who has extended the limits of practice in the area of child and adolescent care. The titles Pediatric Nurse Associate and Pediatric Nurse Practitioner are used interchangeably.

Family nurse practitioner: a registered nurse licensed in Arizona who has extended the limits of practice to provide health care management of the family unit within the limits prescribed.

Adult nurse practitioner: a registered nurse licensed in Arizona who has extended the limits of practice to provide health care management for adult persons of the family unit.

Obstetrical/gynecological nurse practitioner: a registered nurse licensed in Arizona who has extended the limits of practice to provide obstetrical and gynecological health care for women primarily in ambulatory health care settings.

School nurse practitioner: a registered nurse licensed in Arizona whose practice provides health care management for children and adolescents.

STATE-BY-STATE DEFINITIONS OF ADVANCED NURSING PRACTICE
(continued)

Neonatal nurse practitioner: a registered nurse licensed in Arizona who has extended the limits of practice to provide health care management to the newborn in both short- and long-term care.

ARKANSAS

Nurse anesthetist: any nurse registered under the provisions of this state's Professional Nurse Act who holds a diploma or certificate evidencing his or her successful completion of the educational program of a school of anesthesia duly accredited by the Council on Accreditation of Educational Programs of Nurse Anesthesia or other nationally recognized accrediting body and who holds a current certificate of certification from the Council on Certification of Nurse Anesthetists or the Council on Recertification of Nurse Anesthetists or other nationally recognized certifying body may give or administer anesthetics in this state in the presence and under the supervision of a licensed physician or dentist.

Nurse practitioner: any person licensed or possessing the qualifications to obtain a license as a registered nurse under the provisions of this Act who holds a certificate and/or academic degree evidencing his or her successful completion of the educational program of an accredited school of nursing or other nationally recognized accredited program recognized by the state board of nursing as meeting the requirements of a nurse practitioner program may be licensed as a registered nurse practitioner in accordance with the rules and regulations promulgated by the state board of nursing.

Registered nurse practitioner: a registered nurse duly licensed in this state, who has been authorized by the state board of nursing to deliver health care in collaboration with a licensed physician. Such persons, under the direction of a licensed physician, shall be authorized to engage in activities recognized by the nursing profession and specified in the Arkansas state board of nursing rules and regulations relating to registered nurse practitioners. Nothing herein is to be deemed to limit a registered nurse practitioner from engaging in those activities which normally constitute

the practice of nursing or those which may be performed by persons without the necessity of the license to practice medicine. Nor shall this Act preclude hospital-employed professional paramedics from administering medication for diagnostic procedures under the direction of a physician.

CALIFORNIA

Nurse-midwife: the certificate to practice nurse-midwifery authorizes the holder, under the supervision of a licensed physician and surgeon, to attend cases of normal childbirth and to provide prenatal, intrapartum, and postpartum care, including family-planning care, for the mother, and immediate care for the newborn.

As used in this chapter, the practice of nurse-midwifery constitutes the furthering or undertaking by any certified person, under the supervision of a licensed physician and surgeon who has current practice or training in obstetrics, to assist a woman in childbirth so long as progress meets criteria accepted as normal. All complications shall be referred to a physician immediately. Nurse-midwifery does not include the assisting of childbirth by artificial, forcible, or mechanical means, nor the performance of any such version.

As used in this article, "supervision" shall not be construed to require the physical presence of the supervising physician.

A nurse-midwife is not authorized to practice medicine and surgery by the provisions of this chapter.

Nurse anesthetist: a person who is a registered nurse, licensed by the board of nursing, and who has met standards for certification from the board. In the certification and recertification process, the board shall consider the standards of the Council on Certification of Nurse Anesthetists and the Council on Recertification of Nurse Anesthetists and may develop new standards if there is a public safety need for standards more stringent than the councils' standards.

Nurse practitioner: a registered nurse with additional preparation and skills in physical diagnosis, psychosocial assessment, and management of health/illness needs in

(continued)

STATE-BY-STATE DEFINITIONS OF ADVANCED NURSING PRACTICE
(continued)

primary health care, who has been prepared in a program conforming to board standards. The nurse practitioner shall function within the scope of practice as specified in the Nursing Practice Act as it applies to all registered nurses.

COLORADO

Advanced practitioner of nursing: a professional nurse who by reason of postgraduate education and additional nursing preparation has knowledge, judgment, and skill beyond that required of a professional nurse and who has completed a nationally accredited educational program for preparation as an advanced practitioner of nursing or who has passed a national certification examination of a nationally recognized accrediting agency accepted by the board.

CONNECTICUT

Certified nurse practitioner: any registered nurse licensed under chapter 378 of the general statutes who has completed a formal educational nurse practitioner program and is certified by the American Nurses' Association, the National Board of Pediatric Nurse Practitioners and Associates, or the Nurses Association of the American College of Obstetricians and Gynecologists.

Certified psychiatric-mental health clinical nurse specialist: any registered nurse licensed under chapter 378 who has completed a formal educational program as a psychiatric-mental health clinical nurse specialist and is certified by the American Nurses' Association.

Certified nurse-midwife: any individual certified as nurse-midwife pursuant to public act 83-441.

DELAWARE

Advanced registered nurse practitioner: a currently licensed registered nurse who has gained added knowledge and skills through an organized postbasic program of study and clinical experience, who has met national certification requirements as approved by the board of nursing, and who is designated to perform advanced or specialized nursing practice. Advanced registered nurse practitioner shall include, but not be limited to, pediatric nurse practitioner, family nurse practitioner, maternal/gynecological nurse practitioner, clinical specialist in psychiatric-mental health nursing, nurse anesthetist, and gerontological nurse practitioner.

FLORIDA

Advanced or specialized nursing practice: in addition to the practice of professional nursing, the performance of advanced-level nursing acts approved by the board which, by virtue of postbasic specialized education, training, and experience, are proper to be performed by an advanced registered nurse practitioner. Within the context of advanced or specialized nursing practice, this practitioner may perform acts of nursing diagnosis and nursing treatment of alterations of the health status and may also perform acts of medical diagnosis and treatment, prescription, and operation which are identified and approved by a joint committee of members of the board of nursing and of the Board of Medical Examiners.

GEORGIA

Certified registered nurse anesthetist: any person who is authorized by this article to practice nursing as a registered professional nurse in this state who has successfully completed the education program of a school of nursing approved by the board in accordance with this article or has successfully completed an educational program outside the state or the United States which meets criteria similar to and not less stringent than those established by the board, who has successfully completed the educational program of a school for nurse anesthetists accredited by the American Association of Nurse Anesthetists (AANA), and who either is certified as a registered nurse anesthetist by the American Association of Nurse Anesthetists or has an application pending for such certification.

STATE-BY-STATE DEFINITIONS OF ADVANCED NURSING PRACTICE
(continued)

HAWAII

(To be adopted in 1987)

Advanced practice nurse: a registered nurse who possesses a current Hawaii license and who is a graduate of a master's degree program with a clinical specialty or is currently certified by a nationally recognized certifying body to practice in a specialized area of advanced nursing, or both, may use the designation.

IDAHO

Nurse practitioner: a licensed professional nurse having specialized skill, knowledge, and experience (and) authorized, by rules and regulations jointly promulgated by the Idaho state board of medicine and the Idaho board of nursing and implemented by the Idaho board of nursing, to perform designated acts of medical diagnosis, prescription of medical therapeutic and corrective measures, and delivery of medications.

ILLINOIS

None.

INDIANA

Nurse practitioner: a registered nurse qualified to practice nursing in a specialty role based upon the additional knowledge and skill gained by the registered nurse through a formal, organized program of study and clinical experience or equivalent as determined by the board of nursing which does not limit but extends or expands the function of the nurse in the area of primary health care, which care may be initiated by the client or provider in settings which shall include but not be limited to hospital outpatient clinics and health maintenance organizations.

IOWA

Advanced registered nurse practitioner (ARNP): a nurse with current active licensure as a registered nurse in Iowa who is prepared for advanced nursing practice by virtue of additional knowledge and skills gained through an organized post-basic program of nursing in a specialty area approved by the board of nursing. The advanced registered nurse practitioner is authorized by rule to practice advanced nursing or physician-delegated functions on an interdisciplinary health team.

The specialty areas of nursing practice for the advanced registered nurse practitioner which shall be considered as legally authorized by the board are as follows:
- nurse anesthetist
- nurse-midwife
- pediatric nurse practitioner
- family nurse practitioner
- school nurse practitioner
- obstetric/gynecologic nurse practitioner
- psychiatric-mental health nurse practitioner.

KANSAS

Advanced registered nurse practitioner (ARNP): a professional nurse who holds a certificate of qualification from the board of nursing to function as a professional nurse in an expanded role, and this expanded role shall be defined by rules and regulations adopted by the board.

KENTUCKY

Advanced registered nursing practice: the performance of additional acts by registered nurses who have added knowledge and skills through an organized postbasic program of study and clinical experience and who are certified by the American Nurses' Association or other national organizations or agencies recognized by the board of nursing to certify registered nurses for advanced nursing practice. The performance of such acts shall be consistent with the certifying organizations' or agencies' scopes and standards of practice recognized by the board by regulation.

(continued)

STATE-BY-STATE DEFINITIONS OF ADVANCED NURSING PRACTICE
(continued)

"Advanced registered nurse practitioner" shall mean one who is registered and designated to engage in advanced registered nursing practice including but not limited to the nurse anesthetist, nurse-midwife, and nurse practitioner.

LOUISIANA

Advanced practitioner of nursing: a health care provider who is currently licensed as a registered nurse in Louisiana and who, by virtue of additional educational preparation, has gained knowledge and skills in a specialty area of nursing.

Primary nurse associate (also known as nurse practitioner) is a registered nurse who provides direct nursing care to individuals, families, and other groups in a variety of settings, including homes, institutions, offices, industry, and schools and other community agencies. The nursing service provided by the primary nurse associate is aimed at the delivery of primary acute or chronic care which focuses on the maintenance, achievement, and restoration of optimal functions in the population. The primary nurse associate engages in nursing decision making. The primary nurse associate also participates in making decisions with other health care professionals regarding the needs of clients, and functions under the direction of a physician. By virtue of and consistent with additional educational preparation, knowledge, and clinical skills, a primary nurse associate may perform appropriate nursing functions, including:

• assess and develop a comprehensive health data base (including the elicitation of a comprehensive health history and performance of physical assessment, using skills of observation, inspection, palpation, percussion, and auscultation, as well as basic instruments and indicated screening procedures) for the purpose of reporting abnormal findings to the physician
• plan, implement, and evaluate nursing care consistent with medical treatment and care prescribed by a physician
• evaluate, plan, implement, and re-evaluate nursing care of individuals requiring emergency nursing measures
• initiate or modify medical treatment when and to the extent authorized by the treating physician within established plan of medical and nursing protocol

• assist the consumer in identifying and using the community resources available for follow-up health care service
• create and maintain accurate records, appropriate legal documents, and other reports of client care consistent with the law
• develop individualized client teaching plans based on assessed nursing needs
• counsel individuals, families, and groups about health and illness and promote health maintenance
• recognize, initiate, and participate in the development and implementation of professional and community educational programs related to health care.

Certified nurse-midwife: a registered nurse who, by virtue of added knowledge and skill gained through an organized program of study and clinical experience recognized by the American College of Nurse-Midwives (ACNM) and subsequent certification by the ACNM, has extended the limits of her practice into the area of management of care of mothers and babies throughout the maternity cycle so long as progress meets criteria accepted as normal. A nurse-midwife never works as an independent practitioner, but always as a member of a physician-directed health care team. She functions within the framework of medically approved criteria, policies, and standing orders. She may:
• assume responsibility for the management and complete care of the essentially healthy woman and newborn related to the childbearing process
• develop with the woman an appropriate care plan attentive to her interrelated needs
• participate in individual and group counseling and teaching throughout the childbearing process
• manage, through mutual agreement and collaboration with the physician, that part of care of medically complicated women which is appropriate to the skills and knowledge of nurse-midwives
• collaborate with other health professionals in delivery and evaluation of health care
• assess own professional abilities and function within identified capabilities
• assume responsibility for own self-determination within the boundaries of professional practice
• maintain and promote professional practice in concert with current trends
• utilize standards for evaluation of nurse-midwifery procedural functions in development and evaluation of practice

STATE-BY-STATE DEFINITIONS OF ADVANCED NURSING PRACTICE
(continued)

- promote the preparation of nurse-midwifery students and assist with the education of other health care personnel
- support the philosophy and official policies of the ACNM.

Certified registered nurse anesthetist: a registered nurse who renders anesthesia care and meets the requirements of Louisiana R.S. 37:930. A certified registered nurse anesthetist works under the direction and supervision of a physician or dentist who is licensed to practice under the laws of the State of Louisiana. She may:
- conduct a preanesthesia visit and assessment with appropriate documentation
- develop an anesthesia care plan
- induce anesthesia
- maintain anesthesia at the required levels
- support life functions during the perioperative period
- recognize and take appropriate action for untoward patient responses during anesthesia
- provide professional observation and management of the patient's emergence from anesthesia
- conduct postanesthesia visit and assessment with appropriate documentation
- participate in the life support of the patient for whatever cause.

Clinical nurse specialist: a registered nurse holding a master's degree in a specific area of clinical nursing. The advanced knowledge, skill, and competence of this nurse is made available to the public through the provision of direct nursing care to individuals. These services are further extended through the planning, guiding, and directing of care given by other nursing personnel.

The primary responsibility of the clinical nurse specialist is patient care delivery to a select population in a specialty area. The role functions of the clinical nurse specialist are: direct nursing care, indirect nursing care, research, change-agent, teaching, and consultation.
- *Direct nursing care:* Utilize a broad base of advanced scientific knowledge, nursing theory, and skills in assessing, planning, executing, and evaluating those aspects of health and nursing care of individuals who require this specialized competence.
- *Indirect nursing care:* Plan, guide, evaluate, and direct the nursing care given by other personnel associated with the nursing functions.

- *Research:* Create and test methods of nursing intervention and health care in the area of specialization.
- *Change-agent:* Act as a catalyst and/or initiator of change by applying new scientific knowledge in nursing practice and disseminating new knowledge and its application in nursing practice; work with agencies or groups of health personnel to change nursing practice and the system of health care delivery.
- *Teaching:* Utilize theories and skills of communication and teaching-learning to increase the knowledge or functioning of individuals and groups, nursing personnel, students, and other members of the health care team.
- *Consultation:* Act as a resource, utilizing advanced health knowledge and skills, to those who are directly and indirectly involved in nursing care.

MAINE

None.

MARYLAND

Certified nurse practitioner: shall be a registered nurse, complete a nurse practitioner program approved by the board of nursing, and meet the other requirements that the board sets.

MASSACHUSETTS

Nurse-midwife: designated by the board of nursing to engage in the practice of midwifery; provided, however, that the nurse-midwife functions as a member of a health care team which includes a qualified physician licensed to practice medicine in the commonwealth; and provided further, that deliveries by a nurse-midwife take place in facilities licensed by the department of public health for the operation of maternity and newborn services.

MICHIGAN

None.

(continued)

STATE-BY-STATE DEFINITIONS OF ADVANCED NURSING PRACTICE
(continued)

MINNESOTA

Advanced nursing practice: the performance of health services by certified registered nurse anesthetists and certified nurse-midwives as defined in Minnesota.

MISSISSIPPI

None.

MISSOURI

None.

MONTANA

Nurse practitioner practice: the management of primary health care of individuals, families, and communities, with ability to:
• assess the health status of individuals and families through health history taking, physical examination, and defining of health and development problems
• institute and provide continuity of health care to clients (patients), work with the client to ensure understanding of and compliance with the therapeutic regimen within established protocols, and recognize when to refer the client to a physician or other health care provider
• provide instruction and counseling to individuals, families, and groups in the areas of health promotion and maintenance, including involving such persons in planning for their health care
• work with other health care providers and agencies to provide and, if appropriate, coordinate services to individuals and families.

Nurse-midwifery practice: the independent management of care of essentially normal newborns and women, antepartally, postpartally, and/or gynecologically.

Nurse anesthetist practice: the performance of or the assistance in any act involving the determination, preparation, administration, or monitoring of any drug used to render an individual insensible to pain for surgical and other therapeutic procedures.

NEBRASKA

Nurse practitioner: meets the following qualifications:
• has acquired additional knowledge and skills within a particular clinical area designed to enable him or her to practice
• has completed an approved basic program in nursing prior to and in preparation for licensure as a registered professional nurse
• is currently licensed as a registered professional nurse in the State of Nebraska
• has successfully completed an advanced course of study which prepares the participant for certification in a specific expanded role in nursing and which provides additional knowledge and skills in physical and psychosocial assessment and management of health and illness needs of a specialized population
• has met the certification requirements and is currently certified with the approval of the boards.

Certified registered nurse anesthetist or **nurse practitioner-anesthetist:** a currently licensed registered professional nurse holding a current certificate as a nurse practitioner in the specific expanded role of the practice of anesthesia.
Practice of anesthesia shall mean: the performance of or the assistance in any act involving the determination, preparation, administration, or monitoring of any drug used to render an individual insensible to pain for procedures requiring the presence of persons educated in the administration of anesthetics, or the performance of any act commonly the responsibility of educated anesthesia personnel. Such term shall include the use of those techniques which shall be deemed necessary for adequacy in performance of anesthesia administration when those acts fall within the domain of professional nursing practices for which such nurse bears independent responsibility and those medically delegated functions of an anesthesiologic nature.

Certified nurse-midwife: a person certified under the Nebraska Certified Nurse-Midwifery Practice Act to practice certified nurse-midwifery in the State of Nebraska. Nothing in the act is intended to restrict the practice of registered nurses.

STATE-BY-STATE DEFINITIONS OF ADVANCED NURSING PRACTICE
(continued)

NEVADA

Certified registered nurse anesthetist: a person who has completed a nationally accredited program in the science of anesthesia who, when licensed as a registered nurse under the provisions of this chapter, administers anesthetic agents to a person under the care of those persons licensed by the State of Nevada to practice dentistry, surgery, or obstetrics.

NEW HAMPSHIRE

Advanced registered nurse practitioner: a registered nurse who presents certifying credentials from a program acceptable to the board of nursing, as indicative of having had specialized preparation as determined by the board, shall be identified on the license issued as an advanced registered nurse practitioner, or ARNP. The nurse certified as such shall be qualified to function in collaborative relationships with physicians as well as in private practice.

NEW JERSEY

None.

NEW MEXICO

Advanced nursing practice: the expanded practice of the registered nurse who has completed a recognized program of study in the expanded practice area or its equivalent as determined by the board.

Certified nurse practitioner: a registered nurse, licensed to practice in this state, who must have satisfactorily completed a postgraduate program designed for the education and preparation of nurse practitioners.

Certified registered nurse anesthetist: a person licensed as a registered nurse under the Nursing Practice Act who is a graduate of an approved school of nurse anesthesia.

NEW YORK

None.

NORTH CAROLINA

None.

NORTH DAKOTA

Clinical nurse specialist: The board of nursing shall restrict use of the title *clinical nurse specialist* and the abbreviation "CNS" to the registered nurse with a master's degree in nursing who has submitted evidence of specialization within a defined area of nursing practice.

OHIO

None.

OKLAHOMA

Nurse practitioner: a registered nurse who has successfully completed a formal program of study approved by the Oklahoma Board of Nurse Registration and Nursing Education which is designed to prepare registered nurses to perform in an expanded role in the delivery of primary health care, including the ability to:
• assess the health status of individuals and families through health and medical history taking, physical examination, and defining of health and developmental problems
• institute and provide continuity of health care to patients (clients); work with the client to ensure understanding of and compliance with the therapeutic regimen within established protocols; and recognize the need for referral of the client to a physician or other health care provider
• provide instruction and counseling to individuals, families, and groups in the areas of health promotion and maintenance, including involving such persons in planning for their health care

(continued)

STATE-BY-STATE DEFINITIONS OF ADVANCED NURSING PRACTICE
(continued)

• work in collaboration with other health care providers and agencies to provide and, where appropriate, coordinate services to individuals and families.

OREGON

Nurse practitioner: a registered nurse who has been certified by the board of nursing to practice in an expanded specialty role within the practice of nursing.

PENNSYLVANIA

Certified registered nurse practitioner: A registered nurse duly licensed in this Commonwealth who is certified by the boards in a particular clinical specialty area and who, while functioning in the expanded role as a professional nurse, performs acts of medical diagnosis or prescription of medical, therapeutic, or corrective measures in collaboration with and under the direction of a physician licensed to practice medicine in this Commonwealth.

The incorporation of physician supervision to the certified registered nurse practitioner's performance of medical acts in the following ways:
• immediate availability of a licensed physician through direct communications or by radio, telephone, or telecommunications
• a predetermined plan for emergency services which has been jointly developed by the supervising physician and the certified registered nurse practitioner
• a physician available on a regularly scheduled basis for referrals; review of the standards of medical practice incorporating consultation and chart review; establishing and updating standing orders, drug and other medical protocols within the practice setting; periodic updating in medical diagnosis and therapeutics; and cosigning records when necessary to document accountability by both parties.

RHODE ISLAND

None.

SOUTH CAROLINA

A professional nurse may perform additional acts requiring special education and training which are recognized jointly by the medical and nursing professions as proper for such nurse to perform if licensed under this chapter and recognized by the board of nursing through its rules and regulations.

School nurse practitioner: a registered nurse (RN) who has advanced skills in assessing, monitoring, and managing the physical and psychosocial health/illness status of individuals, families, or groups. The school nurse practitioner performs these skills and other acts as part of the activities within the school health program.

Occupational health nurse practitioner: an RN who has advanced skills in assessment, monitoring, and management of physical and psychosocial health/illness status of adults in the occupational setting. The practitioner performs these skills and other acts which are agreed upon jointly by medicine and nursing.

Pediatric nurse practitioner: an RN with advanced skills in assessing and managing the physical and psychosocial health/illness status of children, families, or child-related groups.

Family planning nurse practitioner: an RN who has advanced skills in assessing, monitoring, and managing physical and psychosocial health/illness status of individuals, families, and groups in a variety of settings. This nurse performs acts related to family planning and human sexuality.

Community health clinical nurse specialist: an RN with advanced skills in the assessment, monitoring, and management of physical and psychosocial health/illness status of individuals, families, or groups in a variety of community settings.

Family nurse practitioner: an RN who provides diversified health care and is prepared to assist in giving comprehensive, continuous personalized care of individuals, principally in primary care settings. They facilitate entrance of individuals into the health care system and provide continued care to them as ambulatory patients/

STATE-BY-STATE DEFINITIONS OF ADVANCED NURSING PRACTICE
(continued)

clients. To coordinate the comprehensive care of the clients, activities within secondary and tertiary settings often fall within the scope of their practice. Family nurse practitioners have advanced skills in assessment of the physical and psychological health/illness status of individuals and families. They are capable of managing common episodic and chronic illnesses in collaboration with the physician and other health care workers. They are skilled in health teaching and counseling. The focus of practice is family centered and stresses health screening, supervision of the well, and disease prevention.

Certified nurse-midwife (certification by the American College of Nurse-Midwives): a registered nurse who has extended the limits of her practice into the area of management of care of mothers and babies throughout the maternity cycle so long as progress meets criteria accepted as normal. Nurse-midwifery also includes interconceptional care for family planning, immediate care of the newborn at delivery, and well-child supervision. The nurse-midwife may practice in partnership with a physician or group of physicians rendering care within the provinces of obstetrics, preventive gynecology, and family planning. The physician–nurse-midwife team will offer care throughout the maternity cycle to patients receiving care in a variety of settings—private offices, outpatient, health department clinics, and hospitals.

Certified registered nurse anesthetist: a registered professional nurse who has graduated from a school of nurse anesthesia accredited by the American Association of Nurse Anesthetists. After graduation, each anesthetist must evidence individual competency by passing a rigid qualifying examination administered by the American Association of Nurse Anesthetists. The graduate nurse anesthetist is then eligible for certification as a certified nurse anesthetist by the American Association of Nurse Anesthetists.

Advanced practice in psychiatric-mental health nursing: performed by a clinical nurse specialist, a registered nurse who practices professional nursing and who, through additional educational preparation and supervised experience, has achieved a high level of knowledge, skill, and competence in the psychiatric-mental health clinical area.

SOUTH DAKOTA

None.

TENNESSEE

Nurse practitioner: the board of nursing shall issue a certificate of fitness to nurse practitioners who meet the qualifications, competencies, training, education, and experience sufficient to prepare such persons to write and sign prescriptions and/or issue drugs within limitations noted.

A nurse who has been issued a certificate of fitness as a nurse practitioner has not been automatically given the right to write and sign prescriptions and/or issue drugs, but such person shall be given such privileges as provided for by Tennessee Code Annotated, only when the certificate of fitness of the nurse practitioner and the recommendation of the Primary Care Board for the site at which the nurse practitioner is practicing has been recorded and filed.

The registered nurse may perform, in addition to the foregoing, those acts which require additional education which shall be authorized by the board through its rules and regulations.

Certified registered nurse anesthetist: in addition to performing all those functions within the scope of practice of a registered nurse as provided in this chapter, may accept the delegation of and perform the following medical functions:
- develop an anesthesia care plan
- induce anesthesia
- maintain anesthesia at the required levels
- support life functions during the perioperative period
- recognize and take proper action for untoward patient responses during anesthesia
- provide professional observation and management of the patient's emergence from anesthesia during the immediate postoperative period
- conduct postanesthesia visit and assessment when appropriate
- participate in the life support of the patient for whatever cause.

The medical functions shall be performed only under the supervision of a licensed physician responsible for the medical care of the patient.

(continued)

STATE-BY-STATE DEFINITIONS OF ADVANCED NURSING PRACTICE
(continued)

TEXAS

Advanced nurse practitioner: a registered professional nurse, currently licensed in Texas, who is prepared for advanced nursing practice by virtue of knowledge and skills obtained through a postbasic or advanced educational program of study acceptable to the board. The advanced nurse practitioner is prepared to practice in an expanded role to provide health care to individuals, families, and/or groups in a variety of settings including but not limited to homes, hospitals, institutions, offices, industry, schools, community agencies, public and private clinics, and private practice. The advanced nurse practitioner functions in a collegial relationship with physicians and other health professionals, making independent decisions about nursing needs and interdependent decisions with physicians regarding health regimens, and assumes dependent responsibilities in carrying out delegated medical acts.

UTAH

Registered nurses with advanced or specialized preparation who meet the criteria set forth in the rules and regulations and pay any additional fees provided for application for special licensure, shall have their professional nursing licenses designate their advanced or special category of practice including, but not limited to:
• nurse practitioner
• nurse anesthetist
• nurse specialist.

VERMONT

Nurse practitioner: an RN, practicing in the expanded role, who has completed advanced educational preparation in order to provide health care in various settings.

Collaboration: The nurse practitioner acts independently in dealing with the nursing needs of the individual and jointly, with a physician who holds a current license and engages in active clinical practice, for all related medical functions.

The term *nurse practitioner* will describe all the categories of registered professional nurses practicing in the expanded role, including but not be limited to:
• adult nurse practitioner
• certified nurse-midwife
• certified registered nurse anesthetist
• family nurse practitioner
• ob/gyn nurse practitioner
• pediatric nurse practitioner
• clinical specialist in psychiatric and mental health nursing.

The nurse practitioner accepts the responsibility, accountability, and obligation to practice in accordance with the accepted standards of nursing as defined by the profession. Nurse practitioners practice in accordance with current standards and functions as defined by the Scope of Practice statements for each specialty area and as developed by national professional nursing organizations.

Functions: The nurse practitioner practices professional nursing pursuant to Title 26, V.S.A., Chapter 28, § 1572 (2). The nurse practitioner performs medical acts within approved protocols mutually agreed on by the nurse practitioner and collaborating physician. The collaborating physician has responsibility for medical acts under Title 26, 1354, Chapter 23, but the nurse practitioner and collaborating physician take joint responsibility for medical acts performed under written protocols. These protocols must be reviewed and signed annually by both parties. Initial protocols will be on file in the workplace and the board office. The board will be apprised of any changes in the protocol or collaborating physician. Nurse practitioners practicing in the expanded role and employed by an institution will develop protocols with the medical staff of that institution. These protocols will be reviewed and signed annually by both parties.
• Prescriptions may be written and signed by the nurse practitioner for those drugs covered in current protocols and in compliance with all other state laws and regulations. A current list of endorsed nurse practitioners will be made available to the Vermont Board of Pharmacy.
• Nurse practitioners may write orders in hospitals under the same protocols and according to hospital policy.
• Nothing herein is to be deemed to limit the scope of practice or prohibit a nurse from engaging in those activities which normally constitute the practice of nursing.

STATE-BY-STATE DEFINITIONS OF ADVANCED NURSING PRACTICE
(continued)

VIRGINIA

Certified nurse practitioner: a registered nurse currently licensed in Virginia who has satisfactorily completed an approved program specifically designed to prepare nurses as nurse practitioners, and has been duly certified by the joint boards of medicine and nursing.

Categories:
- adult nurse practitioner
- family nurse practitioner
- pediatric nurse practitioner
- family planning nurse practitioner
- ob/gyn nurse practitioner
- emergency room nurse practitioner
- geriatric nurse practitioner
- certified nurse anesthetist practitioner
- certified nurse-midwife practitioner
- school nurse practitioner
- medical nurse practitioner
- maternal/child health practitioner
- neonatology nurse practitioner

Other categories may be determined by the Boards.

Medical acts which may only be performed in accordance with protocols: elicit detailed medical histories and systems review; perform physical examinations; initiate, perform, and interpret selected diagnostic procedures and tests; prepare a recommendation of diagnosis and/or treatment plan for the physician; implement a treatment plan upon the direction of the physician; initiate emergency treatment in the absence of a physician.

WASHINGTON

Advanced registered nurse practitioner (ARNP): recognition document may be issued to any person who meets the requirements of the board. Only persons holding this recognition document shall have the right to use the title "advanced registered nurse practitioner" or the abbreviation "ARNP." This document authorizes the ARNP to engage in the scope of practice allowed for his or her specialty area and is valid only with a current registered nurse license.

WEST VIRGINIA

Nurse anesthetist: in any case where it is lawful for a duly licensed physician or dentist practicing medicine or dentistry under the laws of this State to administer anesthetics, such anesthetics may lawfully be administered by any person (a) who has been licensed to practice registered professional nursing under this article, and (b) who holds a diploma or certificate evidencing successful completion of the education program of a school of anesthesia duly accredited by the American Association of Nurse Anesthetists: Provided that such anesthesia is administered by such person in the presence and under the supervision of such physician or dentist.

Nurse-midwife: a qualified professional nurse registered with the West Virginia Board of Examiners for Registered Nurses who by virtue of additional training is specifically qualified to practice midwifery according to the statement of functions, standards, and qualifications for the practice of nurse-midwifery as set forth by the American College of Nurse-Midwives.

WISCONSIN

Nurse-midwifery: the management of care of a woman in normal childbirth and the provision of prenatal, intrapartum, postpartum, and nonsurgical contraceptive methods and care for the mother and the newborn.

Advanced practitioner of nursing: a registered professional nurse who performs advanced nursing acts and who may perform medical acts in collaboration with a licensed or otherwise legally authorized physician or dentist, in such manner to assure quality and appropriateness of services rendered. This practitioner: performs such acts by reason of postgraduate education and additional nursing preparation, which provide knowledge, judgment, and skill beyond that required of a registered professional nurse; has completed a nationally accredited educational program for preparation as an advanced practitioner of nursing; or has passed a national certification examination of a nationally recognized accrediting agency accepted by the board.

Practicing politics to influence policy

On first thought, nursing and politics may seem incompatible. But politics are inherent in any system, and the health care industry is certainly no exception. For nurses, politics means one thing: influencing powerful people to make policy decisions that promote quality patient care. This involves influencing those in government who decide how nursing is defined and regulated, as well as influencing policymakers to secure nursing's fair share of diminishing health care resources.

Policy decisions that affect your ability to provide quality patient care are made on unit; departmental; institutional; and city/community, state, and federal governmental levels. Today's rapidly changing health care environment, in its state of flux, demands that nurses expand their scope of influence to all of these levels—even the highest.

Principles of politics

The art of politics is really the art of influencing people. Whether the people you need to influence are in nursing management, on your hospital's medical staff, or on the state senate's health financing committee, the art of influencing people can be summed up in six basic principles. Following these principles can help you develop your political skills fully, so you can have a greater say in decisions that influence the way you practice nursing and, ultimately, nursing care and the nursing profession.

• *Principle 1—Identify the people in power.* Identify all the people who have the power to make decisions that affect nurses and their practice. First, identify the decision makers in your own organization—the administrators at executive and middle-management levels, department heads, and board members. At governmental levels, identify city council or county representatives, and state and federal legislators.

• *Principle 2—Get to know those in power.* Central to the art of influencing people is getting to know those in power and developing friendly relationships with them. Seemingly minor acts like congratulatory or thank-you notes, compliments, and simple favors can go a long way in solidifying beneficial relationships. Then, when you need the influence of such people, they'll be more likely to deliver favors.

• *Principle 3—Develop or join a special-interest group.* Team up with others to gain more influence. Cultivate groups within your workplace by recruiting and supporting associates who share your concerns about nursing and quality patient care. Join your state nurses association and specialty nursing organizations. Become active on committees at work and in professional and community organizations. In addition, cooperate with community health care groups to keep consumers aware of your work and thereby mobilize public opinion in your favor. Whenever possible, teach the public about nursing and related health care issues through news releases, workshops, and presentations to community organizations and citizens' groups.

• *Principle 4—Target your issues carefully.* Use your time and energy to best advantage by focusing your efforts on those issues on which you can have some potential impact. Be realistic; don't waste your efforts on issues that you have no hope of influencing.

• *Principle 5—Build alliances.* Cultivate relationships with other groups, departments, or organizations that share your group's interest in a particular issue. Join forces with these groups for more power in influencing this issue.

• *Principle 6—Return favors.* Be sure to recognize and reward policymakers and legislators who have been helpful to your special-interest group. You can do so, for example, by serving on a committee to help a hospital administrator, formally acknowledging the person's support with a letter or award, or doing campaign work for or contributing campaign funds to a legislator.

Following these six basic principles can help you influence policymakers at any level. It's never too late to start building your political clout. Begin today, so you can make a difference tomorrow.

BRENDA L. LYON, RN, DNS

New sources of burnout

Even though the word burnout first appeared in the nursing literature only 8 years ago, it's now universally recognized as one of nurses' special problems. And it's easy to see why.

The very nature of nurses' daily work puts them at risk of being overwhelmed by others' problems. By definition, our profession demands caring involvement. So regardless of the unit on which staff nurses work, they are subject to a variety of potential stressors. Unfortunately, changes in today's health care environment now conspire to impose many additional stressors on nurses in virtually every practice setting. Whether these stressors contribute to burnout depends on nurses' views of them and on the effectiveness of nurses' coping strategies.

New stressors
The widespread effects of the new federal prospective payment system, based on Diagnosis-Related Groups (DRGs), have had enormous impact on every aspect of the health care system. Indeed, learning to live with DRGs has been difficult for everyone—but probably most difficult for nurses. As hospital budgets shrink and doctors hospitalize only the most acutely ill

patients and for shorter lengths of stay, nurses are caring for sicker patients in less time and with less help of every kind. As patients are discharged to complete their recovery at home, nurses' responsibility for teaching them self-care and continued treatment has become critically important. Again, nurses have acquired more responsibility for more difficult and complex work, without additional time in which to do it.

The nursing profession itself, through its determination to push for professional advancement, is also a source of stress for many nurses. For example, many practicing nurses who do not have baccalaureate preparation feel threatened and insecure in their jobs.

Other potential stressors include feeling trapped in one's job, lack of communication, feeling powerless, and working in an environment perceived to be demanding, frustrating, and/or unrewarding.

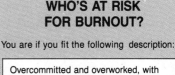

WHO'S AT RISK FOR BURNOUT?

You are if you fit the following description:

Overcommitted and overworked, with pressure to succeed

Focused mainly on work; see yourself as "the only one who can do the job"

Woman under age 30

Passive, unassertive, and lacking self-confidence

Lacking autonomy and control; feeling helpless, powerless, and trapped

Recent BSN graduates who may lack extensive clinical preparation.

STAGES OF BURNOUT

STAGE 1

Emotional and physical exhaustion associated with various physical complaints—colds, GI problems, and aches and pains. The nurse dreads going to work and spends as little time as possible with patients.

STAGE 2

A negative and cynical attitude toward people, including patients and staff. The nurse begins to feel that patients deserve their problems.

STAGE 3

Terminal burnout, resulting in the nurse feeling disgust with herself and humanity; she perceives her life to be out of control. (Burnout rarely reaches this stage.)

Clearly, stress is an inescapable and universal part of nursing and will surely continue to be so. But it doesn't necessarily lead to burnout. Your individual response determines whether job stress will be overwhelming and eventually lead to burnout, or whether it will become an occasion for personal growth.

Coping strategies

Dealing effectively with stress requires multiple coping skills that are based, first of all, on self-knowledge. Before you can cope effectively, you must identify the stressor. You must know exactly what it is that makes you feel bad and evaluate it. Identify the specific events that make you feel stressed and what you do to cope with them. To do this, try keeping a daily log. While at work, quickly jot down the stressors as they happen and how you dealt with them. After a few days, such a log will clearly show the recurring stressors as well as any coping strategies. It will show if you use only one or two or many strategies and whether your strategies are

effective. Typically, nurses who cope easily have a wide repertoire of strategies, including a variety of backup strategies. No single strategy can conquer all stressors. You must develop your own list of strategies appropriate to your individual situation, usual techniques, and temperament. You can start by considering the following general guidelines:

• *Develop a sense of humor.* It relieves tension, keeps things in perspective, and prevents us from taking ourselves too seriously.

• *Learn to communicate openly, individually and in groups.*

• *Plan to grow.* Make and take advantage of opportunities for personal and professional growth.

• *Learn and develop assertiveness skills.*

• *Develop on-the-job support groups.* These have been found to be very successful in preventing burnout. They may start out as gripe sessions in which nothing is solved. But after group members have vented their feelings, they can turn to problem solving. Such a group works best with a leader who can be objective.

• *Take time out.* Take coffee and lunch breaks without talking about work. Take vacations and vary work assignments. If working with a particular patient is stressful, swap assignments for a couple of days. If you feel you need a permanent change, think about transferring to another nursing unit. But, before you transfer, identify the stressors on your current unit so you won't request transfer to another unit with the same ones.

• *Set both short- and long-term objectives.* While objectives give us a definite aim in life, they're not "written in stone." They can and will change as you continue to grow and develop personally and professionally.

• *Develop effective time-management skills.* Set priorities, stick to them, and use a daily "to do" list.

• *Develop a "decompression" routine.* Choose an after-work activity that helps you relax and leave the stressors at work.

• *Engage in an enjoyable physical activity.* Be sure to choose an activity that you really like because an unpleasant one will become a stressor.

• *Develop new interests unrelated to work.* Avoid having your work become the center of your universe.

• *Give the people you work with positive feedback.* People who feel needed and appreciated for their efforts become more pleasant to work with.

• *Eat nutritionally balanced meals.* Good nutrition is essential to physical and emotional well-being.

High costs of burnout

Burnout is costly to the individual nurse, the patient, other staff, the hospital, and ultimately the nursing profession itself. When a nurse feels chronically frustrated and angry, she may withdraw emotionally from her patients, dehumanizing them and seeing them as diseases or surgical procedures, as mere objects for the performance of technical skills.

Burnout is infectious and can sweep through a nursing unit. As nurses resign, fewer nurses are available for patient care, which increases stress on the remaining staff. In turn, orientation of new staff becomes an added stressor. Widespread burnout can adversely affect the status and future of our profession. Who would want to join a profession so fraught with problems that its members leave? And, in changing how an individual nurse feels about herself, burnout changes the image of nurses and nursing; it can adversely affect how society and the consumers of nursing care see our profession.

We can't afford burnout, so we must accept individual responsibility for preventing it. For, as Hans Selye said, "None of us can expect others to look after us more than after themselves." This doesn't mean being recklessly selfish. But it does mean being responsible to and for ourselves.

EDWINA A. McCONNELL, RN, MS

Collaborative practice in nursing

As nursing's role changes, nurses are changing their relationships with doctors and other health care professionals. More and more, we enjoy a collegial relationship with these other professionals, with whom we share responsibility for patient care. Nurses, doctors, dietitians, social workers—all health care professionals—share the same ultimate goal: improving the patient's mental and physical health. Each profession pursues this goal in its own way and develops its own treatments. These different treatments help the patient most when they come together as compatible, mutually supportive parts of an organized and coherent effort. Such closely integrated treatment can make the difference between success and failure, but it's possible only in a setting that provides policies and procedures for interprofessional, or collaborative, practice. In such a setting, each professional can collaborate with and depend on the others, to everyone's mutual benefit—especially the patient's.

For a nurse, whose primary goal is the patient's well-being, the ability to communicate effectively and work productively with doctors and all other health care professionals is critical. Often, a nurse's effectiveness is directly related to her ability to influence the other members of the health care team to work together in the patient's behalf. One of the best ways of gaining such influence is through structured collaborative practice with doctors, nurses, and other health care professionals.

Collaborating with doctors

As nurses have taken on wider clinical responsibilities, the traditional nurse-doctor relationship has changed in many ways. Nurses are now taking a much more active role in identifying and treating patient problems, through nursing diagnosis and other steps of the nursing process. Though functioning as patient advocates, we need not feel that we are doctors' adversaries. Such antagonistic relationships are always mistakes, for they will undermine, not promote, good patient care. To help our patients the most, nurses and doctors need to respect each other as professionals and work together in a true collegial spirit.

For nurses and doctors, collaborative practice generally takes one of three forms: collaboration between a patient's primary nurse and his doctor, joint practice between a clinical nurse specialist (CNS) or nurse practitioner (NP) and a doctor in a hospital or office setting, or collaboration among a primary nurse and a CNS or NP and doctor in joint practice.

Here are some examples that show how nurse-doctor collaborative practice can work in a hospital setting:

• *Daily nurse-doctor patient rounds,* in which the patient's primary nurse and his doctor (and possibly a CNS or NP in joint practice with the doctor) check on his condition together. This allows the nurse(s) and doctor to compare observations and insights and discuss interventions, plans, and goals of treatment to develop a coordinated medical and nursing care plan. It also enables comprehensive patient teaching, with no conflicting or overlapping information, and presents a unified care team, which promotes confidence and trust in the patient and his family.

• *Nurse-doctor educational exchange,* both formal and informal. Formal interdisciplinary educational forums held on a monthly basis, for example, give doctors and nurses the chance to discuss case studies and jointly evaluate the effectiveness of the medical and nursing care provided. Informal educational exchange between nurses and doctors is continuous. As nurses gain more clinical expertise, doctors rely more and more on their input in such areas as patient assessment, patient

teaching, and discharge planning. Accordingly, nurses should take every opportunity to familiarize doctors with nursing practice—an area in which most have little knowledge. Doctors who understand the nursing process, nursing standards, and nursing theory are generally more supportive and respectful of nurses, which leads to better collegial relationships.

• *Exchange of documentation* between nurses and doctors. As you know, nurses find the doctor's patient chart and progress notes a valuable source of information on the patient's condition. In a collegial relationship, doctors want access to nurses' notes for the same reason—to benefit from the nurse's insight into the patient's condition and progress.

• *Joint practice committees,* composed of an equal number of staff nurses and doctors. Such a committee meets regularly to discuss common problems and issues that affect medical and nursing practice. Since each member of the committee has an equal voice, the committee's recommendations and decisions reflect the concerns of both disciplines and represent a unified position to hospital administration.

• *Medical-nursing management committees,* composed of head nurses, the nursing director, and the medical director. Such a committee meets regularly to share information, provide mutual and staff support, and develop strategies for dealing with common management concerns.

Collaborating with other health care professionals

In the past, a doctor and a few staff nurses typically provided most or all of a hospitalized patient's care. But as health care has grown more specialized and complex, many other health care specialists—including dietitians, social workers, psychologists, radiologists, laboratory technicians, physician's assistants, and respiratory, physical, and occupational therapists—often contribute to a patient's care. Unfortunately, as the number of team members increases, so does the potential for fragmented, overlapping, or discordant care. To ensure coherent patient care, the multidisciplinary health care team should promote collaborative practice as illustrated by the following examples:

• *Multidisciplinary team planning.* A doctor, primary nurse, CNS, social worker, nurse discharge planner, and several allied health care professionals meet regularly, once a week, to plan strategies for reaching patient goals. The doctor, primary nurse, and CNS provide information on the patient's condition gained from their practice. The social worker and nurse discharge planner assist with nursing home placement and home care needs, as necessary. Allied health care workers provide information on the patient's capabilities and suggestions for continuing therapy after discharge.

• *Care conferences.* Scheduled as frequently as the patient's needs require, to cope with the patient's special problems or changing condition. Coordinated by the patient's primary nurse, these conferences involve the entire health care team and sometimes the patient and his family as well.

Collaborating with other nurses

As the patient's chief care provider, the primary nurse directs and coordinates the nursing team and acts as liaison between the patient and other care providers. To make sure the patient gets quality care, the primary nurse must collaborate not only with doctors and other health care professionals, but also with all the nurses who care for the patient. Effective collaboration requires the following key elements:

• *Integrated nursing care plans.* Based on a nursing assessment and nursing diagnosis, the nursing care plan becomes a permanent part of a patient's medical records. A recently developed integrated nursing care plan model recognizes independent, dependent, and collaborative nursing interven-

tions. In such a care plan, nursing interventions require coordination with nursing, medical, and allied services' plans and goals to ensure coordinated, consistent patient care.

• *Peer review,* both formal, at regularly scheduled intervals, and informal, in day-to-day practice. All nurses caring for a patient need to share and evaluate all information and observations on the patient's condition to help develop an integrated and effective nursing care plan.

• *Access to nursing resources* to provide the clinical expertise, experience, and leadership necessary for quality nursing practice. For example, a more experienced nurse or a CNS can help a primary nurse develop specialized assessment and diagnostic information, suggest specific nursing care measures, and provide appropriate patient teaching.

JOYCE A. KUNKEL, RN, MS, CNRN
JOHN K. WILEY, MD, FACS

Power: It's changing hands and moving your way

You're all aware of the dramatic changes that prospective payment systems have brought about in the health care industry since the fall of 1983. Like it or not, these systems are here to stay. The Diagnosis-Related Group model is just the first. Experts predict this model won't last, but other forms of prospective payment will be with us for a long time.

Prospective payment systems have changed the goal of health care from *cost containment* to *cost reduction.* As a result, they've created significant shifts of power within the health care industry. Nursing needs to respond to these power shifts that are taking place and turn them to its advantage.

Shift from providers to payers

The most fundamental change is this: because of prospective payment, power is shifting from those who provide health care (such as hospitals, doctors, and nurses) to those who pay for it (such as the government, insurance companies, and consumers).

Nobody wants to pick up the bill anymore. The government has passed it on to hospital corporations, the consumer, and industry (by allowing negotiations with insurance companies for cost-effective health care packages). Industry, in turn, is pressuring employees to shop around for the cheapest health care services and to examine bills carefully for errors. Following Washington's lead, insurance companies are refusing to pay more than a predetermined amount for medical bills. Consequently, consumers must be more selective in choosing a hospital, and hospital administrators must watch each dollar spent on patients.

The implication for nursing is clear. Since the consumer is going to have more power, we have to work harder at selling ourselves to the public. We need to polish our image so that we look and sound like the professionals we are. Above all, we have to let people know just how much nurses do—what services we provide and how they can get those services cheaper from us than from other health care workers. For example, in a recent review of nearly 30 studies, the American Nurses' Association and the National Association of Pediatric Nurse Associates and Practitioners pointed out how clinical nurse specialists and nurse practitioners often provide more efficient care than doctors. In fact, couldn't we agree that most of this nation's primary health care needs can be met by nurses?

This is no time for nurses to be modest. We've always been closest to the patient, so we have an advantage in getting our message out. That message is simple and direct: No other group of health care professionals does more for sick people than nurses do. We help them get better; we help them get out of the hospital as quickly as possible; we help them get on with their lives.

Making peace with doctors

Playing off this shift in power from health care providers to those who pay for it are other changes within the power structure of hospitals. One of the most important is the power drain that doctors have suffered as a result of prospective payment systems. Like nurses, doctors too have been stung by cost-reduction measures. In the past, they operated pretty much on their own; but today, it's different. Consumers no longer trust doctors the way they did. They're asking questions. And because of the current glut of doctors, consumers have the luxury of looking around first before choosing a doctor they can trust—and afford.

All this has led to some changes in medical practice, such as making rounds twice a day and making house calls and courtesy phone calls. Some doctors have even started sending flowers to patients, as reported in news stories.

What does this mean for nursing? It means we now have the opportunity to do something we should have done a long time ago—align ourselves with doctors. Making them our enemies was a political error; we cut ourselves off from a power source. Now is a good time to make peace. Doctors are nervous about all these changes. Nervous people do things they've never done before—like cooperate with former adversaries.

Despite their loss of power, doctors will always be influential. If nursing is to strengthen its power base, we'll need them on our side.

Nursing education must change

Power is also shifting from nursing educators to nursing administrators. In the past, administrators took a laissez-faire attitude toward nursing education. Now their attitude is changing. They're looking for nurses with clinical

HOW POWER IS SHIFTING IN HEALTH CARE

The arrows in this graphic representation of the health care industry show the direction in which power is shifting. The most fundamental power shift is from health care providers (hospitals, doctors, nurses) to those who pay for it. But within the hospital itself and within nursing, power is moving toward nursing administrators and eventually toward staff nurses.

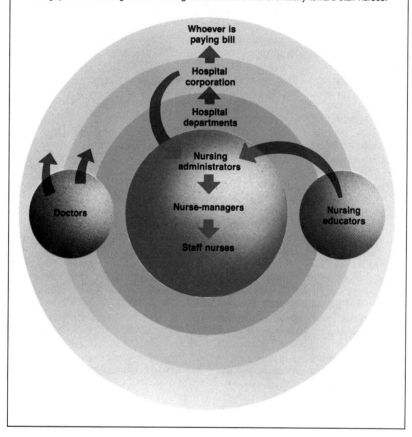

skills and a sophisticated, businesslike appearance. That's what they're promising the public in their marketing programs. One hospital on the West Coast, for example, is offering its nurses courses in "looking good" and "sounding good" during interactions with patients, family members, and colleagues. Many nursing school graduates have had trouble finding jobs as hospital staff nurses during the past 2 years. To meet the challenge of supplying hospitals with marketable graduates, nursing educators must adjust their curricula to reflect the demand for more business-oriented graduates.

Few people grasp the significance of nursing degrees—a BSN, even an MSN. They just don't mean that much to the business people moving into power roles in today's hospital corporations. They don't know our language and they don't care to learn it. So we have no choice but to learn theirs. It shouldn't be that hard; the language of the business world is concrete, specific, and quantitative. A lot of people speak it. People in power speak it. We have to learn to speak it.

Remember that our goal is adequate reimbursement for our services. Nursing departments must become profit centers. To do that, we need nurses who fit into the corporate picture. Nursing educators need to take this into account when preparing students for the new realities of hospital nursing. Today, it's our business skills—not our clinical skills, unfortunately—that are going to sell nursing.

Nurse-executive: A power position

In reorganizing under the corporate umbrella, many hospitals have created a new top-level nurse-executive—the vice-president of nursing—and given her responsibility not only for nursing but for other departments as well. In one Pennsylvania hospital, for example, the nursing department now oversees the pharmacy; another hospital has made its nursing department responsible for social services, respiratory therapy, and housekeeping. That's a real vote of confidence for our leaders.

So here we have a new power base within the hospital corporation—the nurse-executive, whose responsibilities go far beyond those of a director of nursing. This trend illustrates how the prospective payment revolution has allowed nursing to enter the upper echelon of the corporate hierarchy.

What these vice-presidents of nursing must concentrate on now is maneuvering for power in the non-nursing world. For example, it's important that a nurse-executive's office be located near that of the chief executive officer (CEO), instead of being off by itself in the nursing department. Just by being physically close to the people who make things happen in a hospital, nurse-executives will find their prestige rising dramatically. Both formal and informal invitations will come their way—opportunities to sit on powerful committees and to talk with

hospital board members, for instance.

Looking farther down the road, nurse-executives should aspire to be CEOs someday. Their success will be nursing's success.

Staff nurses gaining power

As part of the overall movement toward decentralization in hospitals, nurse-executives must relinquish certain responsibilities formerly held by directors of nursing and middle-level supervisors. For example, the power to hire and fire, to prepare unit budgets and staff-development programs, to make staffing decisions—these matters will now be handled by nurse-managers. And nurse-managers, in turn, will be handing over more and more of their traditional responsibilities to the staff nurse—the RN care giver—who remains at the heart of the profession, the single most important person in the whole system.

Staff nurses have been clamoring for years—and rightfully so—for more power. They feel they're the people who are best qualified to make the major decisions concerning patient care. And they want a bigger say in running their units, in choosing equipment and supplies, and so forth. That's exactly what they're going to get. Decisions that were made in the past by nurse-managers will now be made by the nurse who works at the bedside. But to make the decisions in the cost-conscious environment of the modern hospital, the staff nurse needs more than clinical skills. She needs to understand the business of nursing. The hospitals that survive—maybe even thrive—under prospective payment systems will be those that are staffed by nurses who combine both skills.

Seeing the big picture

These power shifts are affecting the entire health care industry, not just nursing. If you keep the big picture in mind, you'll be better able to see where nursing fits in—where *you* fit in. And you'll have a better idea of how to maneuver successfully in the business climate that permeates today's hospitals. No one can represent nursing's best interests as well as we can. Instead of running scared, we must seize the initiative and act aggressively to show the corporate powers-that-be what we can do—how we can run our units efficiently, how we can help hospitals save money and *make* money.

Nursing will always be around. What we have to make sure of is that the nursing of tomorrow is the nursing *we* want, not what someone else wants. To do that, we have to get down to business today.

PATRICIA NORNHOLD, RN, MSN

CLINICAL PRACTICE

Trends and issues in geriatric nursing

If you know anything about current demographics, you know that the population of this country is aging. Today, more than 23 million Americans are over age 65; by the year 2000, this figure will probably rise to 32 million. As you can imagine, this trend is profoundly influencing all areas of health care, including nursing, both in hospitals and in other health care settings. After all, elderly persons are the group most in need of medical and nursing care.

Other health care trends affecting geriatric nursing include the new prospective payment systems for health care funding and the shifting focus of long-term care from hospitals to extended-care facilities and home care.

But just how are these trends affecting geriatric nursing? Here's a look at what's happening.

Geriatric nursing in hospitals

If you work in a hospital, you've probably seen the effects of these trends already. In some parts of the country, well over half of acute care hospital patients are over age 65. Rising acute care costs and new limits on third-party reimbursement for these costs—the result of prospective payment systems—are forcing hospital administrators to take a new approach to the care of these elderly patients. Basically, the changing economic climate has resulted in shorter hospital stays, with patients being discharged earlier to extended-care facilities or to home.

To make sure these patients are prepared for discharge, hospitals are beginning to deal with restorative aspects of care designed to help the patient regain the ability to perform normal activities of daily living. Many hospitals have formed geriatric units for this purpose; some have developed geriatric assessment teams, in which a nurse, doctor, social worker, and perhaps an occupational therapist work together to help the elderly patient regain functional ability before discharge.

Even if they're not part of a geriatric assessment team, nurses who work in acute care settings can help prepare elderly patients for early discharge. Adopting some practices, principles, and equipment used in long-term care—for example, providing practical aids such as raised toilet seats and walkers, and becoming more sensitive to the special physical and emotional needs of the elderly—can make a big difference in promoting an elderly patient's recovery and adjustment to discharge to an extended-care facility or to home.

The hospital nurse can also help elderly patients cope with early discharge by taking a more active role in discharge planning. This should begin on admission, with a physical and psychological assessment to obtain information on the patient's condition and his life-style, focusing on his age-related disabilities and how they inter-

REVIEWING PHYSIOLOGIC CHANGES IN THE ELDERLY

When assessing an elderly patient, you must take into account the physiologic changes that normally accompany aging. This chart reviews these typical changes and the physical problems they commonly cause.

ORGAN OR SYSTEM	NORMAL CHANGES	POSSIBLE PATHOLOGIC RESULTS
Brain	• Diminished number of brain cells or brain weight • Atherosclerotic changes • Lowered activity of endorphins and increased activity of monoamine oxidase (MAO) enzymes	• Poor short-term memory, possibly senile dementia • Multi-infarct dementia • Mental depression
Circulatory system	• Arteriosclerotic and atherosclerotic changes in blood vessels • Increased peripheral resistance with decreased vessel elasticity • Decreased blood volume	• Occlusion of arteries and capillaries, resulting in diminished blood supply to all organ systems • Hypertension, decreased pulse, and increased cardiac work load • Azotemia
Ear	• Anatomic changes in inner ear and cochlea • Diminished activity of cilia	• Presbycusis • Impacted ear canals, decreased sound transmission
Endocrine system	• Decreased estrogen levels, with diminished ovarian function • Decreased response to insulin • Decreased metabolic clearance rate • Decreased pituitary gland function; lowered thyroid-stimulating hormone secretion	• Osteoporosis • Postmenopausal loss of secondary sex characteristics • Hyperglycemia • Decreased sodium reabsorption, leading to hyponatremia • Hypothyroidism in women
Eye	• Increased lens density • Change in aqueous kinetics • Change in lens elasticity • Decreased ability to perceive various intensities of light; loss of binocular vision	• Cataracts • Glaucoma • Presbyopia • Accidents: falls, medication errors
Gastrointestinal tract	• Decreased motility • Decreased endocapillary membrane diffusion • Decreased absorption of calcium • Decreased sensitivity to thirst • Possible diminished hydrochloric acid secretion	• Constipation • Malabsorption • Osteoporosis • Dehydration • Poor absorption, especially of drugs
Heart	• Decreased cardiac muscle mass • Increased calcification of heart valves and skeleton	• Diminished cardiac output; increased risk of congestive heart failure • Conduction defects, irritability of heart muscle, endocarditis, dysrhythmia, valve stenosis or insufficiency

REVIEWING PHYSIOLOGIC CHANGES IN THE ELDERLY *(continued)*		
ORGAN OR SYSTEM	**NORMAL CHANGES**	**POSSIBLE PATHOLOGIC RESULTS**
Immune system	• Decreased T cell function	• Increased incidence of infection and autoimmune disease
Lungs	• Decreased elasticity and increased size of alveoli • Diminished activity of cilia and decreased cough reflex • Lowered diffusion across the alveolocapillary membrane	• Chronic obstructive pulmonary disease • Increased incidence of pneumonia, secondary to impaired bronchoelimination • Hypoxia
Musculoskeletal system	• Diminished mean muscle mass, increased fat mass • Decreased synthesis and absorption of bone calcium	• Increased serum levels of water-soluble drugs; fatigue • Osteoporosis, with accompanying bone fractures • Osteoarthritis, with joint pain and stiffness
Renal and urologic system	• Diminished renal blood flow, glomerular filtration rate, and tubular function; decreased size of kidneys and number of glomeruli • Decreased bladder size	• Tendency toward transient or permanent renal insufficiency and drug toxicities • Incontinence and urinary frequency
Skin	• Diminished sensitivity to pain and temperature changes • Decreased subcutaneous fat • Atrophy of sweat glands	• Accidents, burns • Decubitus ulcers • Heatstroke, hypothermia

fere with his daily activities. Of course, this assessment should be ongoing; new findings can require significant changes in the care plan and, consequently, can prolong or shorten the length of stay. The information from this assessment helps the nurse develop an effective care plan and set a realistic discharge date. It also helps the nurse anticipate and prevent problems after discharge that could result in a return to the hospital.

For discharge planning is only as good as the care the patient receives when he leaves the hospital. One of the most important things the hospital nurse can do for an elderly patient is to communicate with those who will care for him after he leaves the hospital. Effective coordination with outpatient staff, the patient's family, and outside agencies and community services can help ensure a smooth discharge and, what's more important, ensure effective continuing care for the elderly patient.

Geriatric care in other settings

The evidence is clear: Increasingly, geriatric health care means home care. The number of available community programs and services intended to support home care for the elderly is increasing rapidly. Visiting nurse services, home care aides, senior citizen's centers, Meals on Wheels, social welfare services, and the like all help elderly persons cope with health problems at home. One relatively new service, geriatric day care, can be a valuable part of the home health care plan for many elderly patients. In this program, the patient spends all or part of the day at a day-care facility, where he receives medical supervision and nursing care and has the opportunity for recreational activities and social contact with peers. Day care is especially beneficial for an elderly person whose disability interferes with social interaction and leads to isolation.

Besides normal patient care responsibilities, the home health care nurse is also responsible for identifying and linking the patient with available and appropriate community resources.

Of course, home care isn't appropriate for every elderly patient. Often, an extended-care facility, such as a nursing home, is the best alternative. In these facilities, levels of nursing, once split into health-related and skilled nursing categories, are becoming increasingly blurred as these facilities admit more chronically ill patients and struggle to control the spiraling costs of care. This means more opportunities for registered nurses and nurse specialists to practice in these facilities.

Whatever the setting, geriatric nursing is becoming more and more important as the population ages and as changes in the health care industry affect the very fabric of health care in this country. Nurses who care for the elderly have a unique opportunity to help patients who really need help—and to work in an area of nursing that will only expand as time goes by.

ALAN T. STURM, RN, GNC

Nursing diagnosis and the nursing process

You know that nursing diagnosis is a vital part of the nursing process. As the step that follows identification of the patient's problems, nursing diagnosis expresses your professional judgment of the patient's clinical status, his responses to treatment, and his nursing care needs. You perform this step so you can carry out your nursing care plan. In effect, nursing diagnosis actually *defines* the practice of nursing.

What it is

A nursing diagnosis is a statement of a health problem that a nurse is licensed to treat, a problem for which she will assume responsibility for therapeutic decisions and accountability for the outcomes. It states a synthesis of our ability to recognize the presenting signs and symptoms and to make a professional judgment about an actual or potential health problem.

Data gathering and assessment

Although continuous and careful patient observation is second nature to most nurses, putting observations in writing isn't always so natural. But you'll find writing nursing diagnoses easier if you follow these simple steps. First, collect information from your patient on his health, cultural, religious, environmental, and social background; on his daily living habits; and on his coping mechanisms. Find out what his personal health goals are, how he feels about his present problems, and on whom he relies for support. Add information from your own observation and assessment.

These assessment data, which are necessary for an accurate nursing diagnosis, contain both subjective and objective information. Subjective data, which are reported to you verbally, identify a health problem through a primary source (the patient's description of his own symptoms) or a secondary source (any other informant). Be sure to record all subjective data as a direct quote. Remember that it may be important to record the patient's denial of a problem—for example, when a patient with peripheral neuropathy denies pain in an ulcerated or edematous area.

Objective data, which are also derived from primary and secondary sources, include any facts or observable information about the patient. Primary data include written notes or observations from the patient himself (for example, a daily record of insulin dose that a patient keeps for the community health nurse). Secondary sources are those written notes or observations from any source other than the patient. They include your findings at physical assessment (the results of inspection, palpation, percussion, auscultation, and olfaction) as well as the results of diagnostic tests, operative reports, and/ or a review of the relevant literature.

Generating a problem list

The next step, developing a problem list, helps you clarify your thinking about the assessment data you've collected. Less formal in structure than a fully developed nursing diagnosis, it describes your patient's problems or needs. It's easy to generate such a list if you use a conceptual model or an accepted set of criterion norms. Examples of such norms include normal physical and psychological development, Maslow's hierarchy of needs, and Erikson's stages of development. Thus, you can identify the patient's problems and needs with such simple phrases as low circulation, high fever, or low hydration. The next step is to prioritize the problems on the list and then develop the working nursing diagnosis.

Nursing diagnosis defined

The term nursing diagnosis implies the identification of a patient's problem and that part of its treatment that a nurse is legally empowered to manage. Thus, the nursing diagnosis implies the major legal difference between medicine and nursing. Though the identification of problems often overlaps the two disciplines, their treatments are clearly different. Medicine focuses on curing pathology; nursing focuses on holistic care that includes cure and comfort. Nurses can independently diagnose and treat the patient's response to illness, certain health problems, and the need

for patient education. We comfort, counsel, and care for patients and their families until they are physically or emotionally ready to provide self-care.

Writing a nursing diagnosis

Some nurses are confused about how to document a nursing diagnosis because they think the language is too complex. But the formula for this is so simple that it can soon become second nature to you. Use the method recommended by the North American Nursing Diagnosis Association (NANDA). This group generated a list of diagnostic headings (see *Approved Nursing Diagnoses*, pages 186 and 187) that, when combined with individual findings and suspected etiology, gives a clear picture of the patient's needs. Thus, for clarity in charting, start with one of the NANDA categories as a heading for the diagnostic statement. The category can reflect an actual or potential problem. Then, using the PES format, state your patient's specific problem (P), followed by its possible etiology (E) and the patient's signs and symptoms (S). Let's look at a sample diagnosis:

Heading: Impaired physical mobility
Problem: Decreased ambulation
Etiology: Related to a fracture of the right hip; status post–surgical hip replacement.
Symptoms and signs: "I can't walk without help." Patient has not ambulated since surgery on (give date and time). Range of motion limited to 10 degrees flexion in the right hip. Patient is unable to walk 3' from the bed to the chair without the help of two nurses.

This format links the patient's problem with the etiology without stating a direct cause-and-effect relationship (which may be hard to prove).

Avoid common errors

One major pitfall in developing a nursing diagnosis is writing one that nursing intervention can't treat. Errors can also occur when nurses take shortcuts in the nursing process, either by

APPROVED NURSING DIAGNOSES

Listed below are the diagnoses approved in 1986 by the Sixth Conference on Classification of Nursing Diagnoses. They're listed under headings that show emotional and physical responses to disease. Many new diagnoses have been added in 1986, as indicated by an asterisk.

EMOTIONAL PROBLEMS

Anxiety
Coping, Family: Potential for Growth
Coping, Ineffective Family: Compromised
Coping, Ineffective Family: Disabling
Coping, Ineffective Individual
Hopelessness*
Fear
Grieving, Anticipatory

Grieving, Dysfunctional
Post Trauma Response*
Spiritual Distress (distress of the human spirit)
Violence, Potential for: Self-Directed or Directed at Others
Rape Trauma Syndrome

IMPAIRED FUNCTIONING

Airway Clearance, Ineffective
Body Temperature, Potential Alteration in*
Bowel Elimination, Alteration in: Constipation
Bowel Elimination, Alteration in: Diarrhea
Bowel Elimination, Alteration in: Incontinence
Breathing Pattern, Ineffective
Cardiac Output, Alteration in: Decreased
Communication, Impaired: Verbal
Fluid Volume, Alteration In: Excess
Fluid Volume Deficit, Actual
Fluid Volume Deficit, Potential
Gas Exchange, Impaired
Growth and Development, Altered*
Hyperthermia*
Hypothermia*
Incontinence, Functional*
Incontinence, Reflex*
Incontinence, Stress*
Incontinence, Total*
Incontinence, Urge*
Infection, Potential for*
Injury, Potential for (Poisoning, Potential for;

Suffocation, Potential for; Trauma, Potential for)
Mobility, Impaired Physical
Nutrition, Alteration in: Less than Body Requirements
Nutrition, Alteration in: More than Body Requirements
Nutrition, Alteration in: Potential for More than Body Requirements
Sensory-Perceptual Alteration: Visual, Auditory, Kinesthetic, Gustatory, Tactile, Olfactory
Sexual Dysfunction
Sexuality Patterns, Altered*
Skin Integrity, Impairment of: Actual
Skin Integrity, Impairment of: Potential
Sleep Pattern Disturbance
Swallowing, Impaired*
Thermoregulation, Ineffective*
Tissue Integrity, Impaired*
Tissue Perfusion, Alteration in: Cerebral, Cardiopulmonary, Renal, Gastrointestinal, Peripheral
Urinary Elimination, Alteration in Patterns
Urinary Retention*

PAIN AND DISCOMFORT

Comfort, Alteration in: Pain
Comfort, Alteration in: Chronic Pain*

Oral Mucous Membrane, Alteration in

PROBLEMATIC RELATIONSHIPS

Diversional Activity, Deficit
Social Interaction, Impaired*

Social Isolation

APPROVED NURSING DIAGNOSES (continued)

SELF-CARE LIMITATIONS

Activity Intolerance
Activity Intolerance, Potential
Health Maintenance, Alteration in
Home Maintenance Management, Impaired
Knowledge Deficit (specify)
Neglect, Unilateral*

Noncompliance (specify)
Powerlessness
Self-Care Deficit: Feeding, Bathing/Hygiene,
   Dressing/Grooming, Toileting
Thought Processes, Alteration in

STRAINS IN LIFE PROCESSES

Adjustment, Impaired*
Family Process, Alteration in
Parenting, Alteration in: Actual
Parenting, Alteration in: Potential

Self-Concept, Disturbance in Body Image,
   Self-Esteem, Role Performance, Personal
   Identity

omitting or hurrying through assessment, or by basing the diagnosis on inaccurate assessment data.

Planning patient care

After developing the nursing diagnosis, identify long- and short-term goals. The first step, the long-term goal (LTG), should be stated as: "The patient will..." To identify the LTG, convert the nursing diagnosis into a positive statement. Thus, "Impaired mobility: decreased ambulation," when converted into an LTG, would read: "The patient will ambulate independently prior to his hospital discharge." Then you need to assign a date and time when you expect the patient to meet this LTG.

Identifying the short-term goals (STGs) is the second step in planning patient care. STGs should be stated thus: "The patient will be able to...

• walk 3' from the bed to the chair in his room with the assistance of two nurses by (give date and time)."

• increase his walking distance from 3' to 20' with the assistance of two nurses (give date and time)."

• perform quadriceps setting exercises on the right leg three times a day at 9 a.m., 5 p.m., and h.s. during his hospital stay."

The third and final step in planning patient care is to clearly identify the nursing orders or nursing treatment plan. These orders correlate directly with the patient's LTGs and STGs and specify nursing activities directed toward achieving the patient's goals. For example, "The nurse will walk the patient from the bed to the chair in his room (3') at least once a day during his hospital stay." This planning step in the nursing process is a time for expressing your creative thinking about resolving the patient's problems. It's the time to describe exactly what you and your patient would like to have happen, and it becomes the criterion against which you'll judge further nursing actions.

Implementation

To follow through with your care plan, move on to the implementation of your interventions. Implementation is action-oriented. The nurse carries out the nursing orders, and the patient moves toward achieving the stated goals. Documentation of this step describes what happens at the bedside.

Evaluation, the forgotten step

Evaluation reviews whether the interventions were successful and the goals were met. This last step receives little attention and tends to be poorly documented. Your evaluation should ask and answer the following questions:

Was the assessment data adequate for generating a list of actual or potential problems? Did you prioritize the problems and state the working diagnosis clearly and correctly? Did the symptoms and signs support the diagnosis? Were the STGs and LTGs met? Were they realistic? Did the patient show the expected behaviors? Did the nurse perform the nursing actions listed? Does any new data cause you to reconsider the diagnosis, goals, or nursing orders?

Concluding comments

Nursing diagnosis defines what we do and demonstrates convincingly that what we do is distinct from what doctors and other health care professionals do. On a more directly practical level, nursing diagnosis saves time by improving communication among staff members and ensuring consistent care. Once every nurse on the unit develops care plans based on nursing diagnoses, patient care is bound to improve. Then, each nurse who cares for a particular patient will know exactly what his problems and goals are and what must be done to solve those problems and meet those goals.

JUDITH RICCIARDI ERRICKSON, RN, MS
ELISE ROBINSON PIZZI, RN, MSN

Using the scientific approach in nursing

Systematic, scientific research needn't be confined to laboratories and universities. It should be part of every nurse's job. Of course, not every nurse has the time or resources to conduct full-scale research projects. But every nurse should develop a systematic, research-oriented approach to solving the everyday problems of nursing practice.

An inquisitive attitude is an important factor in scientific research. Still, all accurate, useful research requires a scientific approach as well.

The research process consists of the following steps:
• defining the problem
• searching the literature
• selecting a research method
• collecting the data
• analyzing and presenting the findings.

Defining the problem

All meaningful research begins with a problem, which is often stated as a question. Many problems and questions for nursing research arise naturally from daily practice. For instance, at one time nursing care of all patients with myocardial infarctions included cardiac precautions—restricting hot and cold liquids and caffeine, and avoiding rectal temperature-taking and vigorous back rubs. But when nurses began to question the validity of using these precautions, research was done on their effectiveness. The result? Studies found these precautions unnecessary for most patients, and they've since been deemphasized.

Searching the literature

When you have a good question to answer or a problem to solve, the next step is to find out what is already known about it. The best way to do this is by searching the literature. Surveying the existing body of knowledge guides your study and helps place it in that body of knowledge, to ensure that your study is relevant and meaningful.

Selecting a research method and collecting data

Next, you develop a research design—your plan for collecting data for study. Your research design depends on the type of study you're doing (see *Types of Research Designs*).

An experimental study measures the consequences of a particular action on the study participants (for example,

TYPES OF RESEARCH DESIGNS

Research designs fall into two broad categories: experimental and nonexperimental. Experimental research allows the researcher to manipulate the factor being studied, the independent variable; it is either true or quasi-experimental. In true experimental research, a randomized control group is used; in quasi-experimental research, it is not. Nonexperimental research does not manipulate the independent variable and is therefore not as scientifically conclusive as experimental research. Correlational, survey, case study, ethnographic, and grounded theory research designs are nonexperimental. Correlational design attempts to identify relationships between illness or conditions occurring now and factors that have already occurred. Other nonexperimental designs are descriptive research. These designs attempt to observe, describe, and document variables rather than identify relationships between variables. A survey gathers data from a portion of the population by interview or questionnaire to examine characteristics, opinions, or intentions of that population. Case studies investigate individuals or groups in depth to determine why developments occur as they do in the case. Ethnographic and grounded theory, seldom done in nursing, merely describe events in a population and attempt to develop a theory about that population. Quasi-experimental, correlational, survey, and case study are the most common designs used in clinical research, either medical or nursing. The ability of a research design to test or generate a theory exists on a continuum, as shown in the flowchart.

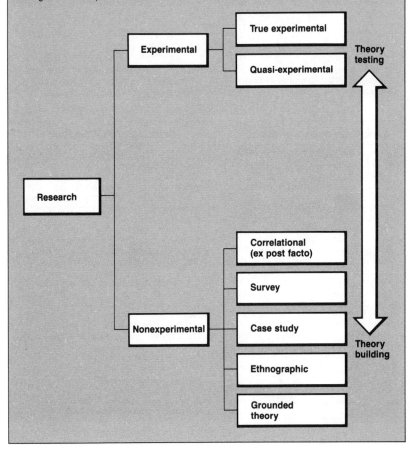

evaluating the effectiveness of a patient-teaching program on patients' compliance with antihypertensive medication regimens). In contrast, nonexperimental research involves collecting data without introducing any treatments or changes to study participants. Nonexperimental research is limited to measurements of existing states, conditions, behaviors, or characteristics (for instance, a study of the correlation between nurses' educational levels and salaries).

When selecting a research design, you also need to specify:
• study group—the population you wish to evaluate
• data collection procedures—the methods you'll use to collect data, such as questionnaires, documents, observation, interviews, or physiologic measurements
• quality controls—methods to control extraneous variables, the factors that can interfere with the accuracy of your study.

Analyzing the findings
A meaningful research study hinges on systematic, accurate data analysis. Statistical analysis—either descriptive or inferential—allows you to quantify the data so that it becomes interpretable and meaningful. Descriptive analysis—means (averages), frequencies, and percentages—directly quantifies your observations and measurements. Inferential analysis—including chi-square, linear regressions, and factor analysis—allows you to identify statis-

---

REVIEWING SAMPLING METHODS

A sound sampling method is crucial to the validity of any research study. Ideally, the sample group should closely reflect the makeup of the target population; unrepresentative sampling will invalidate results. Sampling methods are classified into two categories: probability sampling and nonprobability sampling.

Types of probability sampling	Types of nonprobability sampling
• *Simple random sampling.* In this type of sampling, the researcher picks subjects, using random methods. The sample population should be representative of the target population. • *Stratified random sampling.* The researcher chooses subjects randomly from certain population strata, such as urban and rural dwellers, men and women, or different age-groups. This method should prevent underrepresentation of any group in the target population. • *Multiple-stage cluster sampling.* The researcher picks subjects after the target population has been stratified several times. This method tends to yield a very representative sample group. • *Systematic probability sampling.* The researcher chooses subjects at a fixed interval (for example, every tenth name on a list of subjects) from a sample group that's representative of the target population.	• *Convenience sampling.* In this method, the researcher picks subjects from a convenient group that shares certain characteristics with the target population. The sample derived from this method may not be representative if the group is too homogenous, however. • *Snowball sampling.* The researcher first chooses subjects by convenience sampling; then, if he needs additional subjects, he has the initial subjects recruit friends for the study. Like convenience sampling, this method also tends to yield a homogenous sample group. • *Quota sampling.* The researcher picks subjects by the convenience method at first, until he fills a quota for a certain characteristic; then, he chooses subjects with a different characteristic until he fills the next quota, and so on. • *Systematic nonprobability sampling.* The researcher chooses subjects at a set interval (such as every tenth name on a list of subjects, as in systematic probability sampling) from a convenience sample.

tically significant relationships among the variables studied.

After analyzing your research data, you need to interpret it and examine it in a broader, more practical context. Did your findings answer the research question or solve the research problem? Were they statistically and clinically significant? How do they relate to existing knowledge? What further research is needed? Your answers determine the value of your research.

Presenting the results

The final step in the research process is to communicate your findings, so that other nurses can use them to provide better patient care. Publishing your findings in a professional journal is a good way to reach large numbers of practicing nurses. Your research report must be clear, concise, and objective and, above all, must link the findings with practical implications for nursing.

MARGARET FISK MASTAL, RN, MSN, CNAA

Avoiding legal risks in the OR

All surgery, especially under general anesthesia, carries a risk of unpreventable death. (See *Dealing with Death in the OR*, page 192.) However, working in the operating room (OR) or recovery room (RR) presents its own special legal risks. Nursing malpractice in the OR or RR commonly takes one of two forms: *failing to perform nursing procedures correctly* or *following incorrect or inappropriate orders*. Here's a closer look at both forms of malpractice and the best ways to protect yourself from lawsuits.

Failing to perform procedures correctly

Malpractice lawsuits can arise from:
• *failure to check the chart* for a consent form, preoperative test results, or allergy warnings. For example, if your patient has a serious allergic reaction to an anesthetic agent because you failed to check his chart, you'll be held liable along with the surgeon and the anesthesiologist.
• *failure to perform a sponge and instrument count or performing it inaccurately.* Ordinarily, if you skip a sponge or instrument count on a doctor's order, you could be held liable for any resulting harm to the patient. According to standard nursing practice, an OR nurse must do a count for each patient unless doing so risks the patient's life.
• *inadequate postoperative observation* of the patient in the OR or RR, in transit between these two places (where most malpractice lawsuits arise), or in transit to the medical/surgical unit. What's the main culprit? Usually, it's a "pass the buck" attitude:
—The surgeon may have considered his job finished after he closed the patient.
—The anesthesiologist (who's normally responsible for patient transfer) may have decided not to accompany the patient or may have delegated responsibility for the transfer to an OR nurse.
—The OR nurse he asked to accompany the patient may have failed to do so.
—The RR nurse may not have participated in the transfer until she received the patient.

In some hospitals, delegation of patient transfers during the critical postanesthesia period—when the patient is most vulnerable to hemorrhage and respiratory and cardiovascular problems—is left to chance, so unqualified personnel may end up making the transfers. Ideally, all postoperative patients should be accompanied to the medical/surgical unit by an RR nurse. But if tight staffing makes this impossible, an RR nurse should at least accompany high-risk patients—those with chest tubes, for example.
• *anesthesia errors by nurse anesthetists.* In most states, if you're responsible for anesthetizing patients, the

DEALING WITH DEATH IN THE O.R.

Nurses who work with terminally ill patients routinely help the patient and his family come to terms with expected death. They provide support, answer questions, and often just listen as the patient and his family go through the normal grieving process. They are prepared to deal with the patient's death. The situation changes, however, when a patient who's expected to survive dies suddenly in the operating room (OR).

Nurses choose to work in the OR for many reasons, often for the sense of excitement and accomplishment that comes with assisting at a procedure that saves a patient's life or improves the quality of his life. Such nurses tend to think of the OR as a place where sick and broken bodies are mended and made whole, and where things rarely go wrong. If a patient dies unexpectedly on the operating table, even the most competent and experienced OR nurse may feel out of her element. Despite her limited contact with the patient and his family, she may be called upon to deal with the emotional impact of the patient's death on the family. For, although the surgeon informs the family

of the patient's death, he usually spends only a few minutes with the family; often, the OR nurse has to deal with them after the surgeon leaves.

Because dealing with grieving family members is normally outside the OR nurse's realm of responsibility, most OR nurses are generally ill-prepared for this task. Unfortunately, in many hospitals, the OR nurse's responsibilities in such a situation aren't clearly defined. If your hospital has no such guidelines, insist that they be developed. Such guidelines should clarify the following issues: responsibility for notification of death, disposition of the patient's body, provision of an appropriate location for the family to view the patient's body, and responsibility for documenting the events and actions in the OR that led to the patient's death.

Peer support can also help. One useful strategy may be coordination with staff nurses caring for a patient scheduled for high-risk surgery for help in preparing the patient and his family for the possibility of death and in dealing with the patient's family after death.

MARIANNE NETTINA, RN, BS

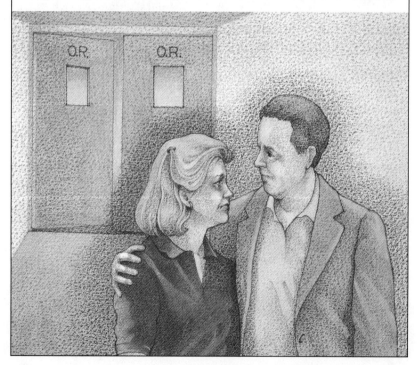

medical standards for anesthesiology apply to your performance. If you don't meet these standards and you harm a patient, you're liable.

Following incorrect orders

As an independent professional, you're accountable for every order you carry out. So you need to evaluate every order for its safety and appropriateness.

If a doctor insists on closing a patient before you do a sponge and instrument count, find out why. If his explanation makes sense to you, abide by his judgment. But if the patient is stable and you know that you have enough time for a sponge and instrument count, stand your ground. By following a doctor's order to skip such a count on a stable patient, you're placing yourself at legal risk. If the patient later needs surgery to remove a hemostat left in his abdomen, your hospital, the doctor, and you will probably be held liable.

If you decide to challenge a doctor's order, be sure to follow these steps:

• *Talk it over.* The first step in questioning any doctor's order is to clarify the order. If he simply has forgotten the order or made a mistake, the issue is easily resolved. But if he insists that the order be carried out as prescribed, you'll have to tell him why, in your nursing judgment, you can't comply. (Before taking such a position, however, be sure you know exactly what your state's nurse practice act permits an OR nurse to do.) Ask the doctor about his rationale for giving the order. His explanation may be reasonable, and knowing his rationale will help you make an informed decision.

• *Report the incident to your manager.* Suppose a doctor orders a patient into the OR before consent forms are signed and, despite your objections, insists on starting surgery immediately. Notify your manager at once.

• *Follow the chain of command.* Most medical staffs have a chain of command or a committee to deal with patient care issues. After you've notified your manager about an incident, she should continue the process. If she won't proceed, you may have to continue up the chain of command—documenting every step—until the issue's resolved. Because this takes time, the quickest solution would be to have the doctor himself perform the procedure in question; thus, he assumes sole accountability for any consequences.

• *Document the incident.* If the issue remains unresolved, document the steps you've taken. Include a detailed description of the incident and the names of any witnesses.

Taking other precautions

Here's some more advice for avoiding legal risks in the OR and RR:

• *Familiarize yourself* with your state's nurse practice act, the nurse practice standards of the Association of Operating Room Nurses, and your hospital's written policies on OR emergencies.

• *Document carefully.* Documentation may not help you avoid legal problems completely, but it can *reduce* your legal risk. Suppose a doctor closed on a patient even though your sponge and instrument count was incorrect. Documenting the corrective measures performed—such as patient X-rays—could reduce your legal risk.

• *Carry adequate malpractice insurance* before setting foot in an OR. Generally, a hospital's malpractice insurance covers both OR and RR nurses. But you may need your own professional liability insurance. Check with your hospital administration for information on their coverage.

• *Don't let yourself be intimidated.* If a doctor gives you an inappropriate order, don't follow it. For example, if a sponge and instrument count doesn't come out right, repeat the count unless such a delay clearly threatens the patient's life. The law requires you to consider the patient's safety first. In fact, by putting your patient's best interests first and standing your ground when you know you're right, you can avoid most legal risks in the OR.

JEAN RABINOW, JD

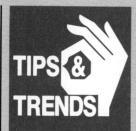

TIPS & TRENDS

GAINING LEGITIMACY

Hypnosis in medicine

Hypnosis, once discredited by the medical establishment, is now gaining acceptance as a legitimate therapeutic tool in surgery, dentistry, pain control, psychology, and the treatment of habit disorders, such as smoking and overeating. Explain to patients that hypnosis involves four stages: preparation, induction, trance, and conclusion. During preparation, the patient answers screening questions. Induction is the transition from the waking to the hypnotic state. Next, during the trance, the therapist attempts to decrease the patient's symptoms. At the conclusion, the therapist gives posthypnotic suggestions to facilitate a return to the normal waking state.

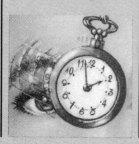

SIGN OF SHIFTING OPINION

New AMA policy on dying

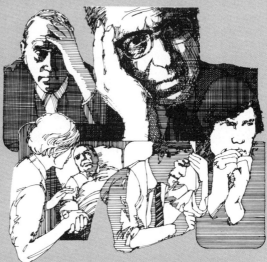

A recent decision by the American Medical Association (AMA) represents another step in the evolution of a broad social policy in the delicate area of dying and death. In March 1986, the AMA's judicial council voted unanimously that it would be ethical for doctors to withhold "all means of life-prolonging medical treatment," including food and water, from a patient in an irreversible coma, even when death is not imminent. The AMA decision doesn't obligate any doctor to withdraw therapy, but is expected in the long run to make such withdrawal more socially acceptable. At present, the decision is of greatest concern to the doctors, nurses, and families of the estimated 10,000 people who are in irreversible comas in institutions throughout the country. Citing ethical standards and fear of criminal prosecution or malpractice suits, many doctors have refused to withhold or withdraw such treatments as respirators or tube feedings despite requests from family members and the previously expressed wishes of the patient. Although the AMA decision has no legal standing, as an indicator of shifting medical and social opinion, it should figure heavily in future legal debates.

Elder abuse

An emerging problem in this country, elder abuse affects an estimated 500,000 to 2 million persons each year. According to recent statistics, white women over age 75 are the most frequent victims, and approximately 85% of elder abuse is committed by a family member—most of whom reside with their victim.

Elder abuse isn't confined to physical violence, the most easily identifiable form of abuse; it also encompasses more insidious forms such as psychological abuse, neglect, theft or misuse of property, and medical mismanagement. Estimates of abuse vary widely, mainly because of underreporting and problems in identifying abuse. Victims may deny abuse for several reasons, including fear of losing family contact, fear of isolation, and feelings of shame or guilt. Another problem: although many states have child abuse legislation, few states have mandatory reporting laws for elder abuse or laws protecting persons who report such abuse.

Recent research has identified several seemingly common characteristics of both abusers and victims. These prevalent traits include a history of physical or mental illness, violent behavior, and substance abuse; low stress tolerance level; financial problems; and social isolation. Perhaps most important, many abusers of the elderly were themselves, as children, abused by their victims.

When caring for an elderly person who has unexplained injuries, particularly bruises or burns, study his history for a pattern of such injuries. A history that shows multiple or recurring injuries should alert you to the possibility of abuse and the need for further investigation by the patient's doctor or an appropriate social service agency.

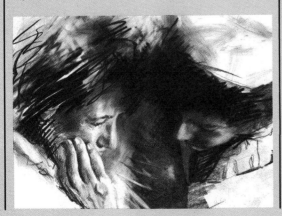

Trust in antitrust

Nurses working in expanded roles will be pleased with a recent decision issued by the U.S. Ninth Circuit Court of Appeals. It ruled that nurses can sue when anticompetitive arrangements between hospitals and doctors exclude nurses from practicing.

The controversy began in March 1983 when Manteca (Calif.) Hospital terminated its contract that had allowed nurse anesthetists to provide anesthesia services. A nurse anesthetist sued the hospital, claiming its policy eliminated competition for anesthesia services and violated antitrust laws.

A federal court dismissed the suit, saying that nurses and doctors don't compete. But the court of appeals reversed this decision, ruling that nurses can sue under antitrust laws when they're excluded from practicing because of exclusionary arrangements between hospitals and doctors. This reversal gives nurses who perform functions also performed by doctors the full protection of federal antitrust laws.

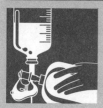

Nursing procedures

Intravascular infusion device

This device is used for administering I.V. or intraarterial drugs and fluids and for obtaining blood specimens. Under a local anesthetic, the infusion device is implanted subcutaneously against the chest wall with a catheter leading into a central vein. Heparinization is necessary every 3 to 4 weeks.

Before using this device in a patient, it's essential to learn how to care for it; how to access the site, utilize the system, prepare the system for a heparin lock, administer continuous or bolus injections, and draw blood; and how to discontinue therapy.

Correctly used, this device decreases the risk of infection. Because it requires fewer supplies (as compared to the external device) and doesn't require daily maintenance, the intravascular infusion device is cost-effective. It's especially useful in patients who require long-term chemotherapy, antibiotics, or fluid therapy.

Equipment

Three alcohol swabs/three povidone-iodine swabs/sterile barrier/sterile gloves/6" (15-cm) extension tubing/two 10-ml syringes/5-ml syringe/20-ml syringe/heparinized saline solution (100 units/ml)/normal saline solution/three-way stopcock/Huber point needle (for heparinization only: 19G to 20G 1" 90-degree needle; for bolus injection: 20G to 22G 1" straight needle; for continuous infusion: 20G to 22G 1" to 1½" 90-degree needle; for drawing blood: 19G to 22G 1" straight or 90-degree needle)/dead-end plug for injection site/I.V. or drug solution/blood tubes and appropriate syringes/sterile 4" x 4" gauze pad.

Preparation of equipment

Before beginning this procedure, review instructions for preparing a ster-ile field. Maintain sterile technique when setting up the equipment and accessing the device. Before starting the procedure, gather all supplies, and make sure that they're functional and that their sterility has not expired.

Essential steps

• Explain the procedure to the patient to reduce fear and anxiety.
• Wash your hands for 2 minutes.
• Prepare a sterile field and open supplies.
• Using sterile technique, don gloves.
• Clean the area to be accessed with alcohol swabs, starting over the portal site and moving outward in a spiral motion to cover a 4" (10-cm) diameter. Discard the swab.
• Repeat the above step with povidone-iodine.
• Drape the patient with a sterile barrier, exposing only the access site.

To assemble and set up equipment

• Attach a stopcock to the female end of the extension tubing.
• Attach the male end of the tubing to the Huber point needle.
• Prepare a 10-ml syringe for normal saline solution and a 5-ml syringe for heparinized saline solution.
• Attach the saline syringe to the stopcock and purge the tubing.

Procedure

• Locate the portal septum by palpation. Hold the port with your index finger and thumb to stabilize it.
• Insert the appropriate needle perpendicularly into the septum until it touches the bottom of the portal chamber.
• Check patency. Flush the system with 5 ml of normal saline solution with slow, even pressure to confirm the position. Aspirate for blood return.
• Turn the stopcock off toward the patient.
• Secure the needle with Steri-Strips and apply gauze or transparent dressing. If the patient is to receive a bolus injection, the site need not be covered.

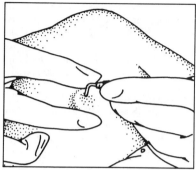

Inserting the Huber point needle into the center of the portal septum

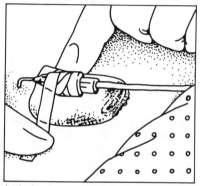

Anchoring the needle with gauze and Steri-Strips

Tape the needle only to stabilize it.

To perform heparinization
• Place the injection port on the female end of the stopcock.
• Flush with 5 ml of heparinized saline solution.

To begin continuous infusion
• Attach I.V. tubing to the female end of the stopcock. If necessary, fold a sterile 4″ x 4″ gauze pad and place it under the needle for support.
• Open the stopcock.

To begin bolus injection
• Attach the syringe with medication to the female end of the stopcock.
• Inject the medication.
• Flush the system with 2 ml of heparinized saline solution.

• Flush with 10 ml of normal saline solution.
• Heparinize the system and remove the needle.

To draw blood
• Attach a 12-ml syringe to the female end of the stopcock.
• Withdraw 6 to 12 ml of blood and discard.
• Withdraw the desired amount of blood.
• Flush with 2 ml of heparinized saline solution.
• Flush with 20 ml of normal saline solution.
• Heparinize the line and remove the needle or maintain the heparin lock.

To discontinue Huber point needle
• Attach the heparinized syringe to the stopcock.
• Flush the system with 5 ml of heparinized saline solution. Maintain positive pressure with the syringe while simultaneously turning the stopcock off toward the patient.
• While simultaneously withdrawing the Huber point needle, press down on the portal septum with two fingers.
• If oozing occurs, apply a bandage.

Special considerations
Use only syringes that are larger than 5 ml. Smaller syringes may cause excess pressure that can lead to disconnection of the device.

Use only Huber point (noncoring) needles to reduce incidence of septal searing. Use straight needles only once, as for heparinization. When drawing blood, use a short needle to facilitate blood flow. For obese patients, use a 1½″ to 2″ (3.75- to 5-cm) needle to ensure penetration.

For patients receiving continuous infusions, change injection ports every 48 hours. If the patient is allergic to povidone-iodine, prepare the site with alcohol.

If the patient's hospitalized, you'll need to heparinize the device every 3 to 4 weeks. (If he's at home, he must

MAJOR COMPLICATIONS OF IMPLANTABLE DEVICES

BLOCKED CATHETER	AIR EMBOLUS	INFECTION
Cause • Clot at end of catheter • Positional catheter tip	**Cause** • Air in system	**Cause** • Bacterial invasion
Prevention • Flush catheter appropriately.	**Prevention** • Tape all junctions.	**Prevention** • Follow good hand-washing technique. • Follow sterile procedure.
Detection • Inability to draw blood	**Detection** • Line disconnected • Shortness of breath, chest pain, cyanosis	**Detection** • Red, swollen, and tender skin • Purulent exudate • Low-grade fever
Treatment • Change patient's position; have patient: —cough —turn head —raise one or both arms —lie flat —assume Trendelenburg's position —take deep breath —do Valsalva's maneuver. • Change needle. • Have chest X-ray taken, as ordered. • Administer urokinase flush, as ordered.	**Treatment** • Stop air from infusing. • Place patient in Trendelenburg's position or on left side with chin and knees to chest. • Call for help.	**Treatment** • Culture site. • Call doctor.

return to the doctor's office to have his device heparinized, or the visiting nurse may perform the procedure.) Also heparinize the device after each infusion, bolus, or drawing of blood.

Not all catheters have a blood return; however, they should be checked for placement (on a chest X-ray) before administering therapy.

Notify the doctor of wound hematoma; redness, swelling, or pus at the implantation site; bleeding; arm and neck swelling; device rotation; and inability to infuse fluid.

Complications

Common problems associated with an intravascular device include blocked catheter, air embolus, infection, and bleeding (see *Major Complications of Implantable Devices*). If the patient goes home with the device, teach him how to detect these problems. Instruct him to contact the doctor if any of these problems occur.

Patients must also be aware of problems that may occur while undergoing radiologic testing. The metal intravascular device may obscure the view on a computed tomography scan and chest X-ray. This problem can usually be avoided by placing the device outside the diseased area. Magnetic resonance imaging examinations are contraindicated since the magnetic field could rotate the device.

Documentation

Document each access to the device, reason for the access, presence or absence of blood return, needle and dressing changes, patient education, and the results of patient education. Document medications on the medication chart. Document I.V. fluids on the parenteral therapy record and intake and output record.

LANA M. WILHELM, BSN, CNSN

Triple lumen catheter

This catheter is used for simultaneous infusion of drugs and fluids requiring separate venous access sites. Patients who can benefit from using the triple lumen catheter are those who require continuous or intermittent fluid or medication, simultaneous administration of potentially incompatible medications, blood administration, central venous pressure (CVP) monitoring, and venous blood sampling.

Each catheter consists of a #7 French catheter stem with three separate lumens or ports: proximal, middle, and distal. The proximal port has the longest pigtail because its end is farthest from the catheter tip. The proximal lumen is 18G and is used for blood sampling and general access. The middle lumen, also 18G, is usually used for intravenous hyperalimentation. The distal 16G lumen is used for CVP readings, administration of blood products, and general access.

Precautions

Caring for the triple lumen catheter is similar to caring for a Hickman or Broviac catheter and a central line, with the exception of fluid administration. Care of the triple lumen catheter also requires these special steps, which differ from care of a central line:

TRIPLE LUMEN CATHETER

The proximal and middle lumens of the triple lumen catheter are 18G and are used for blood sampling, intravenous hyperalimentation, and general access. The 16G distal lumen is used for central venous pressure readings and administration of blood products.

Proximal lumen port

Distal lumen port

Middle lumen port

16G

18G

18G

• Any time a lumen is open to air, the catheter should be clamped.

• When heparinizing the catheter, the lumen should be clamped when the last 0.5 ml of heparin is being infused, to create a positive pressure and thus prevent clotting.

• The adapter should be disinfected for 2 minutes before any injection. Also, the connection between the p.r.n. (intermittent infusion device) adapter and lumen should be disinfected for 2 minutes before disconnection.

• Luer-Lok intermittent injection caps must be changed every 3 days. (*Note:* Clamp the catheter before changing the cap.)

• Only 20G 1″ needles should be used when puncturing a Luer-Lok cap.

• Lumens not in use should be heparinized every 8 to 12 hours. Lumens used for intermittent infusion should be heparinized after each use or at least every 8 to 12 hours.

Equipment
Gather the following equipment.

For insertion of a triple lumen catheter
Shave preparation kit, if necessary/sterile gloves/sterile drapes/masks, povidone-iodine sponges and ointment/alcohol sponges/3-ml syringe with 25G 1″ needle/1% or 2% lidocaine injectable/heparin/two radiopaque inside-the-needle catheters/10-ml syringe with Luer-Lok tip/I.V. solution, with administration set prepared for use/sterile 4″ × 4″ gauze sponges/1″ adhesive tape; sterile scissors.

Some institutions have prepared trays containing most of the equipment necessary for insertion.

For removal of a central venous line
Sterile suture-removal set/sterile gloves/two masks, if necessary, for suspected infection/sterile drape/alcohol sponges/povidone-iodine ointment/sterile 4″ × 4″ gauze sponges/sterile, plastic adhesive-backed dressing/sterile culture tube and sterile scissors for a culture, if necessary.

Preparation of equipment
Before insertion of a central venous line, confirm catheter size with the doctor. Set up the I.V. solution and prime the administration set. As ordered, notify the radiology department that a portable X-ray machine will be needed.

Essential steps
Wash your hands thoroughly to prevent the spread of microorganisms.

To assist with insertion of a central venous line
• Reinforce the doctor's explanation of the procedure, and answer the patient's questions. Ensure that the patient has signed a consent form, if necessary, and check his history for hypersensitivity to the local anesthetic.

• Establish a sterile field on a table, using a sterile towel or the wrapping from the instrument tray.

• Place the patient in Trendelenburg's position to dilate veins and reduce the risk of air embolism.

• For subclavian insertion, place a rolled blanket lengthwise between the shoulders to increase venous distention. For jugular insertion, place a rolled blanket under the opposite shoulder to extend the neck, making anatomic landmarks more visible. Place a linen-saver pad under the appropriate area to prevent soiling the bed.

• Turn the patient's head away from the site to prevent possible contamination from airborne pathogens and to make the site more accessible. Or, if dictated by hospital policy, mask the patient unless this increases his anxiety or is contraindicated because of his respiratory status.

• Cleanse the insertion site with soap and water to remove dirt and body oils. If necessary, shave the area. Then, put on a mask and gloves and cleanse the area around the insertion site with povidone-iodine, working in a circular motion outward from the site to avoid reintroducing contaminants.

• After the doctor puts on a sterile mask

and gloves and drapes the area to create a sterile field, open the packaging of the 3-ml syringe and needle and present it to the doctor, using sterile technique.

• Wipe the top of the lidocaine vial with alcohol and invert it. The doctor then fills the 3-ml syringe and injects the anesthetic into the site.

• Open the packaging of the catheter and the 10-ml syringe. Heparinize each lumen of the catheter with 100 ml of heparin and present them to the doctor, using sterile technique. The doctor then attaches the catheter needle to the syringe, punctures the skin, and inserts the catheter. During this time, prepare the I.V. administration set for immediate attachment to the catheter hub. Ask the patient to perform Valsalva's maneuver while the doctor attaches the I.V. line to the catheter hub. This raises intrathoracic pressure, reducing the possibility of an air embolus.

• After the doctor attaches the I.V. line to the catheter hub, set the flow rate as ordered. The doctor then sutures the catheter in place.

• As ordered, put on sterile gloves, apply povidone-iodine ointment over the site, and apply a sterile 4″ × 4″ gauze sponge.

• After an X-ray confirms correct catheter placement, secure the catheter with tape, reapply the sterile dressing, and tape it to the skin. Label the dressing with the time and date of catheter insertion and catheter length (if not imprinted on the catheter).

To remove a triple lumen catheter

• Explain the procedure to the patient and wash your hands. Note the length of the catheter, which should be imprinted on the catheter or written on the dressing. Open the suture-removal set, and use the inside surface of the wrap to establish a sterile field.

• Using sterile technique, open two gauze sponges and one alcohol sponge and drop them onto the sterile field. Squeeze povidone-iodine ointment onto one gauze sponge. Then loosen and carefully remove the dressing. If a culture of the catheter is to be taken because of suspected infection, put masks on yourself and on the patient before removing the dressing to prevent contamination of the site by airborne organisms.

• Close the flow clamp on the I.V. tubing, and put on sterile gloves.

• Remove any sutures securing the catheter, taking care not to cut the catheter. If you're removing a cutdown catheter, avoid cutting any skin sutures.

• Grasp the needle or catheter hub, and slowly and carefully withdraw it from the vein. If the catheter can't be retracted easily, allow the patient to relax; then try again. Avoid forceful retraction, because venous spasm may be causing the resistance. If resistance continues, tape the catheter in place and notify the doctor.

• After you've removed the catheter, apply pressure with a gauze sponge to stop bleeding. Carefully inspect the tip of the catheter, taking care to prevent contamination. The tip should appear round and smooth. If it's ragged or damaged, notify the doctor immediately, because a severed catheter can cause an embolus. If the catheter appears severed, place it on the sterile field and measure its length.

• After bleeding stops, inspect the insertion site for signs of infection, and collect a specimen of any drainage for culture. Cleanse the area around the insertion site with an alcohol sponge to remove dried blood and adhesive, then apply povidone-iodine ointment to the area. Place a sterile, plastic adhesive-backed dressing to prevent exposure of the incision to the air.

• If a culture specimen from the catheter is required, prepare the insertion site with alcohol before removal of the catheter, as ordered, and use sterile scissors to cut a 1″ (2.5-cm) segment from the tip of the removed catheter. Then place the specimen in the sterile culture tube and send it to the laboratory immediately.

Special considerations

As soon as possible after insertion, check catheter placement with a portable X-ray machine or, depending on his condition, send the patient to the radiology department. If hyperalimentation fluid is ordered, begin this infusion only after the X-ray confirms correct catheter placement because this hypertonic solution could cause problems if the catheter is misplaced. When catheter placement is in doubt, infuse another I.V. solution, such as dextrose 10% in water, until correct placement is assured. Be alert for such signs of air embolism as sudden onset of pallor, cyanosis, dyspnea, coughing, and tachycardia, progressing to syncope and shock. If any of these signs occur, place the patient on his left side in Trendelenburg's position and notify the doctor. Also, after insertion, watch for signs of pneumothorax: shortness of breath, tachycardia, and chest pain. Notify the doctor immediately if such signs appear. Change the dressing and tubing every 24 hours or according to hospital policy while the central venous line is in place. Dressing changes for a central venous line should be done using sterile technique. This is especially important when hyperalimentation solution is being infused.

Complications

With subclavian vein insertion, pneumothorax is the most common complication. With jugular vein insertion, the catheter may be misdirected toward the brain instead of into the vena cava; a chest X-ray will show this. At either site, air embolism is possible.

Catheter breakage may occur from excessive force or usage. In case of breakage, notify the doctor immediately to have the pigtail replaced.

Sepsis is a serious complication. Since the triple lumen catheter is manipulated more frequently than a single lumen, it involves a greater risk of infection.

Air embolism and clotting are other potential complications.

Documentation

Record the time and date of insertion, the length and location of the catheter, the solution infused, the doctor's name, and the patient's response. Also document the time of the X-ray, its results, and your notification of the doctor. After removing the central venous line, record the time and date of removal and the type of antimicrobial ointment and dressing applied. Also note the condition of the catheter insertion site and collection of a culture specimen.

LANA M. WILHELM, BSN, CNSN

Pressure ulcer care update

The growing numbers of acutely ill hospitalized patients have increased the incidence of secondary problems such as pressure ulcers (also called decubitus ulcers). Since numerous factors can cause pressure ulcers, preventing or managing them requires a multidisciplinary team approach. At admission, assess the patient for potential pressure ulcers and identify probable causes. To ensure optimal continuity of care, share assessment findings with other team members, including the doctor, physical therapist, occupational therapist, dietitian, infection control nurse, enterostomal therapist, and pharmacist.

Identifying causes

Preventing pressure ulcers begins with identifying their causes. Primary causes can be categorized as external and internal.

External factors

• *Pressure.* Pressure greater than 32 mm Hg on bony prominences causes capillaries to collapse, resulting in obstructed blood flow. As a result, nutrients and oxygen can't reach cells, and waste material can't be eliminated from cells. Compression of the blood vessels causes ischemia, which leads to tissue necrosis beginning at the bone and advancing toward the skin. When outward signs of necrosis appear, deeper destruction is imminent.

• *Friction.* This is the force created when two surfaces move against each other. Friction occurs when a patient is pulled across bed sheets and when a restless patient thrashes about in bed. Friction wears off the epidermal skin layer and can break skin capillaries that have already been stretched and compromised by shear and pressure.

• *Shear.* This is the sliding of a bony prominence along its adjacent subcutaneous tissue. It occurs when a patient is left in bed too long with the head of his bed elevated too high. The skin over the sacral area remains stationary against the sheet, while the sacrum slides against the subcutaneous tissue. Shear alone does not cause pressure, but it further constricts the capillaries in areas that are already compromised by pressure. As a result, it further reduces blood supply to that area.

• *Excess moisture.* This contributes to skin breakdown by causing maceration and creating a culture medium for bacteria.

Internal factors

• *Poor nutritional status.* If you suspect this, obtain certain baseline data, including the patient's height and weight; hemoglobin and hematocrit levels; and albumin, blood urea nitrogen, and protein levels. In certain patients, especially those who have deep, nonhealing ulcers, iron, folate, and zinc levels are important. Closely observe the patient's dietary intake. Request a nutritional consultation.

• *Decreased activity/mobility.* Whether due to conditions such as a musculoskeletal disorder or decreased level of consciousness, decreased activity exaggerates the risk of developing pressure ulcers. Determine the patient's activity limitations with the help of a physical therapist.

• *Underlying disease.* This can also put the patient at risk. The medical condition itself (for example, edema) may contribute to skin breakdown.

• *Skin dryness.* Aging and certain illnesses, such as peripheral vascular disease and diabetes, can cause the skin to lose natural oils and moisture. This causes dry, flaky skin and intense itching. The patient may scratch himself, causing ulcerations and infections.

Nursing intervention
Vigorously combat external causes.

To decrease pressure

• Use special mattresses: alternating air; static air (Sof-Care, Roho, Foam); water; air-fluidized beads (Clinitron); rotation beds (Rotorest, Kinetic); air support therapy (Mediscus bed, Kenair bed).

• Use wheelchair pads: foam (convoluted, at least 3″ to 4″ [7 to 10 cm] thick); water; gel pads; air (Sof-Care, Roho).

• Reposition the patient as often as necessary but at least every 2 hours. (Higher-risk patients may need position changes every hour.) Remember that the greater the density of the patient's mass, the greater the pressure exerted. Consequently, patients can tolerate a prone position longer than a side-lying position, since the prone position distributes their weight more evenly over bony prominences. Turning schedules can be helpful.

If necessary, use positioning devices: pillows, foam blocks such as Span-aids, splints, bed cradles. Consult a physical therapist and an occupational therapist for proper body alignment techniques. If the patient is able, teach him to do weight shifts, and explain the importance of position changes.

• Provide skin care and massage. Gentle massaging around bony prominences with a moisturizing, pH-balanced skin lotion helps improve and hasten circulation to the area where the patient has been lying. Application of adhesive-backed foam (Reston) over bony prominences disperses pressure, particularly over the lateral malleolus and protrusions over the spinal column. Since the adhesive backing may irritate skin, use it cautiously in patients with known skin sensitivity (apply a skin preparation first to protect the skin). Relieve pressure points on poorly padded casts, braces, and splints. Make sure the patient's bed sheets are free of wrinkles. Check for foreign objects in bedding, such as crumbs, combs, and dentures. Be sure the patient is not lying on a catheter or on oxygen or I.V. tubings.

To prevent shearing

• Use a lift sheet or lifting device to move or transport the patient.
• Use skin sealants (such as Skin-Prep or Protective Barrier Film) when using adhesive tapes. They protect the skin from damage when adhesives are removed by forming a barrier that helps to absorb stress. The barrier keeps epidermal layers in place, preventing stripping and damage. Skin sealants also enhance the holding power of adhesive bandages. Some skin sealants form an aerated membrane that allows moisture to escape and oxygen to enter.
• Use a tape with an acrylate-based, nonallergenic adhesive such as Micropore. The backing should be permeable to air and moisture vapor. Avoid applying tape under tension; this creates shear and causes stripping of skin cells. Use Montgomery straps as applicable.
• Position the patient carefully. A mechanical device such as a trapeze allows the patient to lift himself or to assist with position changes. Foot boards and gel pads help minimize sliding. Lower the head of the bed to less than 40 degrees, unless contraindicated. Educate the patient and his family about basic principles of positioning.

To prevent friction

• Use a lift sheet or lifting device such as a trapeze, Hoyer lift, Jed-sled, or Davis roller.

• Use genuine sheepskin in good condition.
• Apply elbow and heel protectors.
• Lower the head of the bed to less than 40 degrees, unless contraindicated.
• Apply skin sealants and skin barriers such as transparent dressing. They act as a "second layer of skin" to protect the epidermis.

To prevent exposure to excess moisture

• Practice good skin hygiene. Use pH-balanced skin care products, such as Sween and UniDerm skin cleansers and lotions. (*Note:* The skin is in its healthiest state when its acid mantle is 4.5 to 5.5 pH.) Most ordinary soaps are alkaline.

Keep the skin clean and dry. In obese patients, pay particular attention to the perineal area and skin folds. Use whirlpool baths to cleanse and improve circulation. Avoid use of powders, which can cake and irritate. A light dusting of cornstarch can help reduce skin friction in skin folds under pendulous breasts, in groins, and on abdominal skin.
• Use incontinence devices. Proper use of condoms, diapers, incontinence pads, and moisture barrier ointments can reduce excess moisture. Better-quality incontinence pads contain special layers that absorb moisture from the skin surface and trap it in inner layers.
• Develop bowel and bladder training programs.
• Adjust bathing schedules. Use mild soaps; avoid bubble baths and bath salts. Remember, it isn't necessary to use soap on all skin surfaces every day.
• Apply emollient creams frequently.
• Be sure the patient's nutritional and fluid intake is adequate. If oral intake is inadequate, provide parenteral or enteral support. Provide supplements according to the dietitian's recommendations.
• Work with the physical therapist to provide exercises to improve circulation and mobility. Consult the doctor

regarding the underlying disease. Involve others (for example, an infection control nurse) as indicated. Contact the enterostomal therapist for suggestions regarding mattresses, pressure-relieving devices, and skin care.

Ulcer assessment

If the patient has an existing ulcer, assess it as to:
- stage (see *Assessment of Pressure Ulcers: Stages and Healing*)
- size and depth
- shape
- surrounding inflammation/edema
- exudate
- crater content: clean, granular, necrotic. (*Note:* Wounds with eschar can't be staged because the depth of the wound can't be determined until the eschar is removed.)

Contributing factors should then be identified and corrected or modified. Cleansing the wound is of utmost importance and should be done with each dressing change to remove surface debris and bacteria and to assess the wound's progress. Use sterile gauze moistened with normal saline solution, as ordered. If other solutions, such as hydrogen peroxide or povidone-iodine, are used for cleansing, always follow with a normal saline solution rinse. Never use peroxide or povidone-iodine full strength; these solutions can irritate and inhibit wound healing.

Observe the wound daily or with each dressing change for signs of in-

---

ASSESSMENT OF PRESSURE ULCERS: STAGES AND HEALING

STAGE/CHARACTERISTICS	HEALING
Stage I • Redness of epidermal layer • Blanching upon pressure • Ischemia • Superficial break in the epidermis	Once pressure is relieved, redness disappears in several hours; ischemia in about 36 hours.
Stage II • Partial-thickness ulcer (may include superficial open area—abrasion, excoriations, blisters—or opening into dermal layer) • Localized, painful lesion • Redness • Edema	Once treatment begins, regeneration is complete in 10 to 14 days.
Stage III • Full-thickness ulcer (may extend into subcutaneous layer) • Moderate drainage • Varying amounts of necrotic tissue in base	Healing takes 3 weeks to 3 months or longer.
Stage IV • Ulcer extends beyond subcutaneous layer (may involve muscle, bone, cartilage) • Large amounts of drainage • Possibly wide, undermining skin edges • Possibly purulent, foul-smelling necrotic base	Healing is difficult and unpredictable.

Diagram labels: Epidermis, Dermis, Subcutaneous tissue, Muscle, Bone

fection, such as cellulitis or redness around the wound's edges; odor; and greenish, purulent exudate. Elevated body temperature and elevated white blood cell count are also indications of infection. Mild induration and inflammation, signs of the body's natural response to skin injury, don't necessarily indicate infection.

If you suspect infection, obtain a culture. Remove the dressing and gently cleanse heavy exudate with normal saline solution. Gently press around the wound edges, then swab the wound bed with a sterile applicator and culture according to hospital protocol. Send the culture to the laboratory promptly.

Ulcer treatment

Various products are available for pressure ulcer care. Always follow the manufacturer's recommendations for each product. The pharmacist and enterostomal therapist may also provide some helpful advice. When using any of the products mentioned below, keep the following tips in mind:

• Debrisan. This medication is indicated for all secreting wounds. It absorbs fluid; it does not debride, as its name may imply. Remove all old Debrisan before applying a new layer. For best results, irrigate the wound. Mix beads with glycerin to form a paste.

• Acetic acid. This astringent, bacteriostatic medication is usually used in 0.25% solution. It's effective against gram-positive and gram-negative organisms but may not be effective against staphylococci or anaerobic bacteria. Acetic acid tends to cause excoriation of skin around wound edges, so protect them with an ointment.

• Hydrogen peroxide. Use it half strength for irrigation and dilute it just before using. Use it within a day of opening. Hydrogen peroxide is incompatible with povidone-iodine. Always rinse the wound well with normal saline solution after irrigating with hydrogen peroxide. Discontinue its use when granulation is present, since hy-drogen peroxide will destroy healthy epithelium.

• Dakin's solution. This is a dilute sodium hypochlorite (Clorox) used to clean wounds and counteract odor. If stored too long, it loses strength.

• Povidone-iodine. This antiseptic has rapid germicidal activity and is effective against gram-positive and gram-negative organisms, including staphylococci and anaerobic bacteria. *Do not use with debriding enzymes,* since povidone-iodine will render them ineffective. Dressings become white when antiseptic action has stopped.

• Enzymes (Elase, Santyl, Travase). These enzymes provide chemotherapeutic debridement when surgical debridement is not feasible. Topical antibacterials can be used with enzymes to treat infection. *Do not use with iodine preparations.* Use zinc oxide paste to protect skin around wound edges. When the ulcer is free of necrotic tissue and pink granulation is present, discontinue enzymatic therapy.

• Score area. The crosshatch marks made with a scalpel on eschar help soften the wound when enzymes or continuously moist dressings are used.

• DuoDerm. This oxygen-occlusive, hydroactive dressing can be used in healing Stages I, II, and III of pressure ulcers. It can also be used to cover superficial abrasions, first- and second-degree burns, and skin donor sites. Because it's weather-repellent, it's particularly effective against skin breakdown in the sacral area, especially in incontinent patients.

• Vigilon. This is a moist, gel-like polyethylene oxide wound dressing. It is air-permeable and can absorb up to its own weight in wound exudate.

Documentation

Document the ulcer's location, stage, size, shape, and appearance. Also record the presence of contributing factors. Finally, indicate treatment and the patient's response to it.

TERRY E. JAROS, RNC, BSN
CAROL A. HUNEKE, RN, ET

HOW TO MANAGE PRESSURE ULCERS

Management of pressure ulcers depends on thorough assessment. Specific treatments are based not only on staging of pressure ulcers, but on certain other characteristics as well. When assessing an ulcer, remove pressure from the area and cleanse the ulcer to remove dead tissue and old drainage. Inspect the skin to determine if the epidermis and dermis are intact or denuded. If the epidermis is intact, the lesion is at Stage I and can be treated with simple topical therapy. If the epidermis is denuded but the dermis is

INSPECTION

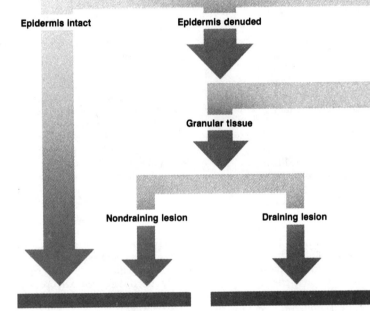

Epidermis intact

Epidermis denuded

Granular tissue

Nondraining lesion

Draining lesion

STAGE I

When the lesion is uncomplicated by incontinence, apply creams such as Sween or UniDerm, barriers such as Granulex Spray or United Skin Prep, a transparent dressing such as Tegaderm or Op-Site, or gelatins such as DuoDerm. When the lesion is complicated by incontinence, use barriers, transparent dressings, gelatins, or ointments such as UniSalve, Peri-Care, or zinc-containing products.

STAGE II, III, IV

To carry out mechanical cleansing and debridement, irrigate the lesion with half-strength hydrogen peroxide or dilute Dakin's solution and rinse with normal saline solution.

Then apply Debrisan beads/paste, karaya powder, DuoDerm granules, or Vigilon dressing to absorb drainage and cleanse the lesion. If the lesion is infected, soak it with an antimicrobial solution, such as 0.25% acetic acid or half-strength povidone-iodine. Remember to consult the doctor.

intact, the lesion will have a granular appearance; you must then determine if it is draining or nondraining to decide treatment. If the dermis is denuded, determine if the lesion is granular or necrotic as well as draining or nondraining to decide treatment. Remember to consult with the patient's doctor when treating Stage III and IV ulcers, when using products that require a doctor's order, and when an ulcer isn't responding to treatment. Also, take care to apply all products according to the manufacturer's instructions.

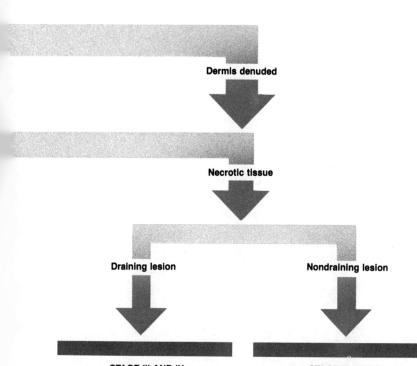

Dermis denuded

Necrotic tissue

Draining lesion

Nondraining lesion

STAGE III AND IV
Irrigate the lesion with half-strength hydrogen peroxide, or apply enzyme ointments such as Travase. Also apply Debrisan beads/paste, Karaya powder, DuoDerm granules, and/or gauze dressings to absorb drainage and debride the lesion.

If the lesion is infected, soak it with an antimicrobial solution such as 0.25% acetic acid or half-strength povidone-iodine. Be sure to consult the doctor.

STAGE III AND IV
Remove all pressure from the involved area, and apply continuous normal saline moist dressing or Tegaderm dressing to soften eschar tissue. Consult with the doctor about surgical debridement or crosshatch incision of the lesion. Once drainage starts, apply treatment for a necrotic draining lesion.

Biliary catheter care

Insertion of a transhepatic biliary catheter allows for safe, effective decompression of the liver in patients with biliary obstruction. The catheter also helps alleviate pruritus and abdominal pain, improves nutritional status by decreasing GI distress, and can shorten hospitalization.

Percutaneous transhepatic biliary drainage may be used preoperatively to temporarily relieve the obstruction caused by biliary stricture until surgery can be performed. Such drainage is commonly indicated in patients with nonresectable malignant biliary obstruction, such as pancreatic cancer and bile duct malignancy.

A transhepatic biliary catheter is also effective in acute suppurative cholangitis or biliary sepsis. Each condition causes an inflammatory response in the area of the porta hepatis that can make operative localization of the common bile duct unsafe or difficult. Biliary drainage helps to effectively decompress the biliary system and to combat infection.

After successful placement of a biliary drainage tract, other therapeutic procedures may be performed, such as balloon dilatation of strictures, endoprosthesis (insertion of a permanent internal stent in patients with nonresectable biliary tract obstruction), and disintegration of bile duct stones.

Insertion
Since catheter insertion can be uncomfortable, the patient usually receives a local anesthetic and, often, a narcotic analgesic before the procedure. Ini-

---

BILIARY DECOMPRESSION

After being passed through an obstruction in the common bile duct or biliary tree, the transhepatic biliary decompression catheter allows bile to drain into the duodenum.

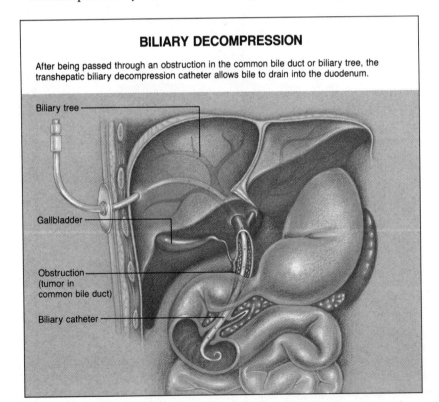

Biliary tree

Gallbladder

Obstruction
(tumor in
common bile duct)

Biliary catheter

tially, he undergoes a percutaneous transhepatic cholangiogram to identify the problem area and opacify the biliary system. Under fluoroscopy, a needle covered by a Teflon sheath is inserted percutaneously from the midaxillary line into the intrahepatic duct. The sheath is kept in place and the needle removed. Once bile is seen coming through the sheath, a guide wire is threaded into the common bile duct, bypassing the area of obstruction into the duodenum. A #8 or #10 French ring catheter is then inserted over the guide wire, replacing the sheath. The catheter is then sutured to the skin surface. A three-way stopcock may be attached to the catheter tip to facilitate irrigation and to help maintain a closed drainage system. The three-way stopcock is then attached to a drainage bag to allow for external drainage. The drainage bag is secured to the patient's leg.

For a few days after catheter insertion, edema of the biliary tree is normal because of the procedure's invasiveness. Once this has resolved (usually in 3 or 4 days) and there are no signs of sepsis, the catheter can be clamped to permit internal drainage. However, if the common bile duct is tortuous or an obstruction is present, internal drainage may not be feasible. Then, external drainage must be continued.

With external drainage, nursing management of the catheter becomes important in terms of maintaining the catheter's patency, maintaining a closed drainage system to prevent infection, and using aseptic technique during dressing changes and irrigations. Should the patient be discharged with an external drainage catheter, he must know proper catheter care and the signs and symptoms of catheter malfunction and infection.

Equipment
For catheter irrigation
Two sterile syringes/bacteriostatic saline solution/needles/three-way stopcock (usually already attached).

For dressing change
Sterile gloves/hydrogen peroxide/antibacterial ointment/sterile gauze/tape/Stomahesive (optional: see "Special considerations," page 212).

Preparation of equipment
Before beginning irrigation, check the doctor's order to make sure it specifies the type and amount of irrigant as well as the frequency of irrigation. If the patient returns from X-ray with a dressing over the insertion site and the catheter clamped, obtain a drainage bag. Keep in mind that the catheter can easily dislodge if it's not adequately secured to the patient. The stopcock should be open to the patient and drainage bag and closed (off) to the extra port. The remaining port must be covered with either a small sterile syringe or cap. Tape a padded tongue blade to the catheter tip with the stopcock; secure this to the patient's skin with additional tape. Be sure there are no kinks in the catheter, which would disrupt proper drainage.

Essential steps
For catheter irrigation
● Inform the patient before beginning irrigation that he may experience some discomfort during the procedure. After catheter placement, the patient may complain of pain and tenderness at the insertion site. The mere motion of irrigating the catheter, therefore, may be irritating to the liver bed and bile ducts, especially if cholangitis or edema is present.
● If a stopcock is not used, the drainage bag must be disconnected before proceeding with irrigation.
● If a stopcock is used, remove the stopcock cap. Insert a sterile syringe. Turn the stopcock so it's open to the patient and closed (off) to the drainage bag. Aspirate a few milliliters of bile. Return the stopcock to its original position. Discard the aspirate.
● Draw the prescribed amount of saline solution (usually no more than 10 to 20 ml), and gently flush the catheter.

Check for bile leakage around the site during irrigation. Aspirate the same amount as was instilled. Reapply the stopcock cap and turn the stopcock so that it's again open to the patient and drainage system.

For dressing change
• Change the dressing daily or as needed, using hydrogen peroxide to cleanse the area around the point of catheter insertion.
• Apply an antibacterial ointment to reduce skin irritation from the sutures.

Special considerations
After catheter insertion, the radiologist may thread the external portion of the catheter through a plastic, transparent piece called a Mulnar disk and suture it to the skin to stabilize the catheter at the insertion site.

If the Mulnar disk is used, the radiologist may not dress the site. However, application of a small, dry, sterile dressing or a piece of Stomahesive may help protect the sutures, reduce infection and local skin irritation, and promote patient comfort.

If the patient complains of abdominal cramping or pain during catheter irrigation, the biliary tree may be overdistended from too much irrigant. Notify the doctor and inform him how much irrigant was used for each irrigation so he can reevaluate the volume. If the patient's pain becomes worse or is accompanied by signs and symptoms of bowel perforation, peritonitis, or intraabdominal bleeding, notify the doctor immediately and prepare your patient for possible emergency cholangiography.

Inability to aspirate the amount of saline solution instilled, bile leakage, or resistance while attempting to irrigate suggests catheter occlusion. *Never* forcibly irrigate the catheter. Notify the doctor immediately if any of the above occur.

The liver normally produces 600 to 1,000 ml of bile per day. Excessive drainage (1,500 ml/day or greater) indicates a backward flow of duodenal contents and may result in severe bicarbonate losses. Patients with external drainage will lose the bile salts and electrolytes that normally enter the GI tract. If the patient becomes lethargic or if his mental attitude changes, consider hyponatremia. Check with the doctor concerning additional laboratory work and fluid and electrolyte replacement. Undigested food particles in the drainage bag may indicate small-bowel obstruction. The patient will probably need additional X-rays.

Complications
Fever, chills, and hypotension suggest catheter sepsis, which may result from catheter occlusion, cholangitis, or liver abscesses. Blood in the catheter may mean the catheter has been dislodged from its original position and has become lodged in a major hepatic vessel.

Dislodgement of sutures at the catheter site may cause the catheter to move or fall out. If this happens, the catheter must be reinserted promptly before the drainage tract created by the initial catheter placement has a chance to narrow. Otherwise, catheter reinsertion will be difficult. External visualization of the side holes of the catheter may also suggest catheter malposition. Excessive catheter drainage may cause severe dehydration and electrolyte abnormalities. Inflammation, swelling, or pain at the catheter site may indicate a wound infection. Recurrent jaundice or bile leakage around the catheter may result from catheter occlusion by a clot or sediment, catheter malposition, or worsening biliary obstruction.

Documentation
Maintain a strict intake and output record. Record the date and time of each dressing change and catheter irrigation. Be sure to specify the type and amount of irrigant used and the condition of the insertion site. Describe any complications concisely and accurately, and carefully document whom you notified and at what time. Record

any instructions you gave the patient and family and their response.

Document the patient's self-care abilities relative to catheter care, awareness of potential complications, and maintenance of adequate nutrition. Specify discharge planning and follow-up care intended upon discharge.

CYNTHIA ANN LaSALLA, RN, BSN

Ileoanal reservoir

The ileoanal reservoir is the latest surgical advancement for patients with ulcerative colitis and familial polyposis. In a two-staged surgical procedure, the colon is removed, the rectal mucosa is stripped, a reservoir is constructed of ileum, and the ileum is sutured into the rectal stump at the end of the anal opening. Since the sphincter muscles remain intact, feces are eliminated in the usual manner. Several techniques are used to construct the reservoir where stool is stored until evacuation is possible. The reservoir can be "S-" or "J-" shaped.

Because the reservoir is internal, this procedure preserves the patient's body image and a near-normal pattern of defecation. It eliminates stomal catheterizations associated with the Kock pouch. In addition, it reduces the incidence of sexual dysfunction.

However, some disadvantages are possible. This procedure may leave some residual rectal mucosa, or rectal mucosa may regenerate, allowing recurrence of inflammation. The patient may find differentiating among gases, fluids, and solids in the rectum difficult. In addition, he may experience tenesmus, fecal urgency, nocturnal incontinence, diarrhea, and perianal skin denudation. Finally, the procedure is considered difficult to perform.

Despite these possible difficulties, the potential benefits to the patient make the ileoanal reservoir preferable to earlier surgical treatments of ulcerative colitis and familial polyposis. These diseases are associated with a high incidence of colorectal cancer. In patients who have had ulcerative colitis for 10 years or more, the risk of colorectal cancer is significantly increased; in all patients with familial polyposis, eventual colorectal cancer is certain. Removal of the colon and rectum cure the disease and remove the risk of cancer. However, since colectomy results in an ileostomy, for many patients this treatment seems worse than the disease itself or the possibility of cancer.

Consequently, new surgical techniques attempted to prevent incontinence in patients requiring total colectomy. One technique, the Kock pouch (or continent ileostomy), uses an internal reservoir constructed of ileum with an external stoma. The pouch must be intubated for evacuation of the stool. The Kock pouch is an improvement over the conventional ileostomy stoma and external pouch; however, it doesn't utilize the sphincter muscle and requires an abdominal stoma. And, some of the same problems commonly associated with conventional ileostomy—the patient's inability to accept the stoma, the change in body image, and regular intubation of the stoma—limited the effectiveness of the Kock pouch.

For many years, ileoanal anastomoses were performed after removal of the colon and rectum. Children tolerate this procedure better than adults. Its major disadvantages are diarrhea and incontinence.

Candidates

Candidates for the ileoanal reservoir include patients with ulcerative colitis or familial polyposis who have a normal anorectal sphincter mechanism and minimal disease of the rectal mucosa. In addition, the patient must be motivated, mature, and in good physical condition.

Patients who are ineligible for an ileoanal reservoir include those with decreased sphincter control; those with a short mesentery, which would prevent surgical construction of the reservoir; and those with cancer of the colon, Crohn's disease, or perianal disease. Obese patients are also ineligible.

Procedure
This surgery proceeds in two stages.

Stage 1
The first step in constructing the ileoanal reservoir is the rectal mucosectomy—the stripping of the rectal segment to form a muscular cuff through which to bring the ileum. The mucosectomy removes rectal mucosa and submucosa for 4 to 6 cm above the dentate line. Rectal muscle layers and anal sphincters are left intact when the primary disease is removed. During the abdominal colectomy, the rectosigmoid is carefully removed to preserve the autonomic nerves on the posterior and lateral pelvic walls. The ileal reservoir is constructed from 30 to 50 cm of the terminal ileum.

In the S-shaped reservoir, three loops of ileum, approximately 12 to 15 cm long, are aligned side by side. The reservoir is constructed by suturing the limbs and opening the segments, thus creating a pouch. A remaining 5-cm segment of ileum forms a spout that is sutured to the dentate line to complete the ileoanal portion of the procedure. In the J-shaped reservoir, the ileum is brought down to the rectal cuff and one limb is looped upward, creating a "J" shape. Then an ileostomy is constructed to divert the stool from the reservoir while healing takes place.

Stage 2
The second stage of surgery involves closure of the ileostomy in a complex, but shorter, procedure.

Nursing intervention
Since the ileoanal reservoir procedure has two surgical stages, prepare the patient preoperatively for each stage.

Stage 1
• Teach conventional ileostomy care.

• Provide skin protection and an effective pouching system.
• Manage fluid and electrolyte levels since high output from the ileostomy is common.
• Provide meticulous perianal skin care since mucous drainage through the anus (which is expected) may be irritating. Skin sealants and vanishing creams may be used to protect the skin. Mini-pads may be worn at night to absorb drainage. Inform the patient that bloody mucous drainage may occur from 10 to 14 days after surgery when sutures are dissolving.
• Instruct the patient to irrigate the reservoir daily to remove mucous drainage.
• Inform the patient that a Gastrografin X-ray is required 6 to 8 weeks after surgery to assess the reservoir, rule out anastomotic leaks, and check the reservoir's anatomic position. Gastrografin is water-soluble and easier to evacuate from the reservoir than barium. Following the X-ray, irrigate the reservoir with 100 to 200 ml of tap water.
• Make sure manometric studies of the sphincter muscle are repeated postoperatively.
• Teach patients Kegel exercises to strengthen sphincter tone:
—Have the patient hold a coin between his buttocks and tighten his sphincter.
—Tape the patient's buttocks together and have him tighten his sphincter.
—Have the patient walk while holding a coin between his buttocks or with his buttocks taped.
—Have the patient squeeze and relax his perianal muscles while he irrigates the reservoir (this helps to assess continence).
• Continue to assess the emotional needs of the patient and his family.

Stage 2
After closure of the ileostomy, patient management requires meticulous perianal care. Residual digestive enzymes present in the mucus and stool are caustic to skin, and bowel movements

ILEOANAL RESERVOIRS

An ileoanal reservoir can be constructed in either an S shape (by aligning and suturing three loops of ileum together) or a J shape (by suturing a portion of the ileum to the rectal cuff and looping the end upward). In the first step of the two-step procedure, a temporary ileostomy is created to allow for stool drainage while the reservoir heals. In the second step, the ileostomy is reversed and stool then drains into the reservoir.

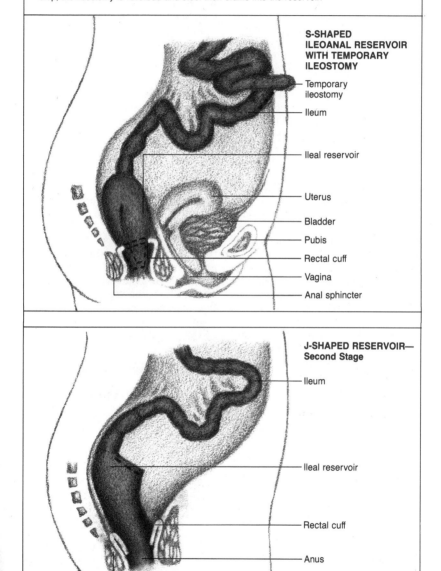

**S-SHAPED
ILEOANAL RESERVOIR
WITH TEMPORARY
ILEOSTOMY**

Temporary ileostomy

Ileum

Ileal reservoir

Uterus

Bladder

Pubis

Rectal cuff

Vagina

Anal sphincter

**J-SHAPED RESERVOIR—
Second Stage**

Ileum

Ileal reservoir

Rectal cuff

Anus

Anal sphincter

are frequent after surgery. In the early postoperative phase, the patient may have as many as 10 to 20 bowel movements in 24 hours (drainage is the same as after conventional ileostomy). As the patient's diet progresses to normal, he may have 6 to 12 bowel movements per day for the first 6 months to 1 year. Thereafter, he averages 3 to 4 bowel movements daily. To minimize discomfort, instruct the patient to avoid skin irritants, such as nylon underwear, harsh or deodorant soaps, and fragrant toilet papers.

• Manage diarrhea with antidiarrheal agents such as psyllium (Metamucil) or loperamide (Imodium). Most patients eat a liberal, regular diet. To help the patient cope with nocturnal leakage of stool and mucus, provide him with mini-pads for bedtime use.

• If the patient complains of perianal pruritus, cleanse the area with Domeboro aluminum acetate solution or Balneol cleansing agents; have the patient take a sitz bath; or apply clotrimazole (Mycelex) cream.

• If the stool becomes thick, intubation and irrigation of the reservoir may be necessary. Instruct the patient in this procedure. Emptying the reservoir is more difficult with the S-shaped than with the J-shaped reservoir. Because the S-shaped reservoir is constructed higher in the pelvis, the levator ani muscles are unable to assist emptying by putting pressure on the reservoir.

Postoperative complications

The most common problems in patients with ileoanal reservoirs are fecal incontinence, nocturnal frequency and/or leakage, diarrhea, perianal skin denudation, perianal pain, and pouchitis, which is irritation or inflammation of the reservoir. The etiology of pouchitis is attributed to bacterial overgrowth in the reservoir. Signs and symptoms include sudden onset of high-volume diarrhea, cramping, and bleeding.

Other possible postoperative complications include adhesions, bleeding, wound infections, anal stenosis, and rectal cuff abscess.

Nursing intervention for complications

• Stenosis of the anal opening requires regular dilation. Teach the patient the following procedure. Using a clean, disposable glove or finger cuff that is well lubricated with a water-soluble gel, gently insert the little finger into the opening. If the stenosis is too tight to admit a little finger, use a dilator, which can be obtained in various sizes.

• Incontinence, nocturnal frequency, and diarrhea usually improve during the first 6 months. The most important nursing function during this period is skin protection. In addition, the patient may become frustrated by the incontinence and frequency. He may limit activities because of his fear of incontinence and lack of control. Provide emotional support to the patient and his family.

• For pouchitis, irrigate the reservoir regularly, provide perianal hygiene, and administer antibiotics as prescribed. Metronidazole (Flagyl) is used effectively. Some surgeons prescribe this drug prophylactically after placement of the ileoanal reservoir.

DEBRA C. BROADWELL, RN, PhD, ET

Patient-controlled analgesia

With patient-controlled analgesia (PCA), a special analgesia pump allows the patient to administer his own I.V. narcotics for pain relief. This technique compensates for variability of drug absorption by different tissues and makes the drug immediately available to the patient. Because the patient receives small increments of I.V. narcotics, he achieves a constant plateau of analgesia without excessive sedation or respiratory depression.

THE PATIENT-CONTROLLED ANALGESIA SYSTEM

The patient-controlled analgesia system (PCA) provides a preset dose of narcotic when the patient pushes the control button. Shown here is the Harvard PCA system by Bard.

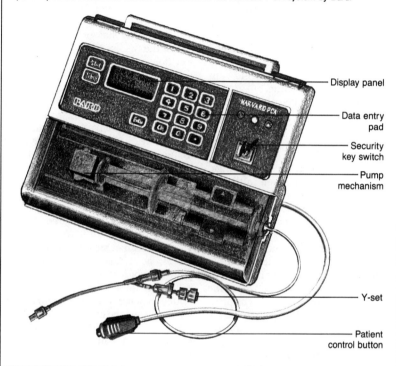

Display panel

Data entry pad

Security key switch

Pump mechanism

Y-set

Patient control button

Studies show that patients who use the pump use up to 31% less narcotic than similar patients on I.M. doses, have fewer postoperative complications related to respiratory depression, and ambulate earlier and more effectively. Patients on PCA are less dependent on the nurse for medication and feel less "lag time" between their awareness of pain and relief from it.

PCA also eliminates tissue breakdown and poor skin turgor at I.M. injection sites. Such tissue trauma contributes to malabsorption of the narcotic and unpredictable pain relief.

Several brands of PCA pumps are available. All operate similarly to the Harvard PCA system by Bard described on page 218.

Candidates

Any patient with an I.V. line who has undergone major surgery or has intractable pain (as from cancer or major trauma, for example) can benefit from PCA. For optimum benefit, the patient should be alert and mentally competent. PCA should be used cautiously in known or suspected drug abusers, patients with respiratory disease, the severely debilitated, and the elderly. Also, acute hypovolemia should be corrected before administering PCA.

Equipment

PCA pump/I.V. catheter with any 2-Y injection port tubing/60-ml Luer-Lok syringe filled with the narcotic ordered by the doctor/48" long (122-cm) arterial pressure tubing/18G needle/alcohol swabs/tape.

Preparation of equipment

• Attach the Luer-Lok syringe to the pressure tubing. (Special Bard tubing may be purchased but is not necessary.)
• Attach an 18G needle to the distal end of the tubing and prime the tubing.
• Turn the security key switch to "unlock" to open the machine.
• Turn the on/off switch to "on" while observing the message panel. The panel should display "okay," the signal that all machine computer systems are operable.
• Prepare the pump for the syringe. Move the pump mechanism to the extreme left; manually spread the "push to release" clips; lay the syringe in the syringe cradle; align the barrel flange with syringe flange slots. Press down on the syringe barrel until both segments of the syringe cradle are in the locked position. Move the pump mechanism to the right until it engages the flange of the syringe plunger. The pressure tubing will exit the pump on the right-hand side. Close the lid and remove the key.
• Press "1" on the data entry pad to select PCA mode. (Available modes on the Bard unit are "continuous infusion" or "PCA mode.")
• Check display panel for date and time. If the information is correct, press "enter." If incorrect, press "clear" and proceed as directed by the display panel.
• Select the PCA dose per injection as ordered by pressing the appropriate numbers, including the decimal. (For example, the doctor will have ordered either morphine sulfate mixed 1 mg/ml or meperidine [Demerol] mixed 5 mg/ml.) To deliver an order of 1 ml per injection, press "1.0." Then press "enter." If you press an incorrect number, reprogram the machine by pressing "clear."
• "Delay" is a safety mechanism to keep patients from overdosing. (The doctor usually orders a delay of 6 minutes between injections with a maximum of 10 injections hourly.) Set the delay by pressing the appropriate numbers on the key pad. If programmed correctly, press "enter." If not, press "clear" and reprogram.
• If the doctor has ordered an initial bolus, the display panel will read "select bolus or PCA mode." Proceed as directed by the display panel.
• Start an I.V. infusion or check the patency of the existing I.V. If functioning, insert the 18G needle into the Y port closest to the patient. Secure with tape. Push "start." The system is now ready for patient use. Place the patient control button within the patient's reach.

Patient preparation

Teach the patient the following:
• why the doctor has ordered PCA
• how PCA works
• safety mechanisms for the patient
• PCA's advantages and individualized pain-control features.

Tell the patient to push the control button whenever he feels pain. If he hasn't pushed the button within the last 6 minutes, a bell will sound and a dose of medication will be released. If he has pushed the button within the last 6 minutes, a bell will sound but no medication will be released.

Don't tell the patient about the delay interval. The bell will act as a placebo. Just tell him to push the button as often as necessary to relieve his pain. Tell him that he may not be completely free from pain, but he should be more comfortable.

Special considerations

Check the patient and the system regularly. Observe how well the patient is controlling his pain and watch for any complications. The patient should be "comfortable" when using PCA within the dose/delay interval. If he isn't, dosage and delay should be reevaluated and adjusted within safe limits. The minimum delay is 3 minutes.

Check for patency and proper functioning of the I.V. system to prevent (or correct) medication delivery and avoid "back infusion" or subcutaneous accumulation of the medication.

Teach the patient to recognize and report signs of infiltration (coolness, swelling at the site). Complications most often arise when the patient is allergic to the narcotic used. Signs and symptoms of toxicity have ranged from nausea and vomiting to uncommon reactions, such as flushing and itching with urticaria.

Never immerse the pump in water. Avoid exposing the pump to temperature extremes.

Troubleshooting
If the patient is uncomfortable while using the PCA pump, check:
• the setting of the PCA dose and delay
• the patency of the I.V.
• the injection mechanism to be sure the syringe is properly installed with the plunger engaged in the pump mechanism
• the patency of all tubing connections.

Documentation
The PCA pump will display historical data of the patient's use of it, including the number of attempts to obtain medication and the number of actual injections received. Chart this data on a separate PCA flow sheet, as specified by your institution. Also chart the drug's effectiveness in relieving pain at the dose administered, the patient's activity level, and how well the patient tolerated the drug.

CYNTHIA BAST, RN, MSN
PAT HAYES, RN, BS

Personality factors

Nursing care of a medical/surgical patient involves more than assessing and managing the signs and symptoms of his disease. To provide effective care, you must understand the personality factors and coping mechanisms that influence how the patient is dealing with his illness. For example, patients tend to regress or more rigidly display existing defense, or coping, mechanisms. A few of the common behaviors you must consider include dependency, denial, and manipulation.

DEPENDENCY
Dependency refers to the patient's transfer of some or all responsibility for his behavior or feelings to his health caregivers.

Assessment
Some dependency is appropriate in normal persons who are stressed by physical illness or surgery. Dependency is sometimes beneficial to both patient and caregiver, since it allows the patient to relinquish control to the caregiver, allowing necessary care. For example, the self-motivated business executive who is a few days post–myocardial infarction (MI) must allow you to provide basic physical care. The dependency that usually occurs with a physical illness helps him accept this potentially difficult situation.

In other patients, dependency is pathological. This kind of dependency is characterized by intense clinging behavior, the need for constant attention, and frequent requests for pain medication. Such overwhelming dependency rarely results from illness alone. Instead, it generally represents a lifelong personality pattern that is exaggerated by the stress of physical illness.

Nursing intervention
Although anger is a normal reaction to difficult, dependent patients, it is rarely effective. The best approach in managing this kind of patient is to support but not encourage his behavior and to appropriately and consistently limit his demands on your time and attention. Communicate these goals to the entire staff to ensure a consistent approach. Openly express your feelings, perhaps during staff meetings, to deal with the

frustration that comes with caring for overly dependent patients.

DENIAL

Denial refers to the patient's unconscious disavowal of information, feelings, or thoughts that are overwhelming or intolerable.

Assessment

Most patients use denial at some point during their illness. For some patients, denial is beneficial. It serves as one of the many coping mechanisms that helps normal individuals to function despite an unpleasant diagnosis or poor prognosis. For example, research has shown that patients who deny their MIs do better than patients who acknowledge them. More research, however, is needed in this area.

Denial is an effective defense against fear and anxiety. In patients who are dying, for example, denial is the first step toward eventual acceptance.

However, denial can interfere with necessary evaluation or treatment of disease. A patient with a chronic illness such as diabetes may demonstrate denial when he refuses to modify his prediabetic high-calorie diet. The patient with an acute MI often expresses denial by attempting to leave the hospital several days after admission. Denial is particularly dangerous in dialysis patients who refuse to continue dialysis treatments.

Some patients express only partial denial. That is, at various times the patient acknowledges aspects of his illness that he had previously denied. Such fluctuation is a normal part of coping.

Nursing intervention

The patient whose denial interferes with treatment compliance can be difficult to manage. In general, don't argue or attempt to prove the patient wrong. Instead, encourage him to use other coping mechanisms. Denial usually gives way to other defenses as the patient begins to accept his situation.

However, when denial persists and causes dangerous noncompliance, call on psychiatric resources to assist both patient and staff.

MANIPULATION

Manipulation is the patient's attempt to satisfy his needs by controlling, without permission, your feelings, thoughts, or behavior.

Assessment

Unlike dependency and denial, manipulation is never beneficial. It is an unhealthy behavior used by an individual who can't satisfy his needs in a more appropriate way. Such a patient, for example, allows only some nurses to attend to his care, complaining that all others are incompetent (a phenomenon referred to as splitting). The patient who, as a means of handling an argument with his wife, threatens an acute exacerbation of his chronic obstructive pulmonary disease is also using manipulation.

Although some manipulators are consciously aware of their behavior and its effects on those being manipulated, many are unaware of the inappropriateness of their behavior and are surprised by the anger they provoke in others. They use manipulation because it is the only coping skill they know.

Nursing intervention

Anger, frustration, distrust, and desire for revenge are common emotions in persons who feel manipulated. Such responses, however, can be detrimental to the nurse-patient relationship. Managing manipulative patients is similar to managing dependent patients. Establish consistent, appropriate limits for the patient's behavior. (These limits are best set by the nursing staff who care directly for the patient.) Make sure that all staff maintain a consistent approach to help prevent splitting. Finally, inform the patient of the effects of his manipulative behavior on others.

BARBARA GROSS BRAVERMAN, RN, MSN, CS

TENS for obstetric analgesia

Relieving labor pain is a special challenge because of the potential hazards of analgesic and anesthetic medication for both the mother and fetus. Currently, transcutaneous electrical nerve stimulation (TENS), a procedure previously used to relieve postcesarean and episiotomy pain, is being used alone or with other pain-relief methods, such as body relaxation and breathing techniques, during labor and delivery. TENS is an acceptable alternative to spinal anesthesia for vaginal delivery in patients with increased risk of uterine rupture. TENS will not mask excessive uterine pain, which could be a warning sign of rupture. TENS can also be used for pain relief during delivery of the placenta and during the immediate postpartum period.

Mechanism of action
TENS is thought to be based in part on the gate control theory of pain. A pulsed alternating current prevents transmission of pain stimuli to the spinal cord. However, recent research suggests that TENS' efficacy may be partly due to a placebo effect.

Nursing interventions
• Teach the patient how to apply and regulate the TENS unit.
• Initiate TENS early in labor. Place electrodes near the sacral column. Allow the patient to adjust the intensity until she becomes uncomfortable and requests assistance.
• Support the patient in her efforts at paced breathing and relaxation.

Special considerations
The use of a TENS unit may interfere with the use of electric fetal monitors. This problem can sometimes be remedied by reducing the amplitude of the TENS unit to minimize interference.

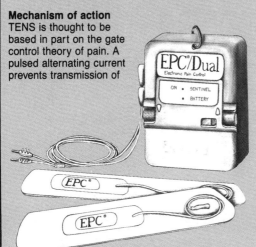

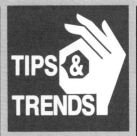

IVH in pregnancy

Intravenous hyperalimentation (IVH) is being used to reverse maternal weight loss and prevent fetal malnutrition. Fetal malnutrition may cause low birth weight (under 2,500 g), congenital anomalies, and impaired mental and motor development.

Maternal malnourishment may be associated with hyperemesis gravidarum, severe eclampsia, inflammatory bowel disease, and pancreatitis.

Nursing interventions
Monitor the patient's weight daily; report any changes. Check urine every shift for glycosuria. Monitor serum glucose and other lab values.
• Provide sterile dressing changes to the central line. Observe the insertion site for redness, swelling, or drainage.
• Teach home IVH care, if applicable.
• Assist with 24-hour urine collection for estriol and nitrogen levels during the 28th week of gestation.
• Culture the exit site and/or blood specimens through the catheter to check for sepsis.

Implantable infusion pump

Patients who require continuous long-term drug therapy can benefit from the Infusaid pump, a small, vapor pressure–powered pump. Implanted under the skin near the desired delivery site, the pump can infuse precisely controlled drug doses to ambulatory patients. It allows site-specific drug delivery (example: intraspinal morphine) for maximum effect, higher doses with fewer systemic side effects, and continuous infusion for as long as 14 days.

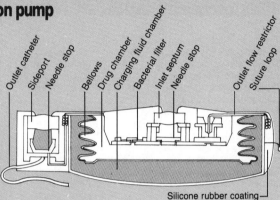

Silicone rubber coating

Nursing interventions
After implantation, delay drug infusion for a few days to allow healing at the site. During this time, check the pump's patency and flow rate—with the bacteriostatic solution placed within it before implantation or with heparinized normal saline solution. During this time, teach the patient about the pump, its operation, the drug, and follow-up care. The guidelines below will help you care for the pump. (Your hospital may offer a certification course on pump care.)
• Learn about the prescribed drug. Review its possible side effects with the patient. Report side effects to the doctor.
• Monitor the patient for signs of infection (low-grade fever, pain, tenderness, redness, swelling, or exudate at insertion site). Report such signs to the doctor before the pump is refilled.

• Review the Infusaid manual before giving care.
• Tell the patient to avoid long, hot baths; prolonged exposure to the sun; and scuba diving.

Pump refill
To assist the doctor in refilling the pump:
• Prepare the drug. Refer to the manual for syringe size.
• Prepare the sterile field.
• Identify the pump by palpating the outer perimeters. Notify the doctor of any inflammation.
• Don sterile gloves.
• Clean the area over and around the pump with alcohol and then povidone-iodine. Drape the area.
• Attach the Infusaid fill set, the angled needle, and an empty 50-ml syringe.
• Insert the needle into the center of the pump (the indented, self-sealing inlet). Empty the pump by placing the syringe barrel below the pump site.
• Record the return volume (add 1 ml to account for tubing) and disconnect the syringe barrel contain-

ing residual solution. If no solution returns, the needle may be misplaced, the chamber may be empty, or the pump may be malfunctioning. Check needle placement by injecting 5 ml of bacteriostatic water. When you release the plunger, the water should return if the needle is placed correctly. Notify the doctor if the pump is not functioning.
• After disposing of the residual solution, attach the drug and purge the system.
• Inject 5 ml of drug into the pump.
• Check the placement. Release pressure on the plunger so that the drug returns to the syringe. Continue injecting the drug.
• Check the placement every 5 ml.
• Remove the needle and apply pressure for several minutes.

Documentation
Note that you have informed the patient about possible effects of the infused drug. Document the refilling procedure.

Sulfamylon sandwich

Direct application of full-strength mafenide acetate (Sulfamylon) can damage newly grafted tissues, and removal requires vigorous, often painful hydrotherapy. For this reason, burn specialists have developed a method that doesn't place the antimicrobial in direct contact with the skin. This dressing, known as the Sulfamylon sandwich, helps promote graft viability, reduce pain, and prevent infection.

The dressing, easily applied at the bedside, consists of several layers of gauze: an inner layer soaked in normal saline solution, which keeps the graft site moist and separates the middle layer from the graft surface; a Sulfamylon-impregnated middle layer, which continuously delivers between 0.6% and 1.2% Sulfamylon to the graft; and a normal saline-soaked outer layer that keeps the entire dressing moist. The middle and outer layers are replaced every 12 hours during the first 72 hours of dressing application; the inner layer, at the end of the first 72 hours. The entire dressing is soaked with normal saline solution every 6 hours to prevent drying.

Sensitivity is rare; a reaction may consist of erythema that clears with a change to a dry dressing such as xeroform gauze.

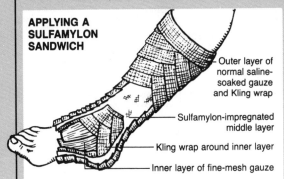

APPLYING A SULFAMYLON SANDWICH

— Outer layer of normal saline-soaked gauze and Kling wrap

— Sulfamylon-impregnated middle layer

— Kling wrap around inner layer

— Inner layer of fine-mesh gauze

1. Apply a layer of normal saline-soaked fine-mesh gauze over the graft site. (Use warm solution for comfort.)

2. Wrap a single layer of normal saline-soaked Kling wrap around the gauze.

3. Next, impregnate a normal saline-soaked Intersorb pad with Sulfamylon, then place it over the Kling wrap. Center the pad in the graft area; don't place it over healed skin.

4. Apply another Intersorb pad, also soaked in normal saline solution, over the Sulfamylon layer. Secure the entire dressing with Kling wrap; soak it in normal saline solution.

Animal companionship therapy

Pet companionship and pet-facilitated therapy (PFT) are currently being used to remedy social isolation among the elderly. Pets appear to encourage communication, a sense of well-being, and a feeling of being loved among this growing, often easily isolated population.

Research

Most animal companionship studies have been conducted among the institutionalized elderly to promote social integration and well-being. This positive effect may result from the companionship the pet provides, the caregiving and exercise it encourages, the sense of safety it instills, and the exchange of touching between pet and owner. In PFT, the pet acts as a bridge between the therapist and the withdrawn, uncooperative patient. Thus therapy extends beyond the usual resources of the institution.

Outreach programs

PFT's success in institutions has led to numerous pet-related outreach programs for the elderly. Unfortunately, pets are often prohibited from retirement homes and other residences for the elderly, where their presence may cause safety, sanitation, and financial problems.

Glossary

The terms listed below were selected from two areas important to current nursing practice: business management and scientific research.

A

Abstract. A noncritical, informative summary of the significant content of a published article or other work.

Accidental sampling. Selecting subjects for a study by availability (convenience sampling).

Analysis of covariance. A statistical method (also known as ANCOVA) for testing effectiveness of therapy on different groups while controlling one or more variable factors (covariates).

Analysis of variance. A statistical method (also called ANOVA) for testing effectiveness of therapy by comparing variability between groups to variability within a group.

Annual budgetary planning (ABP). An organized approach to planning for quality, cost-effective patient care through decentralized nursing responsibility for budget preparation and control.

Assets. The valuable resources, or properties and property rights, owned by an individual or organization. Most assets are tangible (equipment, facilities, and claims on cash); some intangible legal and accounting entitlements (such as patents and goodwill) are also counted as assets.

Attribute variables. Preexisting characteristics of the subject of a study, which the investigator observes and measures.

Attrition. Loss of participants in a study, which can change the composition of the sample and threaten the study's validity.

Average cost. The total costs incurred in the production and/or distribution of a product divided by the number of units produced or distributed. Average costs usually decline with larger volumes of output, reach a minimum level, and increase beyond that volume.

B

Balance sheet. An itemized statement that lists total assets and total liabilities of a business to show its net worth at a given time.

Bargaining strategies. Managing conflict by getting both sides to agree on a compromise.

Basic organization design. The process of specializing jobs in an organization to accomplish work efficiently while ensuring coordination to achieve strategic goals.

Bias. Partiality or prejudice. In scientific research, any factor that distorts the results of a study: a biased sample, for example, doesn't provide equal chance of selection for all members of a population.

Break-even analysis. A method used to determine the point at which a business will neither make a profit nor incur a loss; it is expressed in either the total dollars of revenue exactly offset by total expenses (fixed and variable) or in total units of production, the cost of which exactly equals the income derived by their sale.

Budget. Funds allocated to an organizational unit for future use; an itemized summary of probable expenses and income for a given period. A written, detailed statement of management's goals and plans for sources and uses of money, useful in evaluating organizational and managerial performance.

Bureaucracy. A functional design that divides and assigns work, applies administrative control, and relies on specialization. Standard bureaucracies use external controls; professional bureaucracies use internal or peer controls.

Business portfolio matrix. A classification of a business based on its growth rate and market share, which is used in corporate strategic planning.

Buying center. People who participate in or influence a purchase.

C

Capital budgeting. The process of evaluating proposed investments.

Capital equipment. Equipment used to manufacture a product, to provide a service, or to sell, store, and deliver merchandise; durable goods that are depreciated over many years. Such equipment is not sold in the normal course of business, but used, worn out, or consumed over time.

Career management. The personal and organizational planning of one's work.

Case study. Research method that involves thorough analysis of a person, group, institution, or other social unit.

Cash flow. The actual movement of cash within a business: cash inflow minus cash outflow. A term used to designate the reported net income of a corporation plus amounts charged off for depreciation, depletion, amortization, and extraordinary charges to reserves, which are bookkeeping deductions and not actually paid out in cash; a better indication of capacity to meet obligations and pay dividends than net income.

Causal relationship. Relationship between two variables in which one determines the presence, absence, or value of the other.

Census. A survey that includes all of a population.

Centralization vs. decentralization. The extent to which decisions are made at higher vs. lower levels in the management hierarchy.

Central tendency. Statistical index of the most characteristic set of scores derived from the center of the distribution of scores. The three most common indices of central tendency are the mean, the median, and the mode.

Chi-square test. A test of statistical significance used to assess whether or not a relationship exists between two nominal-level variables; symbolized as x^2. The larger the computed value of chi-square, for specified-size samples, the smaller the probability that the differences are due to random sampling.

Cluster. A subgroup of variables, each of which is more closely correlated with other members of the subgroup than with the other variables in the larger group.

Cluster sampling. A form of multistage sampling in which large groupings (clusters) are selected first (e.g., nursing schools), with successive subsampling of smaller units (e.g., nursing students).

Coding. The process of transforming raw data into standardized (usually numerical) form for data processing and analysis.

Cohort. A set of study subjects who are grouped according to certain characteristics and observed over time. In explanatory studies, these characteristics would be the independent variables.

Cohort study. A trend study that focuses on a specific subpopulation (which is often an age-related subgroup) from which different samples are selected to represent different times (e.g., students graduated in 1986).

Communication networks. Communication patterns designed to experimentally test how the movement of information affects productivity and morale.

Competitive analysis. Analysis of the competitive forces in an industry, including threat of new entrants, bargaining power of buyers and suppliers, and threat of substitute products or services.

Concomitant variation. Consistent variation between two phenomena that may result from a direct cause and effect relationship between the two phenomena or from a third common causal factor.

Concurrent validity. The degree to which an instrument can distinguish individuals who differ on some criterion measured or observed at the same time.

Construct. A concept devised to aid in scientific analysis and generalization. Generally inferred indirectly from observable phenomena, it is an abstraction from reality.

Construct validity. The degree to which a research instrument measures the concept under investigation.

Content validity. The degree to which the items in a research instrument adequately represent the universe of content.

Continuum. Describes the scale for a variable in which the interval between any two values allows a third value.

Control. In research, the process of holding constant possible influences on the dependent variable under investigation. In statistics, treatment of the data to remove the effects of extraneous factors.

Control group. Subjects in an experiment who are measured at the beginning and at the end of a study in the same way as the experimental group, but who do not receive the experimental treatment. Their performance provides a baseline for measuring the effects of treatment.

Convenience sampling. *See* Accidental sampling.

Correlation. A tendency for variation in one variable to be linked to variation in another variable.

Correlational studies. Studies that determine the degree to which variations in one variable are linked to variations in another.

Correlation coefficient. An index that summarizes the degree of relationship between two variables. Correlation coefficients typically range from +1.00 (perfect direct relationship) to 0.0 (no relationship) to -1.00 (perfect inverse relationship).

Cost accounting. The procedure for attributing appropriate cost elements to an activity or a product.

Cost/benefit analysis. Measuring the costs against the benefits realized from a course of action. The essence of managerial decision making, it has received renewed publicity as a tool for governmental decision making. In nonprofit organizations, benefits are often difficult to quantify.

Cost center. Any responsibility center that controls incurred costs. A cost center has no control over sales or revenue.

Criterion-related validity. Validity that compares a test, treatment, or outcome to external standards or criteria.

Cross-sectional design. A type of research design in which data are collected and analyzed from a specific point in time as in a descriptive survey.

Current assets. Cash or other items that will normally be turned into cash within 1 year; assets that will be used up within 2 years.

Current liabilities. Amounts owed that will ordinarily be paid by a firm within 1 year (accounts payable, wages payable, taxes payable, the current portion of a long-term debt, and interest and dividends payable).

D
Data. The pieces of information obtained in the course of a study.

Decision-making research. A study designed to select a course of action from several alternative courses.

Deduction. A process of reasoning that starts with given premises from which it derives valid conclusions. Reasoning from the general to the particular.

Demography. The study of population size, composition, and distribution, and the patterns of change therein. The narrowest definition views demography as the study of vital statistics. In the broadest view, population composition and distribution also include such variables as fertility, mortality, age and sex, marriage, divorce, family size, race, education, illiteracy, unemployment, distribution of wealth, occupational distribution, crime rates, density of population, migration, and other factors.

Directional hypothesis. A hypothesis that predicts direction (positive or negative) of the relationship between two variables.

Direct-mail advertising. Selling directly to customers through the mail.

Diversification. Moving into new and often unrelated lines of business, which may include unfamiliar products or markets.

Double-blind experiment. An experiment in which neither the subject nor the investigator knows the identity of the subjects or controls in the experiment. In clinical experiments, neither the investigator nor the study subject knows which subject receives the placebo and which the experimental treatment. It is used to ensure that the experimental and control groups are identical in every way except in the variable that is being tested.

E
Economics. The discipline concerned with the allocation of resources; one of the social sciences.

• *Macroeconomics.* The study of interaction of economic agents in society and the role of government in affecting their decision-making process.

• *Microeconomics.* The study of the decision-making processes of individual economic agents in producing, distributing, and consuming goods.

Empirical. Capable of being confirmed, verified, or disproved by observation or experiment.

Empirical test. A test of a hypothesis in which the investigator observes the phenomena in question (either under experimental or natural conditions) to determine whether these observations support or disprove the hypothesis.

Entrepreneur. An innovator of a business enterprise who recognizes opportunities to introduce a new product, a new production process, or an improved organization, and who raises the necessary money, assembles the factors of production, and organizes an operation to exploit the opportunity.

Expectancy theory. A theory of work motivation based on the expectations that effort leads to high performance and high performance leads to rewards.

Expense items. Short-lived goods and services that are charged off as they are used—usually in the year of purchase.

Experiment. An arrangement of conditions under which a phenomenon to be observed shall take place.

Experimental group. Subjects who are exposed to the experimental (treatment, stimulus) variable and whose reactions will reflect the effect, if any, of that variable.

Exploratory research. A preliminary study designed to develop or refine hypotheses, or to test and refine the methods of data collection.

External validity. The degree to which the results of a study can be generalized to apply to settings or samples other than the ones studied.

Extrinsic rewards. Rewards from sources outside the job, including pay, promotion, and recognition.

F
Face validity. Validity that is tested by overt inspection.

Factorial design. An experimental design that tests the simultaneous effects of several independent variables on a dependent variable. The design may also involve multiple alternatives for each of the independent variables. This design permits an analysis of the separate main effects of the independent variables and of their interactive effects.

Feasibility study. Determining whether a project is worth doing, often by cost/benefit analysis.

Field study. Collecting data from subjects performing in their normal roles and habitats rather than as subjects in a laboratory study. Data are collected either directly, as in an interview, or indirectly, as in a mailed questionnaire.

Financial planning techniques. Methods for developing goals, objectives, and actions for the financial aspects of a business.

Fiscal policy. Measures under the control of central government policymakers that influence economic activity. Among these are tax policy, the central government budget and its associated surpluses and deficits, and direct stimulus of economic activity through governmental expenditures in target areas.

Follow-up study. A study to determine the subsequent development or condition of the subjects of a study.

F-test. A test of the significance of differences in the values of summary measures, based on the F distribution, which is used in such statistical procedures as the analysis of variance. The F-test is the ratio of:

$$\frac{\text{variance among groups}}{\text{variance within groups}}$$

G
Generalizability. The degree to which findings can be applied from a sample to the entire population.

Goals. The ultimate ends an organization seeks, as opposed to objectives, which are intermediate targets toward meeting those goals.

Growth strategies. Plans for expanding the scope of current business activities in line with market growth.

H
Hawthorne effect. The effect on the dependent variable caused by subjects' awareness of the study. It was first described in the experiments at the Western Electric Hawthorne plant in Chicago during the 1920s and early 1930s. The psychological reaction to the study conditions can be mistaken for the effect of the independent variable and can lead to spurious inferences.

Herzberg's hygiene and motivator factors. Factors that motivate people at work. Hygiene factors are external to the work itself (salary, supervision, company policy); motivator factors occur through work (achievement, responsibility, advancement).

Hierarchy of authority. The vertical levels in an organization. As one moves up in the organization, each level has greater power, decision-making authority, and responsibility than the preceding level.

Historical research. Studies designed to establish facts and relationships concerning past events.

Horizontal integration. Acquiring firms at the same level of activity.

Human resource planning. Strategic and tactical techniques for matching the right people with the right skills, to achieve organization plans.

Hypothesis(es). A tentative explanation of data not yet proved; a tentative deduction; usually the first step in problem solving; a predicted relationship between variables under investigation. Hypotheses lead to empirical studies that seek to confirm or disprove those predictions.

I
Induction. A process of reasoning that proceeds from the particular to the general.

Inference. A judgment or conclusion based on information other than direct observation. Statistical inference is the process of making generalizations from data.

Informed consent. An ethical principle that requires researchers to obtain the voluntary participation of subjects, after informing them of possible risks and benefits.

Interaction effect. The effect on a dependent variable of two or more independent variables acting in combination (interactively) rather than as independent factors.

Internal consistency. A form of reliability referring to the degree to which the subparts of a research instrument measure the same attribute or dimension.

Internal validity. The degree to which the experimental treatment (independent variable), rather than uncontrolled, extraneous factors, is responsible for observed effects.

Interrater reliability. The degree to which two raters, operating independently, assign the same ratings for an attribute being measured.

Intervention. In experimental research, the experimental treatment or manipulation, or the structure the investigator imposes on the research setting before making observations.

K

Key informant. A person who is well informed about the subject of research interest and who is willing to share information and insights with the researcher.

L

Liaison. A position established to coordinate decisions between groups, departments, or jobs.

Likert scale. A composite measure of attitudes that involves summation of scores on a set of items (statements) to which respondents are asked to indicate degree of agreement or disagreement. Typically, each statement has five possible responses: strongly agree, agree, uncertain, disagree, strongly disagree.

Line unit. Any organizational unit whose activities are directly related to the basic objectives of the organization.

Line versus staff. The division of work between workers responsible for accomplishing strategic goals (line) and those who give advice and service to line (staff).

Literature review. A critical summary of research on a topic of interest, to gain information about a research problem.

Longitudinal study. A study designed to collect data on the same subjects at more than one point in time.

M

Management. Defining organizational goals and deciding on the efficient and effective use of resources to ensure high performance.

Management by objectives (MBO). A results-oriented philosophy and system of managing, using mutually established objectives, target dates, and evaluation of performance.

Management information system (MIS). A system, usually computerized, for collecting, storing, and synthesizing information useful for management decision making.

Manipulation. An intervention or treatment introduced by a researcher.

Marginal costs. The additions to total costs necessary to produce one additional item above the prevailing level of output. Marginal costs equal average costs when average costs are at their minimum level and increase above average costs at higher levels of output.

Market. The number of people and their total spending (actual or potential) for your product line within the geographic limits of your distribution ability. The market share is the percentage of sales compared to the total sales of competitors for a particular product line.

Marketing audit. A systematic, critical, and unbiased review and appraisal of the basic objectives and policies of the marketing function, and of the organization, methods, procedures, and people employed to implement the policies.

Marketing plan. A written statement of a marketing strategy and the time-related details for carrying it out.

Matching. The pairing of subjects in one group with those in another group based on their similarity in one or more dimensions, to enhance the overall comparability of groups in an experiment.

Matrix organization. An adaptive organizational structure that provides for interdepartmental and interdisciplinary leadership to achieve common goals; graphically, this structure appears as a grid (matrix) with hierarchical (vertical) coordination through departmentalization and the formal chain of command as well as simultaneous lateral (horizontal) coordination across departments.

Maturation. A threat to the internal validity of a study that results when the passage of time changes factors that influence the outcome measure (dependent variable).

McClelland's need theory. A theory stating that needs for affiliation, power, and achievement are developed (learned) throughout life.

Mean. A statistical measure of central tendency, computed by adding all scores and dividing by the number of subjects or values.

Median. A statistical measure of central tendency representing the exact middle score or value in a distribution of scores; the middle value of a distribution; the 50th percentile. The median is the value above and below which 50% of the scores lie.

Methods (research). The steps, procedures, and strategies for gathering and analyzing research data.

Mode. A statistical measure of central tendency; the score or value that occurs most frequently in a distribution of scores.

Motive power. That element in the working relationship between two or more persons that determines whose plan of action is dominant, marked by an ability to see the broad picture, a desire to change things, and a willingness to be measured by results.

Multistage sampling. A sampling strategy that proceeds through a set of stages from larger to smaller sampling units.

N

N. Often used to designate the total number of subjects in a study (e.g., "the total N was 500").

n. Often used to designate the number of subjects in a subgroup or in a cell of a study ("each of the four groups had an n of 125, for a total N of 500").

Need analysis. Market research to assess interest in a new product.

Net profit. An organization's earnings from its operations during a particular period.

Nondirectional hypothesis. A research hypothesis that does not predict the direction (i.e., positive or negative) of the relationship between variables.

Nonprobability sampling. The selection of subjects or sampling units through nonrandom procedures such as accidental, judgmental, and quota sampling.

Normal curve. A bell-shaped curve that indicates that the majority of the values of the measurements of a variable for a group of study subjects cluster at about the same scale value while fewer and fewer subjects possess values at the extremes of the scale.

Norms. A set of test scores derived from a representative group of respondents, used as standards for evaluating the scores obtained by users of the test.

Null hypothesis. The hypothesis stating that there is no relationship between the variables under study; that the differences obtained in the study happened by chance alone.

Nurse manager. A nurse (such as director of nursing service, head nurse) whose regular job responsibility is the management of personnel.

Nursing audit. A method for assuring documentation of the quality of nursing care in keeping with the organization's standards.

Nursing by objectives (NBO). A results-oriented philosophy and system of managing a nursing department, using mutually established objectives, target dates for completion, and performance evaluation.

Nursing research. A systematic, detailed attempt to discover or confirm facts that relate to specific nursing problems. Its goal is the provision of scientific knowledge in nursing.

O

Observational research. Studies in which the data are collected by observing and recording behaviors or activities of interest.

Operational definition. The definition of a concept or variable in measurable terms.

Opportunity cost. The profits sacrificed by not pursuing the next-best alternative.

Organizational development (OD). A process of creating a climate for change and growth through the development and effective use of personnel and other resources.

Organization chart. Explicit diagram of the formal roles, relationships, and flow of information in an organization.

P

Pairing. A method of matching the individual members of the experimental and control samples with respect to relevant covariables; this helps match groups more closely than randomization alone.

Panel design. A technique in which a selected sample of subjects is interviewed, usually about the same variable (e.g., income), recurrently over an extended time to study the change that has taken place.

Performance evaluation. The regular review and appraisal of personnel performance.

Pilot study. A preliminary study carried out before a research design is complete to assist in formulating the problem, developing the hypotheses, or establishing the priorities. Also called an exploratory study.

Policy. A general guide for behavior or actions.

Politics. Compromising on intermediate goals to reach an ultimate, rational objective. Activities aimed at using the influence of others to reach goals.

Power. The ability to exercise influence over others.

Predictability. The ability to forecast that previously recorded events will recur.

Pre-test. After a research design has been formulated, this test takes place to develop the procedures for applying the research instruments, to test the wording of questions, or to ensure that the specific questions or observations are relevant and precise.

Profit. The excess of the selling price over all costs and expenses incurred in making the sale. Also, the reward to the entrepreneur for the risks in establishing, operating, and managing a given enterprise.

Profit center. An organizational unit that controls both cost and revenue.

Program performance plan (PPP). A long-range schedule of the interrelated steps required to produce a desired result, objective, or goal.

Proposal. A document describing a proposed research study; it communicates the research problem, its significance, planned procedures for solving the problem, and, when funding is sought, how much the research will cost.

Q

Quality assurance program (QAP). A planned approach to aid health care agencies to meet patient care goals through compliance with the standards established by the accrediting agencies and professional groups.

Quasi-experiment. A study in which subjects cannot be assigned randomly to treatment conditions, although the researcher manipulates the independent variable and exercises certain controls to enhance the internal validity of the results.

Questionnaire. A method of gathering self-report information from respondents through self-administration of questions in a paper-and-pencil format.

Quota sampling. The nonrandom selection of subjects in which the researcher prespecifies characteristics of the sample.

R

Randomization. A technique in experimental research to equalize the composition of study groups so they are identical in all pertinent variables. Subjects are assigned to the different study groups according to the laws of chance; also called random assignment.

Random-number table. A table of digits from 0 to 9 set up in such a way that each number is equally likely to follow any other; used in randomization or random sampling.

Random sampling. The selection of a sample so that each member of a population (or sub-population) has an equal probability of being included.

Recruiting. Finding the right people to fill jobs; specifically, balancing the costs of finding the right person against his or her performance potential.

Reliability. A criterion for assessing the quality of data. Data are reliable if they are consistent, accurate, and precise.

Replication. The duplication of research procedures in subsequent investigations to test the validity of earlier results.

Research. Systematic inquiry that uses orderly scientific methods to answer questions or solve problems.

• *Applied research.* Study to obtain new facts or identify relationships among facts for use in solving a practical problem, making a decision, or developing or evaluating a program, procedure, process, or product.

• *Basic or pure research.* Study to establish fundamental theories, facts, or statements of relationships in an area of knowledge not intended for immediate, practical use, to advance scientific knowledge.

• *Descriptive research.* Study that defines the characteristics of persons, situations, or groups, or that measures the frequency of certain phenomena. Sometimes called absolute research.

• *Developmental research.* Study concerned with developing a new procedure, program, or product.

• *Evaluative research.* Study that tests a program, method, procedure, or product to assess the quality, applicability, feasibility, desirability, or worth according to some meaningful measure.

• *Experimental and nonexperimental research.* In experimental research, the investigator controls all elements of the research, often in a specialized research setting such as a laboratory. In nonexperimental research, not all elements of the research are under direct control of the investigator; it is conducted in a natural setting, such as a school, a public health agency, a hospital, or a patient's home. This type of research is frequently retrospective.

• *Explanatory research.* Study that tests a hypothesis about a relationship between an independent variable (causal treatment, stimulus variable) and a dependent variable (effect, response, or criterion variable). The independent variable is manipulated by the researcher.

• *Methodological research.* Study that develops methods, models, tools, products, or procedures for conducting further research or for practical use.

Research design. Plan of the research that is developed before a study begins. The overall plan for collecting and analyzing data, including specifications for enhancing the internal and external validity of the study.

Research problem. The motivation for undertaking a study that consists of a definition of concepts and terms narrowed down from a broadly stated question into one more restricted in scope and related to research findings that have been obtained by others.

Response rate. The rate of participation in a survey; calculated by dividing the number of persons participating by the number of persons sampled.

Responsibility center. Budgetary unit of an organization in which accountability, responsibility, and authority for achieving goals are assigned to a manager.

Retrospective design (or study). In nonexperimental studies, a design in which the dependent variable is observed and then linked to a presumed cause in the past.

S

Sample. A subset of a population selected to participate in a research study.

Sampling. The process of selecting a part of the target population to represent the entire population in a study.

Sampling bias. Distortions that arise from the selection of a sample that is not representative of the population from which it was drawn.

Sampling error (standard error). A measure of the extent to which the sample findings are different from what they would be if all the sampling units in the target population had been studied.

Sampling units. The individual members of a target population: human beings, animals, plants, or inanimate objects.

Score. A numerical value assigned to a scale, test, or other data-gathering instrument to indicate the degree to which the respondent possesses the variable being measured.

Self-report. Any procedure for collecting data that involves a direct report of information by the person who is being studied.

Significance level. The statistical probability, determined by the laws of probability, that an observed relationship could be caused by chance; it is expressed as P (or p) followed by a decimal number. Significance at the P .05 level indicates that the observed relationship could occur by chance only 5 times out of 100.

Skewness. A quality of a set of scores relating to their asymmetrical distribution around a central point.

Span of control. The number of activities (and, therefore, people) supervised by a manager.

Staffing. Providing human resources to carry out an organization's plans for achieving its goals. Analyzing an organization's tasks in terms of meeting human resource needs, recruiting candidates, and selecting candidates to fill the positions.

Staff unit. One that assists and provides services to other units in the organization.

Standard deviation. The most frequently used statistic for measuring the degree of variability in a set of scores.

Standards of care. Clearly defined measures of comfort, techniques, clinical observations, perceptions, interpretations, and judgments used in evaluating nursing actions.

Standards of performance. Written statements that define and measure employees' responsibilities and ability to meet their objectives.

Statistical significance. To test whether or not two or more groups being compared in terms of a summary measure—a mean, a standard deviation, a percentage, or, nonparametrically, in terms of their rank order on a qualitative scale—could be considered to have come from the same target population (i.e., that they are essentially two independent samples from the same population).

Statistics. Summary measures, such as percentages, means, medians, percentiles, and standard deviations, that are computed from measurements obtained from a sample of the total population. Numerical estimates of population parameters, calculated from sample data.

Strategic planning. Deciding how to allocate resources to bring an organization into alignment with its long-term goals and objectives.

Stratified random sampling. The random, independent selection of subjects from two or more strata of the population.

Stratified sample. A sample selected to reflect a known characteristic of the target population, such as age or sex.

Subjects in research. The persons or things from whom study data are collected; study subjects can be human beings, animals, plants, cells, or inanimate objects.

Survey research. Nonexperimental research that obtains information, usually through direct questioning of a sample of respondents.

Systematic sampling. The selection of subjects so that every kth (e.g., every tenth) person (or element) in a sampling frame or list is chosen.

T

Target market. The specific individuals, distinguished by socioeconomic, demographic, and/or interest characteristics, who are the most likely customers for the goods and services of a business.

Target population. The membership of a defined set of subjects in which the researcher is interested and from which a sample of study subjects is selected.

Test-retest reliability. Assessment of the stability of a research instrument by comparing the scores obtained on repeated administrations.

Theory. An abstract generalization that explains the relationships among phenomena. It summarizes existing knowledge, explains observed facts and relationships, and predicts still unobserved events and relationships.

Theory X and Theory Y. Douglas McGregor's sets of the assumptions management makes about employees. Theory X managers assume that most workers lack ambition and need strong direction; Theory Y managers focus on integrating individual and organizational goals.

Theory Z. Assumptions about workers stemming from the influence of Japanese management methods, which include values about group consensus in decision making, workers' dedication, and management visibility.

Total cost. The sum of total fixed and total variable costs.

Total fixed cost. The sum of costs that are fixed in total—no matter how much is produced.

Total variable cost. The sum of changing expenses that are closely related to output.

Trend study. A study in which different samples from a population are studied over time with respect to a selected phenomenon (e.g., serial polls of political preferences).

T-test. A parametric statistical test used for analyzing the difference between two means. It equals the:

difference in sample means minus
difference in population means
standard error of the difference
in sample means

Type-I error. A decision to reject the null hypothesis when it is true (i.e., the researcher concludes that a relationship exists when in fact it does not). Also called alpha error.

Type-II error. A decision to accept the null hypothesis when it is false (i.e., the researcher concludes that no relationship exists when in fact it does). Also called beta error.

U

Uncertainty. In statistics, the possibility of chance, which precludes absolutely conclusive statements.

V

Validity. The degree of reliability with which an instrument measures what it is intended to measure.

Variable. An attribute of a person or object that changes and takes on different values (body temperature, age, heart rate); anything that can change. Variables must have a scale of measurement and must produce statistical data.

● *Dependent variable.* The variable that is observed to determine the effect of experimental manipulation of the independent variable: the criterion, effect, or response variable.

● *Extraneous variables.* The variables that are of minor interest to the researcher but that are present in large numbers in any study involving humans. Including organismic and environmental variables, they may be controlled or uncontrolled.

● *Independent variable.* The variable that is changed or manipulated by the researcher: the experimental, treatment, causal, or stimulus variable.

Variance. A measure of variability or dispersion equal to the square of the standard deviation.

Vertical integration. Acquiring ownership of the natural product source by the user or acquiring services at different levels of business activity.

Z

Zero-based budgeting. A new approach to budgeting. This method gets its name because managers are required to start at zero budget levels every year and justify all costs as if the programs involved were beginning for the first time.

Selected references and acknowledgments

Selected references

Allan, Mark J., et al. "Rapid Dissolution of Gallstones in Methyl Tert-Butyl Ether: Preliminary Observations," *New England Journal of Medicine* 312(4):217, January 24, 1985.

Amelar, R.D., et al. *Current Therapy of Infertility.* St. Louis: C.V. Mosby Co., 1984.

April, Robert. "Neurological Complications of Diabetes," *Practical Diabetology* 4(5):1-3, September/October 1985.

Bagwell, M., and Clements, S. *A Political Handbook for Health Professionals.* Boston: Little, Brown & Co., 1985

Ball, P. "Pancreatic Transplantation: Perioperative Nursing Care," *Association of Operating Room Nurses Journal* 43(3):632-37, March 1986.

Barrett, S. "Commercial Hair Analysis: Science or Scam?," *Journal of the American Medical Association* 254(8):1041-45, August 23/30, 1985.

Beck, Donald. "Principles of Accounting and Finance for the Non-Accountant," *Health Care Supervisor* 2(2):15-26, January 1984.

Bennett, Richard, and Griffen, Ward O. "Patients Controlled Analgesia," *Contemporary Surgery* 23(4), April 1983.

Brucker, M.C. "Nonpharmaceutical Methods for Relieving Pain and Discomfort During Pregnancy," *Maternal and Child Nursing* 9:390-94, November/December 1984.

Cogan, D., et al. "Aldose Reductose and Complications of Diabetes," *Annals of Internal Medicine* 101:82-91, 1984.

Cole, C.H. "Prevention of Prematurity: Can We Do It in America?," *Pediatrics* 76(2):310-12, 1985.

Dailey, Anne Louise. "The Burnout Test," *American Journal of Nursing* 85(3):270-72, March 1985.

Delgado, G., et al. "Intraoperative Radiation in Treatment of Advanced Cervical Cancer," *Obstetrics & Gynecology* 62(2):246-52, 1984.

DeVita, V., et al. *AIDS: Etiology, Diagnosis, Treatment, and Prevention.* Philadelphia: J.B. Lippincott Co., 1985.

Dixon, Jane. "Additional Uses for Relaxation Techniques," *Oncology Nursing Forum* 11(1):16, January/February 1984.

Dodge, D. "Radial Keratotomy," *Association of Operating Room Nurses Journal* 42(2):214-24, August 1985.

Finkler, Steven. *Budgeting Concepts for Nurse Managers.* New York: Grune & Stratton, 1984.

Fleischer, A., et al. "Antepartum Nonstress Test and the Postmature Pregnancy," *Obstetrics & Gynecology* 66(1):80-83, 1985.

Fonkalsrud, E.W. "Endorectal Ileoanal Anastomosis with Isoperistaltic after Colectomy and Mucosal Proctectomy," *Annals of Surgery* 199:151-57, February 1984.

Frankel, Arthur E., and Houston, L.L. "Immunotoxin Therapy of Cancer" in *Immunoconjugate for Cancer Therapy.* Academic Press, 1986.

Frankel, Arthur E., et al. "Prospects for Immunotoxin Therapy in Cancer," *Annual Review of Medicine* 37:125-42, 1986.

Gallacher, D.J., et al. "Nonoperative Management of Benign Postoperative Biliary Strictures," *Radiology* 156(3):625-29, September 1985.

Gerber, A. "The Koch Continent Ileal Reservoir: An Alternative to Conventional Urostomy," *Journal of Enterostomal Therapy* 12(1):15-17, January/February 1985.

Goldstein, J.L., and Brown, M.S. "Familial Hypercholesterolemia: A Genetic Receptor Disease," *Hospital Practice* 20(11):35-46, November 15, 1985.

Hicks, L., and Boles, K. "Why Health Economics?," *Nursing Economics* 2(3):175-80, May/June 1984.

Jaquith, Sharon. "Continuous Measurement of SvO_2: Clinical Applications and Advantages for Critical Care Nursing," *Critical Care Nursing* 5(2):40-44, March/April 1985.

Javid, M. "Efficacy of Chymopapain Chemonucleolysis: A Long-Term Review of 105 Patients," *Journal of Neurosurgery* 62(5):662-66, May 1985.

Jones, S. "New I.V. Catheters That Can Do It All," *RN* 48(2):20-23, February 1985.

Kaplan, E., et al. "The Usefulness of Preoperative Laboratory Screening," *Journal of the American Medical Association* 253(24):3576-81, June 28, 1985.

Kelly, L.Y. *Dimensions of Professional Nursing,* 5th ed. New York: Macmillan Publishing Co., 1985.

Khalsa, D.S. "Stress-Related Illness: Where the Evidence Stands," *Postgraduate Medicine* 78(6):217-21, November 1985.

Kirk, R. and Dunaye, T.M. "Managing Hospital Nursing Services for Productivity," *Nursing Management* 17(3):29-32, March 1986.

LaCamera, D., et al. "Symposium on Infections in the Compromised Host: The Acquired Immunodeficiency Syndrome," *Nursing Clinics of North America* 20(1):241-56, March 1985.

Leavelle, D.E., ed. *Mayo Medical Laboratories Handbook*. Rochester, Minn.: Mayo Medical Laboratories, 1986.

Main, D.M., and Mennuti, M.T. "Neural Tube Defects: Issues in Prenatal Diagnosis and Counseling," *Obstetrics & Gynecology* 67:1-16, January 1986.

McClain, M. "Sudden Infant Death Syndrome: An Update," *Journal of Emergency Nursing* 11(5):227-33, September/October 1985.

Miller, P., and Yardley, S. "White Clot Syndrome: A Complication of Heparin Therapy," *American Journal of Nursing* 85(10):1051, October 1985.

Mittal, V.K., and Toledo-Pereyra, L.H. "Pancreatic Transplantation: The Surgical Process," *Association of Operating Room Nurses Journal* 43(3):620-29, March 1986.

Moldawer, N.P., and Murray, J.L. "The Clinical Uses of Monoclonal Antibodies in Cancer Research," *Cancer Nursing* 8(4):207-13, August 1985.

Nichter, L., et al. "Efficacy of Burned Surface Area Estimates Calculated from Charts—The Need for a Computer-based Model," *Journal of Trauma* 25(6):477-81, 1985.

"Nursing Goes to Market," *American Journal of Nursing* 86(3):324-31, March 1986.

Polit, Denise F., and Hungler, Bernadette P. *Nursing Research Principles and Methods*. Philadelphia: J.B. Lippincott Co., 1983.

Rosenthal, N.E., et al. "Antidepressant Effects of Light in Seasonal Affective Disorder," *American Journal of Psychiatry* 142(2):163-70, February 1985.

Sabin, Sandy. "Rehabilitation Program's Marketing Plan Was Tailored to Fit," *Nursing and Health Care* 6(5):269-71, May 1985.

Soll, B.A., et al. "Treatment of Obstructive Sleep Apnea with a Nocturnal Airway-Patency Appliance," *New England Journal of Medicine* 313(6):386, 1985.

Speciale, J., and Kaalaas, J. "Infuse-a-Port: New Path for I.V. Chemotherapy," *Nursing85* 15(10):40-43, October 1985.

Staley, M., and Luciano, K. "Eight Steps to Costing Nursing Services," *Nursing Management* 15(10):35-38, October 1984.

Suppers, V.J., and McClamrock, E.A. "Biologicals in Cancer Treatment: Future Effects on Nursing Practice," *Oncology Nursing Forum* 12(3):27-32, May/June 1985.

White, K.M. "Completing the Hemodynamic Picture: SvO_2," *Heart & Lung* 14(3):272-80, May 1985.

Whittaker, A.A. "Acute Renal Dysfunction: Assessment of Patients at Risk," *FOCUS on Critical Care* 12(3):12, 1985.

Whittaker, A.A., et al. "Preventing Complications in Continuous Arteriovenous Hemofiltration," *Dimensions of Critical Care Nursing* 5(2):72, March/April 1986.

Winkelman, C. "Hemofiltration: A New Technique in Critical Care Nursing," *Heart & Lung* 14(3):265-71, May 1985.

Acknowledgments

p. 20 Information on Water-Jel dressings provided by Trilling Resource, Ltd. (TRL), Hartsdale, N.Y.

p. 21 Information on heat stress index from Patricia Epifanio, RN, MS, Nurse Coordinator for the Maryland Institute for Emergency Medical Services Systems (MIEMSS), Baltimore, and William Howard, MD, Sports Medicine Center at Union Memorial Hospital, Baltimore.

p. 44 Illustration of electrophysiologic response to antiarrhythmic drugs used with permission of Aspen Publishers, Inc.

p. 47 Photo of ultrasonogram of spina bifida courtesy of Dr. Alfred B. Kurtz, Department of Radiology, Thomas Jefferson University, Philadelphia.

pp. 64-68 Special thanks to Arthur E. Frankel, MD, for reviewing Cancer update: Monoclonal antibody therapy.

pp. 68-71 Special thanks to Michael P. Nunno, MS, Radiation Safety Officer, Radiation Oncology Department, Albert Einstein Medical Center, Northern Division, Philadelphia, for information in Cancer update: Radiation therapy.

p. 69 Photo of Clinac 2500 linear accelerator courtesy of Varian, Palo Alto, Calif.

p. 122 Illustration of the Small Particle Aerosol Generator courtesy of I.C.N. Pharmaceuticals, Inc., Costa Mesa, Calif.

p. 124 Illustration of Recombinant DNA Drug Development courtesy of Genentech, Inc., South San Francisco.

p. 217 Illustration of Harvard PCA System courtesy of Bard Electro Medical Systems, Inc., Englewood, Colo.

Index

Boldface page numbers indicate major entries; i refers to an illustration, t to a table.

B

C

Boldface page numbers indicate major entries; i refers to an illustration, t to a table.

Boldface page numbers indicate major entries; i refers to an illustration, t to a table.

Boldface page numbers indicate major entries; i refers to an illustration, t to a table.

Boldface page numbers indicate major entries; i refers to an illustration, t to a table.

Reye's syndrome, salicylates and, 131
Rheumatoid arthritis, diagnostic testing for, 28-29, 29t
Rheumatoid factor screen, in connective tissue disease test panel, 28, 29t
Rhinovirus, alpha-2-interferon and, 135
Rh isoimmunization pathogenesis of, 24-25i
Rh$_0$ immune globulin dosage in, 23-24
Rh$_0$ immune globulin, determination of dosage of, in Rh isoimmunization, 23-24
Ribavirin, in treatment of respiratory syncytial virus, **121-123**
Rifampin/phenytoin, possible adverse interaction of, 121t
Rubella vaccination, 118-119t

S

Salicylates, Reye's syndrome and, 131
Sample, 231
Sampling, 231
Sampling bias, 231
Sampling error, 231
Sampling methods in research, 190
Sampling units, 231
Schizophrenia, brain scans in, 51
Scientific approach in nursing, **188-191**
Score, 231
Seasonal affective disorder, 112
Security concerns with computerized records, 142
Seizure(s)
subtle, recognition of, **87, 90**
types, differentiation of, 88-89t
Self-pay, as source of income from patient services, 154
Self-report, 231
Serum flecainide, **48-49**
Serum immunoreactive trypsinogen (IRT), 45-46
Serum protein electrophoresis, in autoimmune liver disease test panel, 27t, 28
Serum tocainide, **36-37**

Shaping, as reinforcement technique, 153
Significance level, 231
Silver sulfadiazine, 58
Simultaneous compression-ventilation (SCV) CPR, 6
Sjögren's syndrome, diagnostic testing for, 28-29, 29t
Skewness, 231
Skin grafts, healing aid for, 223i
Skin syndromes in AIDS, 56, 57, 58, 59
Sleep disorder centers, 50
Slow continuous ultrafiltration (SCUF), 14-15i, 15-17
Sodium bicarbonate, new guidelines for administration of, 6-7
Sodium overload, as cause of central pontine myelinolysis, 20
Somatrem, **123, 125-126**
Sorbinil, 126
Span of control, 231
Spasms, from upper motor neuron lesions
classification of, 96
pathophysiology of, 97i
treatment of, **96, 98**
Sperm penetration assay (SPA), 73, 74i, 75
Sphincterotomy, endoscopic, 108, 109i
Spina bifida, protocol for prenatal detection of
by amniotic fluid analysis, 48
by ultrasonography, 47-48
Staffing, 231
Staff management, 149-153
Staff motivation, **149-153**
Staff unit, 231
Stage fright, beta blockers for, 135
Standard deviation, 231
Standard error, 231
Standards of care, 231
Standards of performance, 231
State definitions of advanced nursing practice, 160-171
Statistical significance, 231
Statistics, 231
Stenting, 108, 110
Stevens-Johnson syndrome, **90-91**
Stomatitis in AIDS, 56, 57, 58

Strategic planning, 231
Stratified random sampling, 231
Stratified sample, 231
Stress
definition of, 92
as factor in burnout, 173-174
management of, 94-96
physiology of, 92-94
prolonged, effects of, 94
reaction, 93
response, 92t
factors that influence, 95
Stressors contributing to burnout, 173-174
Stress-related illnesses, **91-96**
preventive measures, 94-96
Subjects in research, 231
Sucralfate/phenytoin, possible adverse interactions of, 121t
Sudden infant death syndrome update, 112
Sulfamylon sandwich, for skin grafts, 223i
Survey research, 231
Sustained-release theophylline, possible adverse reaction to, 121t
Syndromes and disorders, 77-99
Systematic sampling, 232
Systemic lupus erythematosus, diagnostic testing for, 28-29, 29t

T

Target market, 232
Target population, 232
T-cell growth factor. *See* Interleukin-2.
Technologic adjustments, 2-3
Teeth staining, fluoride rinse and, 130
Temazepam dosage for elderly patients, 128t
Temperature-humidity index (THI), 21
TENS for obstetric analgesia, 221
Terminal burnout, 174
Test panels
autoimmune liver disease, **27-28**, 27t
connective tissue disease, **28-29**, 29t
hereditary angioedema, **30-31**, 30t
multiple sclerosis, **31-32**, 32t

Boldface page numbers indicate major entries; i refers to an illustration, t to a table.

Test-retest reliability, 232
Tetanus-diphtheria (adult Td) vaccination, 118-119t
THC testing. *See* Urine tetrahydrocannabinol.
Theory, 232
Theory X and Theory Y, 232
Theory Z, 232
Thioridazine dosage for elderly patients, 128t
Thrombocytopenia, heparin-induced, white clot syndrome and, 98-99
Thrombosis, perinatal, protein C deficiency in, 34, 35
Thyroid hormone dosage for elderly patients, 128t
Tissue oxygen consumption, factors affecting, 11
Tocainide
  possible adverse reactions to, 120t
  serum levels, measurement of, 36-37
Tolazamide dosage for elderly patients, 128t
Total burn surface area, computerized estimation of, 21
Total complement assay, in connective tissue disease test panel, 29t
Total cost, 232
Total fixed cost, 232
Total variable cost, 232
Toxoplasma gondii encephalitis, 56-57, 58
Transhepatic biliary catheter, insertion of, 210-212
Treatment advances, 99-111

Trend study, 232
Triage nursing, **8-11**
  categories, 10t
  deciding factors in, 8
  definition of, 8
  patient history in, 8-9
  physical examination in, 9
Triazolam dosage for elderly patients, 128t
Triple-lumen catheter, **200-203**, 200i
T-test, 232
Type-I error, 232
Type-II error, 232

U

Ulcerative colitis, ileoanal reservoir in, 213
Ultrasonography, in prenatal detection of neural tube defects, 47-48, 47i
Uncertainty, 232
Urgent conditions, criteria for, in triage, 10t
Urinalysis, protocols for, in diabetic nephropathy, 41
Urine tetrahydrocannabinol (THC), **35-36**

V

Validity, 232
Valproate sodium, possible adverse reaction to, 120t
Variable, 232
Variance, 232
Ventilation technique in CPR, new recommendations for, 5
Ventricular tachycardia
  antiarrhythmic drug response in, 44i
  EPS and, 42
Vertical integration, 232
Vice-president of nursing as executive position, 180
Vigilon dressing, in pressure ulcer treatment, 207

W

Warfarin/erythromycin, possible adverse interaction of, 121t
Warfarin/ibuprofen, possible adverse interaction of, 121t
Water-Jel burn dressing, 20
Water-Jel fire blanket, 20
White clot syndrome, **98-99**
Winter depression, 112

Z

Zero-based budgeting, 232
Zona-free hamster egg test, 73, 74i, 75

Malpractice suits.

Think you're covered? Think again.

Ethical time bombs.

A single slip could cost you your career.

Unfair performance evaluations.

How do you challenge a bad review?

Only one journal concentrates 100% on problems like these. Problems that threaten *every* nurse...

NursingLife®

More than 200,000 of your colleagues read every issue of *NursingLife*. Nurses like you who've come to rely on this new journal to help them cope with the tough nursing problems that make getting the job done more difficult.

Join them by entering your own subscription. You'll get expert advice to help you manage your career better and to ease the stress and strains of day-to-day work.

© 1986 Springhouse Corporation

Nursing74®
Nursing75®
Nursing76®
Nursing77®
Nursing78®
Nursing79®
Nursing80®
Nursing81®
Nursing82®
Nursing83®
Nursing84®
Nursing85®
Nursing86®
Nursing87®